Cytopathology of the Breast

ASCP Theory and Practice of Cytopathology 5
William Johnston, MD, Series Editor

The ASCP Theory and Practice of Cytopathology Series

Cytopathology of the Uterine Cervix • *Volume 1*

Cytopathology of the Endometrium • *Volume 2*

Cytopathology of the Central Nervous System • *Volume 3*

Pediatric Cytopathology • *Volume 4*

Cytopathology of the Breast • *Volume 5*

Teaching Slide Sets in the ASCP Theory and Practice of Cytopathology Series

Cytopathology of the Uterus Teaching Slide Set

Cytopathology of the Endometrium Teaching Slide Set

Cytopathology of the Breast

Shahla Masood, MD

Professor and Associate Chair
Department of Pathology
Assistant Dean for Research
University of Florida Health Science Center/Jacksonville
Chief of Pathology
University Medical Center
Jacksonville, Florida

Editor-in-Chief
The Breast Journal

American Society of Clinical Pathologists
Chicago

Publishing Team

Jeffrey Carlson (series design)
Renee Kastar (marketing)
Andrea Meenahan (illustration)
Jennifer Schima (editorial)
Joshua Weikersheimer (acquisitions/development)

Notice

Library of Congress Cataloging-in-Publication Data

Masood, Shahla.
    Cytopathology of the breast/Shahla Masood.
        (ASCP theory and practice of cytopathology ; 5)
    Includes bibliographical references.
    ISBN 0-89189-380-6 (hard cover)
    1. Breast — Cancer — Cytopathology. 2. Breast — Needle biopsy.
    I. Title. II. Series.
    [DNLM: 1. Breast Neoplasms — diagnosis. 2. Biopsy, Needle — methods.
    W1 AS126 v.5 1995 / WP 870 M412c 1995]
    RC280.B8M345 1995
    616.99 ' 44907—dc20
    DNLM/DLC   95-39759
    for Library of Congress   CIP

Printed in Hong Kong

00 99 98 97 96   5 4 3 2 1

To the memory of my parents

and

to my family, Ahmad, Ali, and Sina Kasraeian

▣ Contents

◙ Tables and Figures

Preface

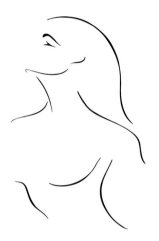

Cancer of the breast remains a medical and social challenge. Despite centuries of scientific inquiry and medical research, little is understood about the etiology, biology, or molecular events underlying the development of breast cancer. The natural history of breast cancer is heterogeneous, ranging from a disease curable by surgery alone to one marked by rapid, metastatic progression refractory to treatment. Breast cancer is not only a systemic disease causing major physical impairment but is also associated with significant psychosexual problems. Identified as a sexual organ, the breast plays an important role in a woman's self-image. For many women, the loss of a breast as the result of breast cancer parallels the loss of their sexual identity.

The magnitude of problems associated with breast cancer has inspired a multidisciplinary effort focusing on early detection of the disease and better management of patients. Attempts have also been made to determine the best possible predictors of prognosis so that appropriate therapy can be selected for each woman who suffers from this devastating disease. With the intensive increase in public awareness of breast cancer and advances in screening mammography, more women can be expected to seek consultation for the evaluation of breast lesions. Because the majority of breast lesions are benign and open biopsies are inconvenient and costly, fine needle aspiration biopsy (FNAB) is becoming an increasingly important diagnostic tool in the evaluation of patients with breast lesions. Fine needle aspiration biopsy is generally regarded as the initial diagnostic procedure of choice for palpable breast lesions. Evidence suggests that FNAB may be just as accurate as open biopsy in the diagnosis of nonpalpable breast lesions, as long as proper measures are in place to reliably localize the lesion and to ensure the precise sampling of the area that appears suspicious on mammography. Stereotactic devices have already shown promise in achieving this goal. However, further investigation and experience are necessary before FNAB can fully replace open biopsy. This can be achieved only through the concerted efforts of experienced clinicians, radiologists, and pathologists.

The widespread use of screening mammography has also led to the detection of more small invasive carcinomas and in situ lesions, as well as an overwhelming number of proliferative breast lesions, which are believed to be associated with an increased risk for the subsequent development of breast cancer. Today, pathologists face a new diagnostic challenge: not only do they have to differentiate between benign and malignant breast lesions, but they must also be familiar with the spectrum of changes occurring in proliferative and premalignant breast lesions. The ability to recognize these changes is crucial, for it affects the management of patients who have a high risk of developing breast cancer. The increased use of cytologic techniques to diagnose breast cancer dictates that pathologists become familiar with emerging techniques that provide prognostic information.

This text is designed to help pathologists improve their technical proficiency and expand their knowledge of the cytomorphology of the various types of palpable and nonpalpable breast lesions. Such knowledge is essential if pathologists are to help patients and clinicians make fully informed decisions regarding available treatment options.

CHAPTER ONE

Introduction to Fine Needle Aspiration Biopsy

History

In 1930, Martin and Ellis,[1] at the Memorial Hospital for Cancer and Allied Disease (Memorial Sloan-Kettering Cancer Center) in New York, were the first to report their experience with fine needle aspiration biopsy (FNAB). Other interested physicians in the United States and Europe began performing FNABs as well, and promising results appeared in the literature.[2,3] However, despite these reports, FNAB was subject to a great deal of criticism. Pathologists were reluctant to diagnose breast carcinoma based solely on the cytologic appearance of individual cells, and surgeons were apprehensive about the possibility of false-positive diagnoses. There was also concern about the spreading of tumors as a result of needle puncture. Tumors growing out of the needle tract had been reported in a few highly influential cases. These reports resulted in a sharp decline in the use of FNAB in the United States. However, needle aspiration continued to be performed in Europe, especially in Sweden. Between 1967 and 1974, Zajicek and Franzen et al[3–5] published the results of their careful and comprehensive work on FNAB, sharing their experience with the rest of the world. Their efforts contributed significantly to a renewal of interest in FNAB in the United States and elsewhere.

Changes in the American medical economy, including a growing emphasis on cost containment, also stimulated interest in breast fine needle aspiration biopsy. The technique of fine needle aspiration was found to be rapid and cost effective when compared with surgical biopsy.[6] It was also shown that the metastatic potential of breast cancer is not influenced by FNAB. Follow-up studies comparing women with breast cancer who had undergone breast FNAB with those who had not showed no significant differences in recurrence or survival rates between the two groups.[7–9] The reawakening of interest in FNAB in the United States resulted in numerous series of reports emphasizing the merits of FNAB in evaluating patients with palpable breast lesions.[10–13]

Meanwhile, it was also recognized that breast cancer prognosis is directly related to the size and stage of the tumor at the time of diagnosis. Detection of breast malignancies before they are clinically apparent has been shown to yield a high rate of in situ and stage I lesions.[14–18] Treatment of such early lesions has been associated with a higher survival rate than treatment of more advanced malignancies.[19,20]

The difficulty remained in the clinical diagnosis of early breast cancer. Traditionally, patients sought medical advice only when they felt a mass, usually by accident. Similarly, physicians looked only for masses in the breast or axilla or for evidence of skin retraction or nipple inversion. Naturally, occult tumors were not diagnosed.

X-ray examination of the breast, or mammography, opened a new window in the detection of abnormalities related to breast cancer. In 1913, Salomon and Beitrage,[21] in Germany, were the first to observe microcalcification in an intraductal carcinoma. Other interested investigators followed this trend by demonstrating the feasibility of detecting occult carcinoma by mammography.[22–24] Today, mammography and ultrasound are the only diagnostic modalities that can reliably detect nonpalpable breast lesions.[17,25–27]

Although mammography is reliable in detecting occult breast lesions, biopsy and pathologic examination are required for definitive diagnosis.[28] Since occult lesions are nonpalpable, they are difficult to localize clinically for diagnostic biopsy. To overcome this problem, percutaneous needle localization excisional biopsy of suspicious lesions detected by mammography was introduced in 1974.[29] Since then, this technique, in conjunction with specimen radiography, has become a standard procedure for sampling clinically occult breast lesions.[17–20,28,29] Unfortunately, the sensitivity of this technique is low. The positive predictive value of mammography ranges from 14% to 38%.[15,30] Thus, many women who undergo unnecessary surgical biopsy for benign breast disease can benefit from other, less invasive alternatives such as FNAB.

If a reliable and consistent method could be found to localize the suspicious lesions detected by mammography, the applicability of FNAB could be extended to the cytologic diagnosis of nonpalpable breast lesions. In 1977, Bolmgren et al[31] developed a stereotactic technique that was later evaluated by Nordenstrom and Zajicek,[32] who performed needle biopsies of nonpalpable breast lesions using a stereotactic compression plate and a screw needle instrument. The study results indicated that this technique has an accuracy comparable to that of excisional biopsy.

Definition

Fine needle aspiration biopsy is a technique for obtaining cellular material using a 21-gauge or smaller needle. Usually, FNAB is performed with a

10-cc or 20-cc syringe using special syringe holders. Diagnosis by FNAB is based primarily on cytologic examination of the aspirate (Image 1.1).

It is important to recognize the difference between FNAB and core (ie, 14-gauge needle) biopsy. In contrast to FNAB, which provides material for cytologic evaluation, core needle biopsy yields tissue fragments for histologic evaluation (Image 1.2). The superiority of FNAB over core biopsy as a means of evaluating palpable breast lesions is already well established. Studies have shown that FNAB is more accurate, has a lower false-negative rate, and is a less painful procedure than the core biopsy.[33-36] The results of core biopsies studied by frozen section are obtained about as quickly as FNAB results but at considerably greater cost. When submitted for frozen section, specimens obtained by core needle biopsy often reveal extensive crush artifact and distorted accompanying fat. Most pathologists who are familiar with both FNAB and core biopsy prefer examining FNAB samples. In addition, the small diameter of the needle used in FNAB allows an easy back-and-forth motion in different directions. Core biopsy, in a single pass, may displace a small, mobile mass and miss the target (Figure 1.1).

Fine needle aspiration biopsy should be performed on all palpable breast lesions. It can also be utilized in assessing mammographically detected nonpalpable breast lesions such as isolated or clustered microcalcifications, ill-defined or spiculated densities, solitary or newly developed well-defined masses, and focal architectural distortions.

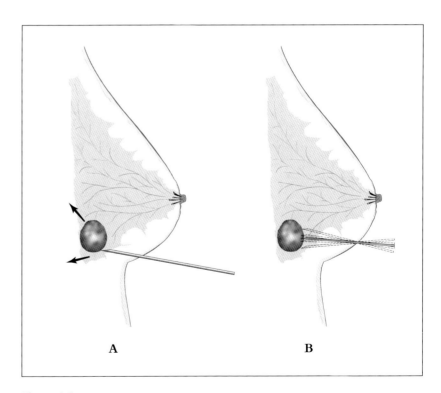

A   B

Figure 1.1
Schematic diagram of different needle biopsy sampling methods. Core needle biopsy displacing a mobile lesion and missing the target (A). Fine needle aspiration biopsy demonstrating motion of the needle in different directions, which permits better, more extensive sampling of the lesion (B).

Advantages of Breast FNAB

Fine needle aspiration biopsy offers several advantages over surgical biopsy. First is its cost-effectiveness. FNAB procedures may cost up to 90% less than an excisional biopsy.[37] By reducing the number of unnecessary breast biopsies, FNAB can maximize the efficiency of hospital bed use.[38] Studies have shown that the major economic benefit of FNAB is not that it replaces excisional biopsy, but that it permits triage: the surgeon can decide which patients should have a one-stage, inpatient procedure and which patients should undergo excisional biopsy as an outpatient under local anesthesia.[39,40] The same studies demonstrated that FNAB would be economically favorable even if its sensitivity fell as low as 37%, its specificity as low as 80%, or if the percentage of cases of cancer in the population biopsied fell as low as 13%.[39,40]

Second, FNAB causes minimal physical and psychological discomfort to the patient. The procedure causes no skin deformity or parenchymal scar that could interfere with follow-up study. In addition, many women find the fine needle aspiration biopsy procedure easy to accept, which may lead to earlier detection of breast malignancies. In my experience, many women delay physician consultation because they fear surgery and breast scars. Fine needle aspiration biopsy relieves this anxiety in patients with benign breast disease. In malignant cases, FNAB allows a woman to actively participate in treatment planning. FNAB also eliminates the need for short-term follow-up mammography of a nonpalpable breast lesion (ie, an indeterminate mass).

Third, FNAB provides rapid results and a potential bedside diagnosis. FNAB may also serve as a therapeutic procedure when a cyst is encountered, and it is an attractive alternative to surgical biopsy in evaluating local recurrences, lymph node metastases, and inoperable conditions.[41,42] Fine needle aspiration biopsy is the only diagnostic procedure considered for presurgical chemotherapy protocol.[43] Fine needle aspirates may also be the only source of tumor sample that can be used for assessing estrogen and progesterone receptors or other prognostic markers.[44–48]

Sequential fine needle aspiration biopsy may provide information regarding the patient's likely response to therapy. When coupled with flow cytometry, FNAB has been shown to be effective in monitoring the response of breast cancer to radiation therapy.[49] Fine needle aspiration biopsy can also facilitate the cytologic identification of clinically occult proliferative breast disease in women with a family history of breast cancer. It provides an effective means of tumor sampling and monitoring of surrogate end-point biomarkers in chemopreventive trials.[50–53]

Advantages of Breast FNAB
Cost-effectiveness
Minimal physical and psychological trauma to the patient
Eliminates two-stage procedure in malignant cases
Eliminates need for repeat mammography of an indeterminate mass
Provides rapid, highly accurate results
Allows women to actively participate in treatment planning
Therapeutic procedure for evacuation of breast cysts
An alternative procedure when surgical biopsy is not possible

An effective means of tumor sampling for prognostic testing and monitoring the effect of therapy

Complications of Breast FNAB

Fine needle aspiration biopsy has a low incidence of complications, although occasionally hematoma formations, bleeding, or infection may occur. Pneumothorax is a very rare complication.[54,55] Vasovagal reactions, ranging in severity from syncope to mild lightheadedness, can occur. Fine needle aspiration biopsy through the areola for central lesions is extremely painful. Tumor implants following an FNAB are extremely rare. However, recent reports have associated stereotaxic core biopsy with malignant seeding from the needle track and epithelial displacement of fragments of breast tissue outside the target lesion.[56,57]

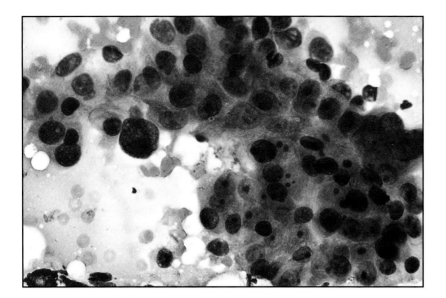

Image 1.1
Cellular material obtained via breast FNAB for cytologic interpretation (Papanicolaou, 400X).

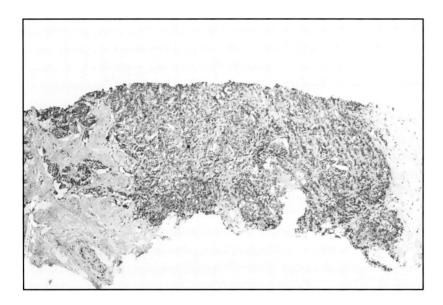

Image 1.2
Fragment of breast tissue obtained via core biopsy for histopathologic examination (H&E, 200X).

References

1. Martin HE, Ellis EB: Biopsy of needle puncture and aspiration. *Ann Surg* 92:169–181, 1930.

2. Saphir O: Early diagnosis of breast lesions. *JAMA* 150:859–861, 1952.

3. Zajicek J, Franzen S, Jackson P, et al: Aspiration of mammary tumors in diagnosis and research: a critical review of 2,200 cases. *Acta Cytol* 11:169–175, 1967.

4. Franzen S, Zajicek J: Aspiration biopsy in diagnosis of palpable lesions of the breast. Critical review of 3,479 consecutive biopsies. *Acta Radiol* 7:241–262, 1968.

5. Zajicek J: Aspiration biopsy cytology, I: cytology of supradiaphragmatic organs. *Monogr Clin Cytol* 4:1–211, 1974.

6. Rosenthal DL: Breast lesions diagnosed by fine needle aspiration. *Pathol Res Pract* 181:645–656, 1986.

7. Berg JW, Robbins GF: A late look at the safety of aspiration biopsy. *Cancer* 15:826–827, 1962.

8. Kline TS: Breast. In: *Handbook of Fine Needle Aspiration Biopsy Cytology*, 2nd ed. New York, NY, Churchill Livingstone Inc, 1988, pp. 199–252.

9. Rosemond GP, Maier WP, Brobyn TJ: Needle aspiration of breast cysts. *Surg Gynecol Obstet* 128:351–354, 1969.

10. Frable WJ: Needle aspiration of the breast. *Cancer* 53:671–676, 1984.

11. Frable WJ: Needle aspiration biopsy: past, present and future. *Hum Pathol* 20:504–517, 1989.

12. Feldman PS, Covell JL: *Fine Needle Aspiration Biopsy and Its Clinical Application: Breast and Lung.* Chicago, Ill, ASCP Press, 1985.

13. Linsk JA, Franzen S: *Breast Aspiration in Clinical Application Cytology.* Philadelphia, Pa, JB Lippincott Co, 1983, pp. 105–135.

14. Proudfoot RW, Mattingly SS, Selling CB, et al: Non-palpable breast lesions: wire localization and excisional biopsy. *Am Surg* 52:117–122, 1986.

15. Marrujo G, Jolly PC, Hall MH: Non-palpable breast cancer: needle localized biopsy for diagnosis and consideration for treatment. *Am J Surg* 151:599–602, 1986.

16. Lefor AJ, Numann PJ, Levinsohn EM: Needle localization of occult breast lesions. *Am J Surg* 148:270–274, 1984.

17. Seymour EQ, Stanley JH: The current status of breast imaging. *Am Surg* 51:591–595, 1985.

18. Poole GV, Chaplin RH, Sterch JM, et al: Occult lesions of the breast. *Surg Gynecol Obstet* 163:107–110, 1986.

19. Azavede E, Fallenius A, Svane G, et al: Nuclear DNA content, histological grade and clinical course in patients with nonpalpable mammographically detected breast adenocarcinoma. *Am J Clin Oncol* 13:23–27, 1990.

20. Werlheimer MD, Castanza ME, Dodson TF, et al: Increasing the effort toward breast cancer detection. *JAMA* 255:1131–1315, 1986.

21. Salomon A, Beitrage Z: Pathologic und klinik der mammar carcinoma. *Arch Klin Chir* 105:573–668, 1913.

22. Kleinschmidt O: In: Sweike P, Payr E, Hurzel S, eds. *Brustdruse in die Klinik der Bosartigeston geschwulste.* Leipzig, 1927.

23. Gershan-Cohen J: *Atlas of Mammography.* New York, NY, Springer-Verlag, 1970.

24. Egan RL: Experience with mammography in a tumor institution. *Radiology* 25:894–900, 1960.

25. Fornage B: Percutaneous biopsies of the breast: state of the art. *Cardiovasc Intervent Radiol* 14:27–39, 1991.

26. Fornage BD, Coan JD, David CL: Ultrasound-guided needle biopsy of the breast and other interventional procedures. *Radiol Clin North Am* 30:167–185, 1992.

27. Fornage BD, Sneige N, Faroux MJ, et al: Sonographic appearance and ultra-sound guided fine needle aspiration biopsy of the breast carcinoma smaller than 1 cm. *J Ultrasound Med* 9:559–568, 1990.

28. Hall WC, Aust JB, Gaskill HV, et al: Evaluation of non-palpable breast lesions: experience in a training institution. *Am J Surg* 151:467–496, 1986.

29. Threatt B, Appelman H, Dow R, et al: Percutaneous localization of clustered mammary micro-calcifications prior to biopsy. *Am J Roentgenol* 121:839–842, 1974.

30. Hermann G, Janns C, Schwartz IS, et al: Nonpalpable breast lesions. Accuracy of pre-biopsy mammographic localization. *Radiology* 165:323–326, 1987.

31. Bolmgren J, Jacobson B, Nordenstrom B: Stereotaxic instrument for needle biopsy of the mamma. *Am J Roentgenol* 129:121–125, 1977.

32. Nordenstrom B, Zajicek J: Stereotaxic needle biopsy and prospective indications of nonpalpable mammary lesions. *Acta Cytol* 21:350–351, 1977.

33. Cheung PS, Yan KW, Alagaratham JT: The complementary role of fine needle aspiration cytology and tru-cut needle biopsy in the management of breast masses. *Aust NZ J Surg* 57:615–620, 1987.

34. Shabot MM, Goldberg IM, Schick P, et al: Aspiration cytology is superior to tru–cut needle biopsy in stabilizing the diagnosis of clinically suspicious breast masses. *Ann Surg* 196:122–126, 1982.

35. Innes DJ Jr, Feldman PS: Comparison of diagnostic results obtained by fine needle aspiration cytology and tru-cut or open biopsies. *Acta Cytol* 27:350–354, 1983.

36. Gonzalez E, Grafton WD, Morris DM, et al: Diagnosing breast cancer using frozen sections from tru–cut needle biopsies. *Ann Surg* 202:696–701, 1985.

37. Kaminsky DB: Aspiration biopsy in the context of the new medicare fiscal policy. *Acta Cytol* 28:333–336, 1984.

38. Salter DR, Bassett AA: Role of needle aspiration in reducing the number of unnecessary breast biopsies. *Can J Surg* 24:311–313, 1981.

39. Silverman JF, Lannin DR, O'Brian K, et al: The triage of fine needle aspiration biopsy of palpable breast masses. Diagnostic accuracy and cost-effectiveness. *Acta Cytol* 31:731–736, 1987.

40. Lannin DR, Silverman JF, Walker C, et al: Cost-effectiveness of needle biopsy of the breast. *Am Surg* 203:474–480, 1986.

41. Malberger E, Edonte V, Toledaro O, et al: Fine needle aspiration and cytologic findings of surgical scar lesions in women with breast cancer. *Cancer* 69:148–152, 1992.

42. Mitnik JS, Vazquez, MF, Roses DF, et al: Recurrent breast cancer: stereotaxic localization of fine needle aspiration biopsy. *Radiology* 182:103–106, 1992.

43. Ragaz J, Baird R, Rebbeck P, et al: Neoadjuvant (preoperative) chemotherapy for breast cancer. *Cancer* 56:719–724, 1985.

44. Masood S: Use of monoclonal antibody for assessment of estrogen receptor content in fine needle aspiration biopsy specimen from patients with breast cancer. *Arch Pathol Lab Med* 113:26–30, 1989.

45. Masood S: Assessment of progesterone receptor immunocytochemical assay in breast fine needle aspirates. *Acta Cytol* 34:735, 1990.

46. Masood S, Frykberg ER, McLellan G, et al: Application of estrogen receptor immunocytochemical assay to aspirates from mammographically guided fine needle biopsy of nonpalpable breast lesions. *South Med J* 84:857–861, 1991.

47. Masood S: Prognostic factors in breast cancer: use of cytologic preparations. *Diagn Cytopathol* 13:388–395, 1995.

48. Masood S, Hart N: Use of fine needle aspiration biopsy specimens in DNA flow cytometry study. *Am J Clin Pathol* 92:535, 1989.

49. Zbieranowski I, Riche JC, Jackson SM, et al: The use of sequential fine needle aspiration biopsy with flow cytometry to monitor radiation induced changes in breast carcinoma. *Anal Cell Pathol* 4:13–24, 1992.

50. Marshall CJ, Schumann GB, Ward JH, et al: Cytologic identification of clinically occult proliferative breast disease in women with a family history of breast cancer. *Am J Clin Pathol* 95:157–165, 1991.

51. Skolnik MH, Cannon-Albright LA, Goldgar DE, et al: Inheritance of proliferative breast disease in breast cancer kindreds. *Science* 250:1715–1720, 1990.

52. Fabian CJ, Zalles C, Kamel S, et al: Biomarker and cytologic abnormalities in women at high and low risk for breast cancer. *J Cell Biochem* 176:153–160, 1993.

53. Masood S: Standardization of immunobioassays as surrogate endpoints. *J Cell Biochem* 19(suppl):28–35, 1994.

54. Catania S, Boccato P, Bono A, et al: Pneumothorax: a rare complication of fine needle aspiration biopsy of the breast. *Acta Cytol* 33:140, 1989.

55. Helvie MA, Ikeda DM, Adler DD: Localization and needle aspiration of breast lesions: complications in 370 cases. *Am J Roentgenol* 157:711–714, 1991.

56. Harter LP, Curtis JS, Ponto G, Craig PH: Malignant seeding of the needle track during stereotaxic core needle biopsy. *Radiology* 185:713–717, 1992.

57. Youngson BJ, Liberman L, Rosen PP: Epithelial displacement in surgical breast specimens following stereotaxic core biopsy. *Mod Pathol* 8:29A, 1995. Abstract.

CHAPTER TWO

Techniques

Palpable Breast Lesions

To sample palpable breast lesions, first prepare the site with alcohol or iodine. Using your free hand to immobilize the lesion, carefully insert the needle into the lesion. After creating a vacuum in the syringe, which is mounted on a special holder, carefully move the needle back and forth until a sample is seen in its hub. Use of a needle with a transparent or translucent hub is suggested. Different parts of the lesion may be sampled, but the needle should be pulled just outside the lesion before changing direction. If gross blood is obtained, the aspiration should be terminated. Adequate sampling of the lesion may require several separate aspirations. Although the first aspiration usually yields the largest sample, aspirating a lesion three or four times provides optimal yield. Lesions larger than 3 cm may require additional sampling of different areas. The vacuum should always be released before withdrawing the needle from the skin. After completing the aspirations, temporary pressure should be applied to the aspiration site to minimize bleeding.

The aspirated material is usually spread on a microscope slide in a thin film using one of several techniques (Figures 2.1 and 2.2). Smears are usually fixed in alcohol for Papanicolaou or special stains. Air-dried smears for stains such as Diff-Quik® or Wright-Giemsa may also be prepared for immediate interpretation (Image 2.1). The material remaining in the syringe and needle after preparation of smears may be placed in Sacco-manno or other fixatives for cytospin preparations or cell block processing (Images 2.2 and 2.3). Any tissue fragments too large for smears should be examined by tissue section from a cell block. Other fixatives or media may

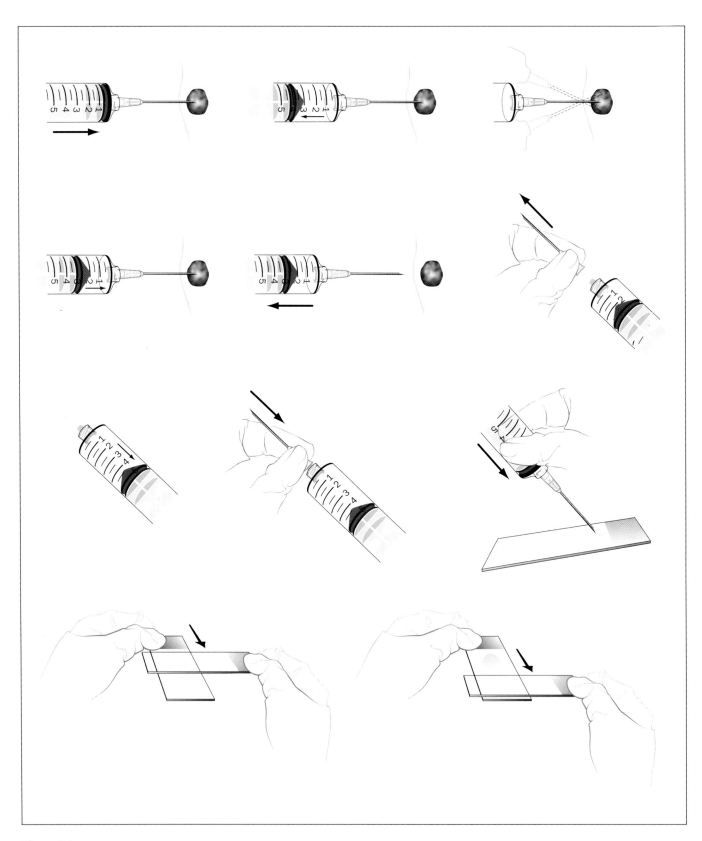

Figure 2.1
Schematic illustration of the technique of FNAB of a palpable breast lesion.

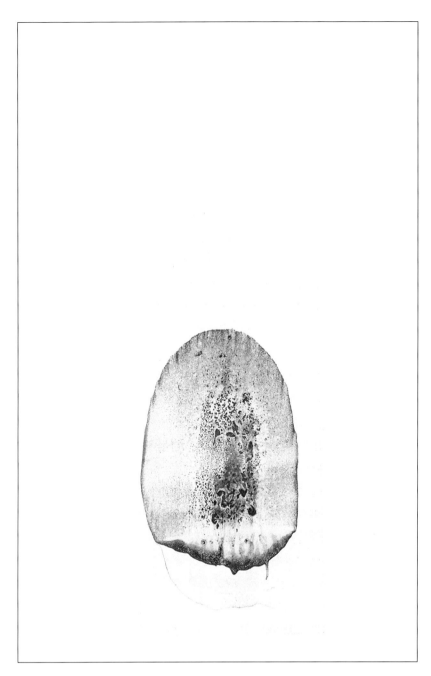

Figure 2.2
An example of the spread of aspirated material on a glass slide in a direct smear preparation.

be utilized for special studies. In my experience, good results can be obtained by using air-dried, Diff Quik–stained and alcohol-fixed, Papanicolaou-stained smears. Pathologists should be familiar with both types of specimen processing and interpretation. Diff-Quik stain is the fastest and most convenient method for evaluating specimens immediately, at the time of aspiration. Papanicolaou stain provides good nuclear details.

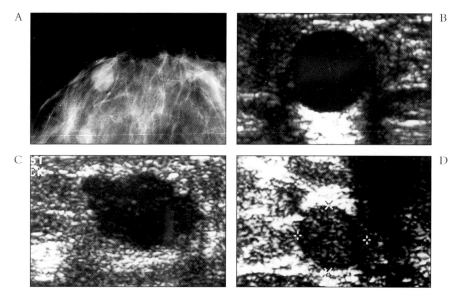

Figure 2.3
Combination of mammography and ultrasound. Mammographic view of an ill-defined mass (A), which can present three different patterns on ultrasound: a cyst (B); a mixed solid and cystic lesion (C); a solid lesion (D).

Nonpalpable Breast Lesions

Patients with nonpalpable breast lesions present with a variety of radiologic abnormalities (Figure 2.3). Mammography or ultrasound are used to localize the lesions. Mammographic localization may be performed using either standard mammographic equipment or a stereotactic device.

Standard Mammography

When a standard mammography unit is used, the breast is usually placed between two compression plates with a localizing device and a scout film is taken. The compression plates have either multiple holes or rectangular windows with centimeter scales along two sides. Compression plates allow the precise positioning of the biopsy needle along the X and Y coordinate axes. Because the target depth has to be estimated from previous mammograms and varies according to the amount of compression used, it may not always be precisely determined. However, compression plates have been reported to have an acceptable accuracy rate in experienced hands. Helvie et al[1] used a fenestrated coordinate grid compression plate, then imaged and biopsied the breast in a single projection. The approximate depth of the lesion was estimated from the original orthogonal view. This technique, applied in 215 cases, demonstrated a sensitivity of 97% and a specificity of 94%. Hann et al[2] performed fine needle apsiration biopsies (FNABs) on 96 women with nonpalpable breast lesions using a standard grid needle localization technique. The depth of the lesions was determined from an orthogonal view with the needle in place. The reported sensitivity and specificity in this series was 91% and 82%, respectively.

My colleagues and I[3] developed a hybrid of these two methods in 1989. Using a standard mammography unit and combining the standard, widely used technique of needle localization with FNAB, we prospectively studied 100 women with nonpalpable breast lesions. This method demonstrated a sensitivity of 85%, specificity of 100%, and overall diagnostic accuracy of 96.7%. Sufficient aspirated material was obtained in 91% of the cases. There were no false-positive results. False-negative results occurred in 3.3% of the cases and included two cases of lobular carcinoma in situ and one case of duct cell carcinoma in situ. These results are comparable to those of FNAB of palpable lesions and to those of open surgical biopsy, and were achieved without the considerable expense associated with stereotactic equipment.[3,4]

The technique we employed involved first obtaining scout, craniocaudal, and lateral low-dose mammograms using a dedicated mammography unit with a localization compression grid attached (General Electric Medical Systems/Milwaukee, WI). This was to establish the position and grid coordinates of the lesion. The skin was then cleaned with antiseptic solution and infiltrated with local anesthesia. The guiding needle from a prototypical coaxial breast localization system (Cook, Inc/Bloomington, IN) was introduced into the lesion and a repeat mammogram was obtained to ensure the positioning of the needle (Figure 2.4). Then, a retractable Homer Mammolok Wire (Namic/Glen Falls, NY) was inserted through the needle to stabilize the needle tip. A 90° companion view was then obtained. The needle tip was judged to be in a good position if it was adjacent to the lesion's margin in both projections (Figure 2.5). The guiding wire was stabilized and the wire removed. A 20-gauge Fransen biopsy needle (Cook, Inc/Bloomington, IN) was then inserted through the guiding needle. A 20-mL plastic syringe placed in a metallic syringe holder (Cameco Precision Dynamics Corp/Burbank, CA) was attached to the biopsy needle (Figure 2.6). The syringe plunger was retracted, creating negative pressure, and the aspiration biopsy performed.

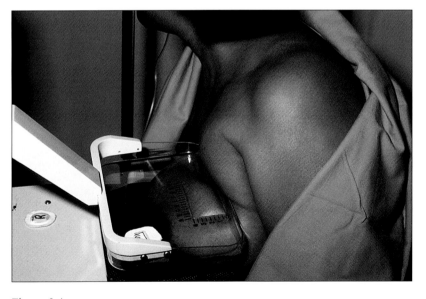

Figure 2.4
Mammographically guided FNAB: the breast is placed between the compression plates and the localizing needle is inserted.

A 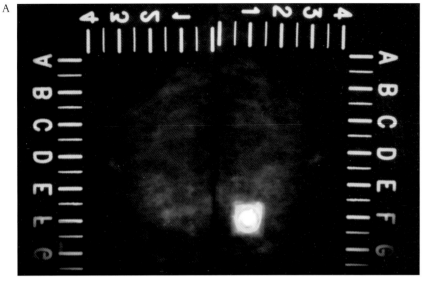 B

Figure 2.5
Compression grid craniocaudal mammographic views establish the position of the suspect microcalcifications (arrow, A). Needle placement is confirmed at the same position (B).

Stereotactic Guidance

Two types of stereotactic devices have been developed: (1) dedicated prone units; and (2) attachments to existing mammography units. The first dedicated stereotactic instrument for FNAB of the breast was introduced in 1977 and subsequently used by Nordenstrom's group[5–7] at the Karolinska Institute in Stockholm. Another early stereotactic instrument, originally

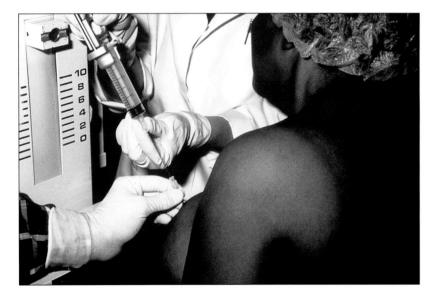

Figure 2.6
Mammographically guided FNAB demonstrating the insertion of the fine needle into the target via the previously inserted localizing needle. Reproduced with permission from: Masood S, Frykberg E, Michum DG, et al: The potential value of mammographically guided fine needle aspiration biopsy for nonpalpable breast lesions. *Am Surg* 55:226–231, 1989.

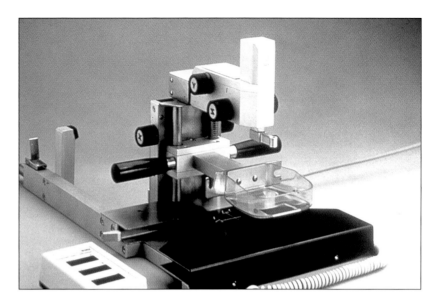

Figure 2.7
An example of a nondedicated stereotaxy unit (courtesy of GE Medical Systems/ Milwaukee, WI).

developed by Bolmgren et al,[8] consisted of an x-ray tube mounted to a hinged arm, a pivoting stand, a patient table compression device with film holder and scale system, a coordinate-controlled puncture device with a separate stand, a biopsy device, and a calculator. Major changes have occurred since the introduction of these early stereotactic devices. Advances in computer science and imaging have resulted in fine stereotaxy devices. Units that attach to standard mammographic units are relatively inexpensive but are time consuming (Figures 2.7 and 2.8).

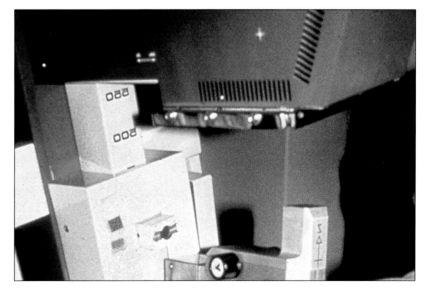

Figure 2.8
Demonstration of the attachment of a stereotaxy device to an existing standard mammography unit (courtesy of GE Medical Systems/Milwaukee, WI).

As in standard mammography techniques, the patient is seated in front of the mammography unit and the breast is placed between perforated compression plates that have an opening to permit introduction of the needle. The breast is positioned craniocaudally and two images are taken at 15° from the vertical area (ie, 75°, 105°). These two projections of the lesion make it possible to calculate the X, Y, and Z coordinates. These coordinates plus two reference lines are entered into a computer that determines how the needle holder should be adjusted for the needle length. An 80 mm, 0.8 mm needle (21 gauge) is used for most aspirates. A 20-mL syringe and a syringe holder are attached to the needle, and the needle is moved within the lesion to improve the yield. The aspirations are usually performed by a radiologist. The amount of time required for the procedure, from preliminary roentgenograms to preliminary cytologic assessment, rarely exceeds 30 minutes.

Computer-assisted dedicated stereotaxy devices have become increasingly popular. Although these devices are more expensive, they are also more practical. The patient is placed in a prone position, which eliminates the discomfort and the vasovagal reflux associated with the stereotaxically guided biopsy procedure (Figure 2.9). Stereotactic guidance is highly accurate, with the needle tip usually placed within 1 to 2 mm of the selected target point (Figure 2.10). The preciseness of this technique readily allows FNAB of lesions smaller than 5 mm.[9]

The limitations of stereotactic guidance include the impossibility of correcting any needle deviation and the length of the procedure, during which compression is maintained and the patient should not move. Also, the technique is not suitable for sampling extramammary lesions, such as lymph node and peripheral lesions, since they cannot be included in the mammographic projection.

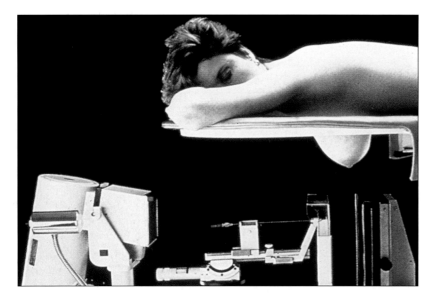

Figure 2.9
Demonstration of a dedicated stereotaxy device: the patient is placed in a prone position and the breast will be placed between the compression plates (courtesy of GE Medical Systems/Milwaukee, WI).

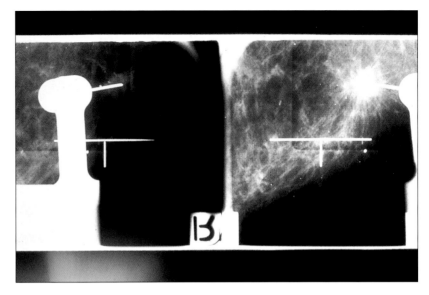

Figure 2.10
Demonstration of the positioning of the needle within the mammographically suspicious area in a stereotaxically guided FNAB (courtesy of GE Medical Systems/Milwaukee, WI).

Ultrasound Guidance

Ultrasonic imaging has become extremely important in evaluating localized breast pathology. Ultrasound is used in combination with physical examination and mammography to determine whether a given lesion is purely cystic, mixed, or solid. The latter two require a definitive diagnosis to preclude malignancy. For the best technical results, the use of a high-frequency (7.5 MHz), hand-held, flat linear array transducer is recommended; its nondiverging beam guarantees an excellent near-field resolution. Use of a local anesthetic is rarely required for ultrasound-guided FNAB. The aspiration is usually performed using a 20- or 22-gauge, 1.5- to 2-inch hypodermic needle attached to a 10-mL or 20-mL syringe and a single-hand aspiration device such as the Cameco® syringe pistol.

There are two different approaches to inserting a needle into a breast lesion visualized by sonography.[10] In the first, the needle is placed in such a way that the target lesion is displaced along the midline of the scan. The needle is then placed so that it is lateral to the midpoint of the transducer and angled obliquely toward the lesion (Figure 2.11). In the second approach, the needle is inserted obliquely, resulting in a continuous display of both the tip and the distal portion of the needle (Figure 2.12). This is the technique of choice for minute lesions or peripheral lesions that are close to the chest wall or to a prosthesis.

One of ultrasound's greatest strengths is its ability to image real-time (ie, dynamically). This enables the user to localize the lesion and confirm needle placement at the time of biopsy. Another advantage of ultrasound-directed FNAB is that it permits needle penetration of mobile targets, such as fibroadenomas, which stereotactic technique can miss. In addition, full real-time monitoring of the sampling process guarantees, in the case of a solid lesion, that the representative sample is extracted from the target and reinforces the diagnostic value of a negative result.

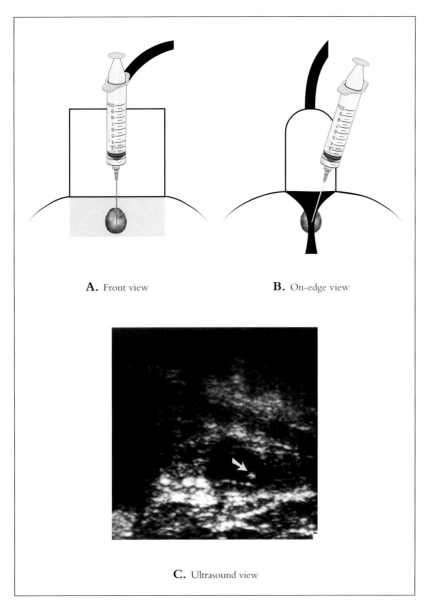

A. Front view   **B.** On-edge view

C. Ultrasound view

Figure 2.11
Technique of ultrasound-guided FNAB. The needle is placed tangential to the lateral aspect of the transducer and oblique to the scan plane. Front view shows the transducer, needle, and syringe (A). On-edge view demonstrates the obliquity of the needle, which is determined from the depth of the lesion measured on the screen (B). The needle tip is seen as a bright echo (arrow) in a scan made during an ultrasound-guided FNAB of a nonpalpable breast lesion (C).

In the case of a cyst, a pneumocystogram can be performed following insufflation of air through the needle[11]; the air reabsorbs in 1 to 2 weeks. Pneumocystography is indicated when wall irregularities are demonstrated on ultrasound, when aspiration of hemorrhagic cyst fluid is required, or when the cyst is the origin of a suspicious density on the mammogram.[12] Ultrasound-guided FNAB is rapid, rarely requiring more than 5 minutes when performed by an experienced practitioner. For minute lesions, the technique requires dexterity and the procedure time may be longer.

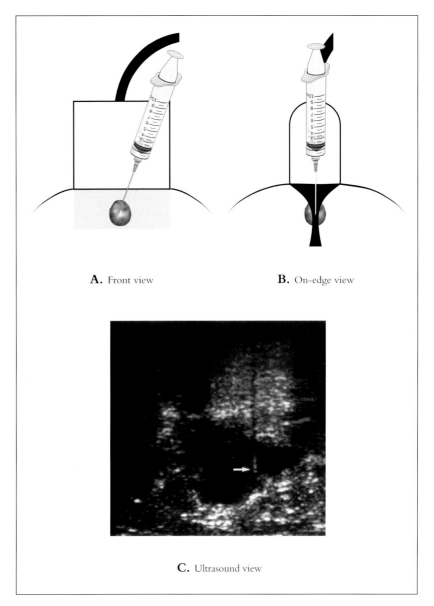

A. Front view   **B.** On-edge view

C. Ultrasound view

Figure 2.12
Another technique of ultrasound-guided FNAB. The needle is inserted oblique to both the transducer and the scan plane. Front view shows the needle placed obliquely in the scan plane (A). On-edge view shows the distal portion of the needle (B). The needle tip is seen in a scan obtained during ultrasound-guided FNAB of an occult breast lesion (C).

Ultrasound vs Mammography

Mammography and ultrasound are complementary imaging modalities in the evaluation of breast lesions, and their indications for use as localizing devices also complement each other. There are many advantages to using ultrasound guidance. These include real-time monitoring of the needle, the shortest needle pathway, rapidity, low cost, and a limited number of passes. For these reasons, patients find ultrasound-guided FNAB highly acceptable. Ultrasound guidance is particularly useful in demonstrating lesions that are not clearly visible on mammograms, such as dense, irradiated, and augmented breast tissue or peripherally located lesions. It is also an attractive alternative for pregnant or lactating women or women who refuse mammography. Ultrasound can also differentiate between cystic and solid non-fatty or noncalcified masses and can depict intracystic neoplasms.[12–14]

Ultrasound's limitations include its dependence on operator experience; the absence of global images of the breast; its inability to visualize minute (smaller than 0.7 cm) carcinomas, microcalcifications, or non-discrete densities; and problems in reproducibility of results and interpretation. Because of these limitations, ultrasound has not been used as a screening modality for detecting nonpalpable breast cancer in asymptomatic women.[12–14]

Mammographic guidance is mandatory for lesions that are not visualized on ultrasound scan. These include isolated microcalcifications, focal areas of architectural distortion, and masses smaller than 0.8 cm. Occasionally, fibroadenomas in a fatty breast may not be visualized by ultrasound.[12–14] Disadvantages of mammographic localization include the length of examination and possible difficulties in penetrating mobile fibroadenomas, lymph nodes, and lesions that are located close to the chest wall or in the lower half of the breast. Also, the needle tip is not visualized during sampling. Sampling is limited to a single axis, and a deviated needle cannot be repositioned.[12–14]

It is best to perform physical examination, mammography, ultrasound examination, and, if needed, fine needle aspiration, during a single visit. If ultrasound fails to visualize the lesion, the patient may undergo mammographically guided FNAB. Clearly, radiologists interested in breast imaging should be familiar with both modalities.

Special Studies

The availability of an immediate microscopic evaluation of breast aspirates is not only an important factor in reducing the number of inadequate samples, but also provides an effective means of triaging the specimen for further studies. To achieve this type of immediate evaluation, a fine needle aspiration biopsy cart can be assembled and either stationed at a clinic or wheeled to the patient's bedside. The cart should contain a microscope, different stains, fixatives, syringes, needles, syringe holders, slides, and the other accessories necessary for performing fine needle aspiration biopsies and processing the aspirated material (Figure 2.13).

Sophisticated ancillary techniques may often be successfully applied to fine needle aspiration biopsies for diagnostic and prognostic testing. Immunocytochemical stains and electron microscopic studies may be used for specific diagnosis of primary neoplasms or to distinguish primary from metastatic cancer. Specific monoclonal antibodies have made hormone receptor studies practical for primary and metastatic breast cancer neoplasms. The use of image cytometry may allow quantitation of hormone receptors as well as the study of ploidy and proliferation rate of tumor cells. Other special studies potentially applicable to fine needle aspiration specimens include flow cytometry and molecular biology, cytogenetics, and microbiology.

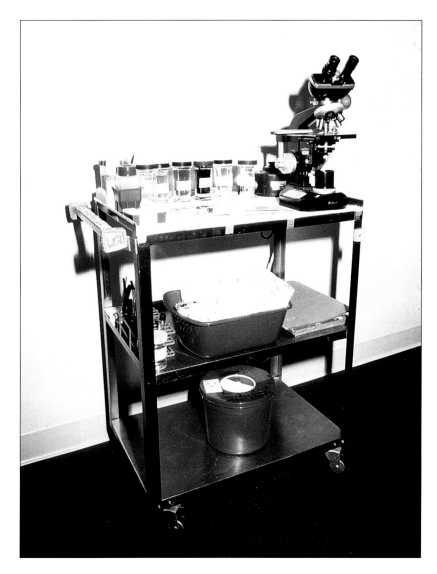

Figure 2.13
An example of an FNAB cart containing a microscope, fixative, and other necessary accessories to be stationed at a clinic or wheeled to the patient's bedside.

How to Establish a Breast Fine Needle Aspiration Biopsy Service

Growing interest in the utilization of FNAB for diagnosing breast lesions has created a need for systems that provide this service effectively. First, it is important to ensure that the physicians who perform FNABs are thoroughly familiar with the technique as well as its indications and interpretation. Aside from traditional training and participation in various workshops, personal experience is the most significant factor contributing to the success of this procedure. Continuous and consistent practice by simulating FNAB on surgical specimens and preparing smears and imprints is the most effective way of developing proficiency in the technique and, subsequently, in the interpretation of fine needle aspiration biopsy. The ability to recognize the differences in the interpretive criteria for exfoliative cytology and FNAB is also essential.

Second, the necessity of establishing an FNAB service has to be justified. The merits and pitfalls of the procedure must be made clear to surgeons, oncologists, and radiologists on the hospital staff. As pathologists, we must convince our colleagues that we are not trying to take away their patients and interfere with their practices. Instead, we are offering an attractive alternative to surgical biopsy that is more convenient for patients. Lectures, interdepartmental conferences, and brochures explaining the merits of FNAB are important marketing efforts.

Third, the physicians who will perform FNABs must be identified—surgeons, oncologists, radiologists, or pathologists. There are many factors that influence this decision, including the geographic proximity of clinic patients and pathologists and the attitudes of the physicians involved.

The debate over who should perform fine needle biopsies started when the procedure was introduced. If politics, which may be an insurmountable problem in any institution, are put aside, the answer seems clear: anyone who is able to obtain a diagnostic specimen is qualified to perform FNABs. However, many investigators have unequivocally shown that pathologists obtain the best FNAB results.[15,16]

At our institution, we strongly believe that FNABs should be performed by the person who examines the smears, ie, the pathologist. Complete familiarity with the clinical picture of the patient and examination of the mass and the gross appearance of the aspirate complements the interpretation of cytologic material when making a definitive diagnosis. An immediate interpretation provided by a pathologist at bedside can significantly reduce the number of insufficient samples and false-negative diagnoses and speed diagnosis and therapy.

Unfortunately, implementation of the system described above may not be feasible in many institutions. An alternative approach is to make sure that the other physicians performing FNAB procedures are adequately trained in all aspects of sampling the lesion and preparing the smears. If possible, they should be provided with a cytotechnologist to assist them in processing the aspirated material. Another alternative is collecting the aspirated material into Saccomanno fixative. This permits the preparation of high-quality smears by trained cytotechnologists no matter who does the aspiration.[17] Howat et al[18] advocate the use of the cytospin method as highly convenient in an outpatient setting. However, direct smears remain the preferred method of preparing breast FNAB specimens.[19]

Initially, surgeons may be reluctant to prescribe a definitive therapy based on cytologic diagnosis alone. For this reason, they should be allowed to challenge the cytologic diagnosis by an excisional biopsy and/or frozen section for a short period of time. Once the trust between pathologist and surgeon is firmly established, the technique of FNAB will be viewed as a reliable diagnostic procedure.

In addition to surgeons and pathologists, several other types of physicians have recently shown interest in FNAB, reflecting ever-increasing concern about breast cancer. These physicians include gynecologists, radiologists, family physicians, and medical oncologists. As part of a teamwork approach to the diagnosis and management of breast cancer, pathologists must tailor their services to the needs of the community of physicians and patients.

Another recently created approach involves performing FNABs of nonpalpable breast lesions under radiologic guidance in the office of the radiologist. This approach results from the increased use of screening mammography and growing interest on the part of radiologists. It permits the diagnosis of deeply seated lesions and small carcinomas, lesions formerly not diagnosed by FNAB. Of course, any physician who examines a woman with a breast mass and performs an FNAB is responsible for ensuring that appropriate and adequate cytologic preparations are available for interpretation and for taking measures to ensure that the patient receives proper referral and follow-up.

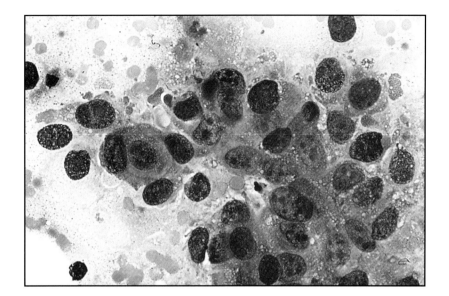

Image 2.1
Slide stained with Diff-Quik for immediate interpretation following FNAB (400X).

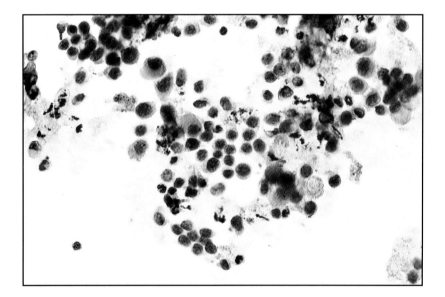

Image 2.2
Cytospin preparation obtained from aspirate of a breast lesion (Papanicolaou, 200X).

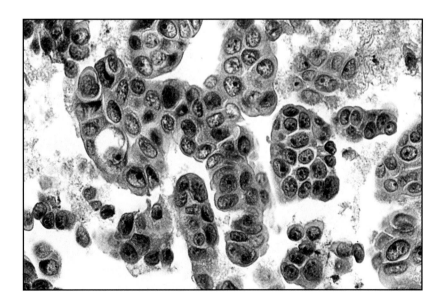

Image 2.3
Cell block preparation of material aspirated from a breast lesion (H&E, 400X).

References

1. Helvie MA, Baker DE, Adler DD, et al: Radiographically guided fine-needle aspiration of nonpalpable breast lesions. *Radiology* 174:657–661, 1990.

2. Hann L, Ducatman BS, Wang HH, et al: Nonpalpable breast lesions: evaluation by means of fine-needle aspiration cytology. *Radiology* 171:373–376, 1989.

3. Masood S, Frykberg ER, Mitchum DG, et al: The potential value of mammographically guided fine needle aspiration biopsy of nonpalpable breast lesions. *Am Surg* 55:226–231, 1989.

4. Masood S, Frykberg ER, Mitchum DG, et al: Prospective evaluation of radiologically directed aspiration biopsy of nonpalpable breast lesions. *Cancer* 66:1480–1487, 1990.

5. Nordenstrom B, Zajicek J: Stereotaxic needle biopsy and preoperative indications of nonpalpable mammary lesions. *Acta Cytol* 21:350–351, 1977.

6. Svane G, Silfversward C: Stereotaxic needle biopsy of nonpalpable breast lesions: cytologic and histologic findings. *Acta Radiol [Diagn] (Stockh)* 24:385–390, 1983.

7. Nordenstrom B, Ryden H, Svane G: Breast. In: Zornoza J, ed. *Percutaneous Needle Biopsy.* Baltimore, Md, Williams & Wilkins, 1977, pp. 43–51.

8. Bolmgren J, Jacobson B, Nordenstrom B: Stereotaxic instrument for needle biopsy of the mamma. *Am J Roentgenol* 129:121–125, 1977.

9. Gent HJ, Sprenger E, Dowlatshahi K: Stereotaxic needle localization and cytological diagnosis of occult breast lesions. *Ann Surg* 204:580–584, 1986.

10. Fornage BD, Faroux MJ, Simatos A: Breast Masses: US-Guided Fine Needle Aspiration Biopsy. *Radiology* 162:409–414, 1987.

11. Tabar L, Pentek Z, Dean PB: The diagnostic and therapeutic value of breast cyst puncture and pneumocystography. *Radiology* 141:659–663, 1981.

12. Fornage B: Percutaneous biopsies of the breast: state of the art. *Cardiovasc Intervent Radiol* 14:29–39, 1991.

13. Fornage BD, Sneige N, Faroux MJ, et al: Sonographic appearance and ultrasound-guided fine-needle aspiration biopsy of breast carcinoma smaller than 1 cm. *J Ultrasound Med* 9:559–568, 1990.

14. Fornage BD, Coan JD, David CL: Ultrasound-guided needle biopsy of the breast and other interventional procedures. *Radiol Clin North Am* 30:167–185, 1992.

15. Cohen MB, Rogers C, Hales MS, et al: Influence of training and experience in fine needle aspiration biopsy of breast: receiver operating characteristics curve analysis. *Arch Pathol Lab Med* 111:518–520, 1987.

16. Lee KR, Foster RS, Papillo JL: Fine needle aspiration of the breast. Importance of the aspirator. *Acta Cytol* 31:281–284, 1987.

17. Young GP, Somers RG, Young I, et al: Experience with a modified fine needle aspiration biopsy technique in 533 breast cases. *Diagn Cytopathol* 2:91–98, 1986.

18. Howat AJ, Stringfellow HF, Briggs AW, et al: Fine needle aspiration cytology of the breast: a review of 1,868 cases using the cytospin method. *Acta Cytol* 38:939–944, 1994.

19. Crystal BS, Wang HH, Ducatman BS: Comparison of different preparation techniques for fine needle aspiration specimens. *Acta Cytol* 37:24–28, 1993.

CHAPTER THREE

Diagnostic Accuracy and Management

In recent years, fine needle aspiration biopsy (FNAB) of the breast has gained significant credibility in the diagnosis of primary and metastatic breast disease. FNAB can also be an adjunct to mammography, enhancing the specificity of mammographic findings. However, limitations exist in the discipline of breast cytology. First, criteria that effectively distinguish between benign, premalignant, and malignant breast lesions are not yet defined. This may reflect lesser but similar difficulties encountered in the histologic interpretation of several types of breast lesions, including premalignant lesions and lesions caused by high-risk proliferative breast disease. Second, the cytologic features of benign and malignant breast lesions overlap. Third, the role of FNAB in the management of breast disease remains controversial. Although several investigators advocate the use of FNAB as an alternative to open biopsy and frozen section,[1-9] others would limit its use to the assignment of patients to different treatment protocols.[10-12]

The fear of an erroneous diagnosis leading to an unnecessary mastectomy is the major reason for existing differences in the practice of FNAB. For this fear to be overcome, the diagnostic accuracy of FNAB must approach that of frozen-section diagnosis. Furthermore, due to the multidisciplinary nature of the FNAB procedure and differences among institutions in their approach to FNAB, it is difficult to interpret the results reported in the literature. This is best reflected in the wide range of reported diagnostic accuracy (50%–95%).[1,10,13–28] Silverman[29] reported similar differences in diagnostic accuracy (77%–99%) when comparing the results of more than 3,000 palpable breast aspirates with their results on histologic follow-up (Table 3.1). In our review of reported results on the diagnostic accuracy of nonpalpable breast lesions in the same number of cases, the figure ranged from 68% to 100%.[30]

Table 3.1
Summary of the Literature on Diagnostic Accuracy of Breast Fine Needle
Aspiration Biopsy in Over 3,000 Cases[*]

Category	%
Diagnostic accuracy	77–99
Senstivity	72–99
Specificity	98–100
Positive predictive value	100
Negative predictive value	87–99
Efficiency of the procedure	89–99

[*]Modified from: Silverman JF: Breast. In: Bibbo M, ed. *Comprehensive Cytopathology*. Philadelphia, Pa,
WB Saunders Co, 1991, pp. 703–770.

Although there are many potential reasons for these variations, experience in performing the FNAB procedure and cytomorphologic interpretation are the most important. Institutional differences can also have a major
impact on statistical results. In an institution where mastectomies are performed based on FNAB diagnosis only, cytopathologists are more conservative about making a conclusive diagnosis of malignancy. In contrast, in a
hospital where FNAB is followed by excisional biopsy, cytopathologists are
more liberal about making a malignant diagnosis. If aspirates suspicious for
malignancy are included in the malignant category there is, naturally, a
greater number of false-positive diagnoses. This is best exemplified by the
reports on European series of FNABs, which are associated with greater
sensitivity and a concomitant higher false-positive rate when compared
with American series.[31] Europeans practice in a less litigious environment,
or perhaps they rely more on confirmatory histologic or frozen-section
diagnosis in all cases positive for malignancy on FNAB. In contrast,
Americans are more conservative, resulting in a greater number of suspicious cases and few or no false-positive diagnoses.[31] The existing differences
in the technique and interpretation of breast FNAB, as well as differences
in breast disease management decisions and the complexity of related
medicolegal issues, create a need for a standardized approach to breast fine
needle aspirates. This can best be achieved through a multidisciplinary
approach, forming networks among individuals interested in the practice of
breast FNAB.

Based on the reports in the literature and our own experience, the
diagnostic accuracy of breast FNAB significantly improves when a pathologist examines the patient and performs the procedure.[1,2,14,17,31,32]
Proficiency in biopsy technique,[14–16,31] smear preparation, and the interpretation of cytomorphologic features is the key to a successful FNAB.[14,33]
The results of a breast FNAB are also influenced by the number of needle
biopsies of an individual lesion. There is strong evidence that the number of
aspirations positively influences the cell yield as well as the diagnostic accuracy of breast FNAB.[34,35] The rates of false negatives and inadequate specimens can be reduced by increasing the number of aspirates and paying
meticulous attention to technique. In one study, the sensitivity of FNAB
increased from 61% with one aspirate to 91% with three aspirates.[35]

In our institution, we recommend performing multiple aspirations (three or four) to ensure sample adequacy. This is particularly important when the breast lesion is large, 3 to 4 cm. In such cases, the presence of a spectrum of changes or multiple entities, such as the coexistence of neoplasia and hyperplasia within the same lesion, may lead to an incorrect diagnosis. For these reasons, additional sampling of different sites is recommended.

Immediate microscopic evaluation of FNAB smears enhances the diagnostic accuracy of the FNAB procedure.[36] Correlating the patient's clinical information with the FNAB results may prompt a repeat aspiration if the specimen is inadequate or if the FNAB results are incompatible with the clinical findings. In addition, recognizing the presence of malignancy via an immediate assessment of the direct smears permits further evaluation of the specimen, including tumor marker studies and prognostic testing.

Adequacy and Suitability of the Aspirated Specimen

Attempts to diagnose breast aspirates that are markedly limited in cellularity or obscured by blood, necrosis, inflammatory exudate, or drying artifact often lead to an incorrect diagnosis.[37–39] For example, low cellularity and poorly preserved specimens resulted in false diagnoses of atypical, suspicious lesions in 1.6% of cases (35 of 3,545 total aspirates) in the series reported by Kline,[38] and in 1.2% of cases (27 of 2,197 breast FNABs) in the series reported by Al-Kaisi.[39] Factors affecting the rate of unsatisfactory aspirates include the experience of the aspirator and the nature of the lesion, including its size and whether marked fibrosis or extensive necrosis are present.[33,37,40]

The standard criteria for a diagnostic aspirate are not yet well defined. Provided that the cells are well preserved and not obscured by blood or inflammatory cells, Kline[38] considers a breast aspirate to be satisfactory when the number of cells is more than three to six epithelial cell groups per slide. Sneige[41] defines adequate cellularity as the presence of more than four to six well-visualized cell groups. The criteria for the adequacy of cytologic specimens from nonpalpable breast lesions are also variable. Dowlatshahi et al[42] recommend that the presence of more than six epithelial clusters of more than 10 cells each be considered a sufficient sample. Layfield et al[43] consider aspirates insufficient when less than 25 epithelial cells are present on each slide.

The application of these criteria to specific, defined entities, including nonproliferative breast tissue with extensive sclerosis, carcinomas with desmoplastic breast reaction, hyalinized fibroadenomas, and lipomas, is limited. In addition, recognition of recurrent or metastatic breast disease via fine needle aspirates requires less restrictive criteria: the presence of one well-preserved cluster of neoplastic cells is sufficient for diagnosis. In our practice, the suitability and adequacy of the specimen is based on the patient's clinical presentation, radiologic findings, whether the lesion is palpable or nonpalpable, the presence or absence of needle resistance during the procedure, and the gross appearance of the aspirate material.

Palpable Breast Lesions

False-Negative Results

Despite efforts to enhance the diagnostic accuracy of breast FNAB, there remains a "gray zone" of diagnostic pitfalls that pose problems in interpreting the cytologic features of breast aspirates. Generally, tumors with extensive necrosis and fibrosis and tumors that measure less than 1 cm give rise to false-negative diagnoses.[33,37,40] Fibrosis is the most important reason for false-negative diagnoses in breast cytology. Fibrosis may be due to desmoplasia, scar tissue, or radiation. A desmoplastic reaction to tumor is commonly seen in lobular carcinoma as well as ductal carcinoma. However, because the cells in lobular carcinoma are small, they may be missed or misinterpreted as lymphocytes. For this reason, an extensive search for these small cells should be made prior to final diagnosis, especially in aspirates from postmenopausal women.

Another cause of false-negative diagnoses is well-differentiated breast tumors, such as tubular, colloid, and papillary carcinoma, and those with insignificant atypia, such as lobular carcinoma and the monomorphic type of ductal carcinoma seen in some elderly patients.[35,37] Malignant tumors associated with a cystic lesion also have a high potential for false-negative diagnosis. These tumors are often characterized by the presence of a hemorrhagic fluid; however, rarely (0.2% of cases), they may show a clear fluid and no residual mass. This is best exemplified by a cystic medullary carcinoma.[44] Therefore, one should recognize the possibility of tumor cells in cystic fluid that contains a conspicuous number of inflammatory cells.

Poor technique resulting in a missed target is an increasingly frequent problem and another important cause of false-negative diagnoses. A review of the literature shows that the rate of false-negative FNABs of palpable breast lesions varies from 1% to 31%,[4,14,15,37,45–49] with an average rate of 10%.[50] This rate can definitely be reduced by gaining experience in the technique of breast FNAB and in the interpretation of breast cytology.

Causes of False-Negative Diagnoses of Breast FNABs

Failure to obtain representative samples from the tumor, which is directly related to tumor characteristics (size, location, degree of fibrosis, histologic type, and degreee of differentiation) and technical factors.

Failure to recognize malignant cells, which is related to the experience of the pathologist who analyzes and interprets the FNAB and the presence of tumors with a monomorphic pattern and insignificant atypia

False-Positive Results

A false-positive diagnosis has dramatic clinical implications, particularly in institutions where no frozen section confirmation is required for positive breast aspirates. A conclusive diagnosis of malignancy in a breast FNAB should be considered only in cases in which the cytologic criteria for malignancy are met and no other explanation for the presence of cytologic atypia exists. It is absolutely essential that the pathologist interpreting breast aspirates be familiar with benign and reactive conditions that give rise to significant cytologic atypia. These include a ruptured cyst, fibrocystic change, fat necrosis, organizing hematoma, atypical fibroadenoma, gynecomastia, granulation tissue, pregnancy-related and lactational changes, papilloma, tubular adenoma, atypical hyperplasia, mucocele-like lesions, changes induced by radiation and chemotherapy, and epithelial hyperplasia in phyllodes tumors.[1,2,6,11,19,39,41,51–58] The rate of false positives has ranged from 0% to 11%.[11] However, when the FNAB is interpreted by an experienced pathologist, the rate has been reduced to 0.1% to 0.2%, which is similar to the rate reported for frozen section examination.[59,60] In a review of 14 series, Feldman and Corell[45] reported an overall false-positive rate of 0.17% (42 false-positive diagnoses of 25,180 breast FNABs).

Causes of False-Positive Diagnoses of Breast FNABs
Incorrect interpretation of atypical lesions
Rendering a diagnosis on inadequate or poorly prepared material

Reporting and Management

The results of FNABs are reported as insufficient, negative (benign), inconclusive (suspicious), or positive for malignancy. "Insufficient" refers to those cases where there is no or minimal cellular material or where the cells are obscured by blood, inflammatory cells, or necrotic debris or are distorted by drying artifact. In these situations, repeat aspirations or excisional biopsy are recommended. Carnoy's solution may be used to lyse the obscuring red blood cells prior to staining. Smears containing an adequate number of well-preserved benign cells are reported as negative or benign. Benign diagnoses should specify the type of lesion, such as the spectrum of fibrocystic change, fibroadenoma, inflammatory conditions, etc. The cytologic findings in negative or benign cases are correlated with clinical and mammographic findings. Some investigators still believe that a negative breast FNAB does not exclude the possibility of malignancy and should be followed by an open biopsy.[4,61] However, evaluations based on the combined findings of physical examination, mammography, and breast FNAB have been shown to increase the accuracy of breast cancer diagnosis. When all three tests are in agreement, a diagnostic accuracy rate of 99% can be achieved.[10,62] Thus, combining physical exam, mammography, and FNAB may help avoid unnecessary surgery, especially in young women. The patient's youth should not, by itself, delay needle biopsy of a breast mass, since carcinoma of the breast may occur in women aged 30 and under.[63–65] On the other hand, when there are any suspicious clinical or mammographic findings, an open biopsy is indicated, despite a negative FNAB.

Breast fine needle aspirates that show cells with significant cytologic atypia or architectural changes but that are quantitatively insufficient for malignancy are reported as inconclusive or suspicious. In these cases, an excisional biopsy or a confirmatory frozen section is needed to establish the final diagnosis. Aspirates that show conclusive cytologic evidence of malignancy are reported as positive (ie, malignant), with specification of the type of lesion and nuclear grading. Proceeding to definitive therapy based on this diagnosis is justified unless the clinical and mammographic findings do not agree with the positive FNAB results. In such cases, confirmation of malignancy by frozen section is recommended prior to definitive treatment (Figure 3.1). Since the distinction between in situ and invasive lesions

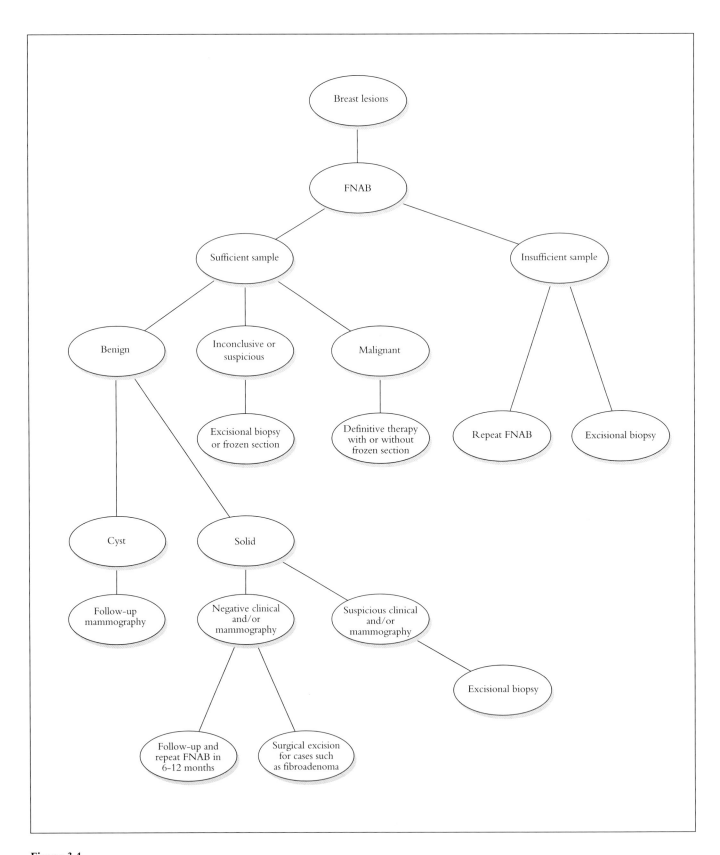

Figure 3.1
Management of patients with palpable breast lesions following FNAB.

cannot be made on breast cytology alone, if the status of tumor invasion is therapeutically important, it can be determined by core biopsy of the lesion or FNAB of the lymph node metastasis if applicable. One point that cannot be overemphasized is that the success of breast FNAB depends on the experience of the pathologist. In pathology practices where the number of breast fine needle aspirates is low or the pathologist is not experienced in the interpretation of breast FNAB, frozen-section confirmation is recommended before any definitive treatment.

Nonpalpable Breast Lesions

Extensive review of the literature, with analysis of the results of 3,000 FNABs of nonpalpable breast lesions with histologic follow-up, shows that when used with a standard mammographic localization device, FNAB has a sensitivity of 68% to 100% (average, 84%) and a specificity of 84% to 100% (average, 96%) for detecting breast cancer[30,66–72] (Table 3.2). In contrast, studies using stereotaxic devices have shown a sensitivity of 77% to 100% (average, 91%) and a specificity of 91% to 100% (average, 97%)[73–81] (Table 3.3) at significantly higher cost.

Reports on the use of ultrasound-guided FNAB of nonpalpable breast lesions are somewhat limited. Fornage et al[82,83] showed a sensitivity of 93% and specificity of 97% for selected cases. In a more recent study, Sneige et al[84] reported the results of ultrasound-guided FNAB on 651 nonpalpable breast lesions. They found ultrasound-guided FNAB to be a reliable, simple, cost-effective alternative to open biopsy, with a sensitivity of 91%, specificity of 77%, and an overall accuracy rate of 84%. These results compared favorably with the best results reported for nonpalpable lesions using mammographic guidance and the best results reported for FNAB of palpable breast lesions (Table 3.4).

I compared the combined results of mammographically and stereotaxically directed FNABs of nonpalpable breast lesions with a similar

Table 3.2
Sensitivity and Specificity of Fine Needle Aspiration Biopsy of Nonpalpable Breast Lesions Using Standard Mammography

Authors	Total Cases (No.)	Cases with Histologic Follow-up (No.)	Inadequate Sample (%)	Sensitivity (%)	Specificity (%)
Arishita et al[66]	61	61	24	87	100
Evans and Cade[67]★	28	28	14	71	100
Hann et al[68]	96	96	36	91	94
Helvie et al[69]	215	74	18	68	97
Kehler and Albrechtsson[70]	182	44	15	100	84
Layfield et al[43]†	71	71	27	78	100
Lofgren et al[71]	215	97	36	92	95
Masood et al[72]‡	100	100	9	85	100
Total or Average	968	571	23	84	96

★A study comparing stereotaxic mammographic localization.
†A study combining stereotaxic (26 cases) with standard (45 cases) mammographic localization.
‡A study using modified technique combining the standard needle localization procedure with fine needle aspiration biopsy.

Table 3.3
Sensitivity and Specificity of Fine Needle Aspiration Biopsy of Nonpalpable Breast Lesions Using Stereotaxic Technique[*]

Authors	Total Cases (No.)	Cases with Histologic Follow-up (No.)	Inadequate Sample (%)	Sensitivity (%)	Specificity (%)
Azavedo et al[73]	2594	567	9	80	99
Bibbo et al[74]	114	114	13	93	94
Ciatto et al[75]	218	115	17	84	96
Dent et al[76]	52	52	—	92	100
Dowlatshahi et al[77]	528	528	10	95	91
Evans and Cade[67]	22	22	27	100	100
Fajardo et al[78]	100	100	—	77	100
Gent et al[79]	490	187	16	97	95
Lofgren et al[80]	219	103	26	93	97
Leiman et al[†]	500	500	23	91	97
Mitnick et al[81]	300	149	2	96	100
Total or Average	5137	2437	16	91	97

[*]A study comparing stereotaxic with mammographic localization.
[†]Unpublished study; personal communication (1995).

number of FNABs of palpable breast lesions reviewed by Silverman[29] and myself.[30] As shown in Table 3.5, comparable results can be achieved with FNAB of nonpalpable breast lesions. This is particularly true when stereotaxy is the localizing technique for FNAB of nonpalpable breast lesions (Table 3.6). The sensitivity range of 77% to 100% (average, 91%) and specificity range of 91% to 100% (average, 97%) with stereotaxic localization technique are superior to the results of mammographically directed FNAB and are comparable to the results reported for FNAB of palpable breast lesions. The rate of inadequate samples ranges from 9% to 36% (average, 23%) with standard mammography and 2% to 27% (average, 16%) with stereotaxic devices.

Overall, it seems that nonstereotaxic techniques have a higher rate of insufficient specimens than stereotaxic procedures. A comparative study by Lofgren et al[80] demonstrated a significant decrease in the percentage of inadequate specimens when a stereotaxic device was used (26% vs 36%). However, when Evans and Cade[67] compared stereotaxic and nonstereotaxic methods of guiding FNABs of nonpalpable breast lesions, they found that use of stereotaxic technique resulted in a higher percentage of inadequate samples (27% vs 14%). They attributed this discrepancy to the fixed

Table 3.4
Sensitivity and Specificity of Fine Needle Aspiration Biopsy of Nonpalpable Breast Lesions Using Ultrasound Technique

Authors	Total Cases (No.)	Cases with Histologic Follow-up (No.)	Inadequate Sample (%)	Sensitivity (%)	Specificity (%)
Fornage et al[82]	36	36	3.6	94	100
Fornage et al[*83]	111	34	3.5	92	93
Sneige et al[84]	651	254	27	91	77
Total or Average	798	324	3.55	92	97

[*]This study includes 60 cases of palpable breast lesions.

Table 3.5

Reported Sensitivity and Specificity of Fine Needle Aspiration Biopsy of Nonpalpable and Palpable Breast Lesions With Histologic Follow-Up

Types of Lesions	Total Cases (No.)	Cases With Insufficient Material (%) Range (Average)	Sensitivity (%) Range (Average)	Specificity (%) Range (Average)
Palpable	3000	4–13 (7)	72–99 (87)	98–100 (97)
Nonpalpable*	3000	2–36 (19)	68–100 (87)	82–100 (96)

*These statistics include the results of both stereotaxic and standard mammographic localization techniques.

needle grid in stereotaxy. My colleagues and I[72] showed that use of a modified nonstereotaxic localizing technique, with immediate microscopic evaluation of the smears, resulted in a lower rate of inadequate samples (9%), with a diagnostic accuracy of 96.7%, sensitivity of 85%, and specificity of 100%. Thus, aside from the differences in localizing devices, accurate needle placement, aspiration technique, the number of passes, and the immediate availability of microscopic assessment of the aspirates are of paramount importance in increasing the cellular yield and accuracy of FNABs of nonpalpable breast lesions.

A certain percentage of cases will always be inadequate, regardless of the type of localizing device used. Hann et al[68] found that 40% of their inadequate cases were from fibrotic and hypocellular lesions that would not be expected to yield cells. The histologic type and the nature of the lesion can also affect diagnostic yield. Usually, medullary, mucinous, and comedocarcinomas are more cellular than infiltrating lobular and scirrhous ductal carcinomas. Benign lesions, such as sclerosing adenosis and hyalinized fibroadenomas, may be associated with a low cellular yield.[68]

The reported false-negative rate for FNABs of nonpalpable breast lesions ranges from 2% to 36%.[30] This may be due to poor localization technique, a small lesion (< 5 mm), or a firm mass, which may deflect the needle. Occasionally, stereotaxically guided FNABs fail due to a missed target, such as a mobile mass or a fibroadenoma.

Sampling error may occur when malignancy is not associated with the abnormality seen on the mammogram. This is best exemplified by lobular carcinoma in situ, which is commonly seen as an incidental finding in tissue adjacent to but not within the lesion on which the biopsy is performed.[79,85,86] Lobular carcinoma in situ also constitutes a major source of false-negative FNABs of nonpalpable lesions, because its bland cellular pattern can be confused with that of benign breast lesions.[84] In situ carcinomas cannot be reliably diagnosed by FNAB because of the necessity of examining their entire histologic architecture to exclude invasion.[30,72]

Table 3.6

Reported Sensitivity and Specificity of Fine Needle Aspiration Biopsy of Nonpalpable Breast Lesions With Histologic Follow-Up

Technique of Localization	Total Cases (No.)	Cases with Insufficient Material (No.) Range (Average)	Sensitivity (%) Range (Average)	Specificity (%) Range (Average)
Standard mammography	571	9–36 (23)	68–100 (84)	82–100 (96)
Stereotaxy	2437	2–27 (16)	77–100 (91)	91–100 (97)

Breast lesions may have a complex structure comprising benign as well as malignant components. Aspiration of such a lesion may produce a cellular yield that represents the benign part of the lesion, resulting in a false-negative diagnosis. Thus, the management of patients with nonpalpable breast lesions should be based on the combined findings of cytologic study and mammography.

The reported false-positive rate of FNABs of nonpalpable breast lesions varies from 0% to 6%.[11,42,43,68,74,76,82,87,88] False positives are usually caused by misinterpretation of atypical lesions, such as those associated with proliferative breast disease, sclerosing adenosis, duct ectasia with inflammation, and intraductal hyperplasia. The number of false positives can be minimized by the application and development of more objective, reproducible interpretation methods.

FNAB's validity as a means of diagnosing nonpalpable breast lesions has been called into question, because it is associated with a high rate of insufficient specimens and cannot be used to distinguish between in situ and invasive carcinoma. In addition, pathologists have failed to show adequate interest in using FNAB to diagnose nonpalpable breast lesions.[89,90] Interest in the use of stereotactic localization and the acquisition of core biopsy specimens with larger (14-gauge) cutting needles has increased, however.[91–93] A dedicated biopsy unit is commonly used in stereotaxically guided core biopsy to minimize patient motion during localization, eliminate vasovagal reaction, and provide more working space for the radiologist during the biopsy procedure (Figures 3.2 through 3.4). This approach provides pathologists familiar with histologic features a core of breast tissue for examination (Image 3.1 and Figure 3.5).

Reports in the radiology literature show that the number of insufficient specimens can be reduced by using stereotactic core biopsy.[90,91] Some investigators advocate the use of the long-throw biopsy gun, outfitted with a 14-gauge needle, and the performance of multiple passes (8–10 samples). In one study, the reported diagnostic accuracy of stereotactic core biopsy vs

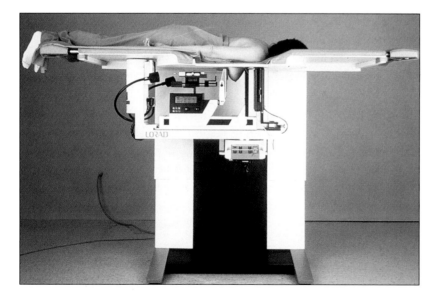

Figure 3.2
Demonstration of a dedicated computer-assisted stereotaxy core biopsy device (courtesy of Kambiz Dowlatshahi, MD).

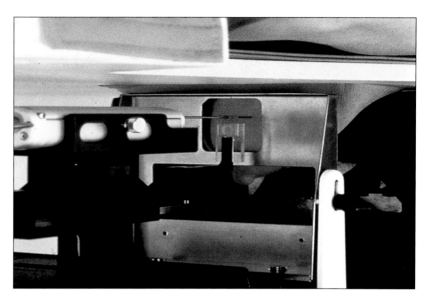

Figure 3.3
Demonstration of the breast being placed between the compression plates for insertion of the core needle (courtesy of Kambiz Dowlatshahi, MD).

surgical biopsy was 96%.[90,91] However, the superiority of core biopsy over FNAB as a means of evaluating nonpalpable breast lesions is not yet established. In a well-designed study, Dowlatshahi et al[92] suggested that needle-core biopsy and FNAB cytology should complement each other in the diagnosis of nonpalpable breast lesions (Table 3.7).

Despite these reports, it remains unclear what needle should be used for sampling occult breast lesions. FNAB is associated with a high rate of insufficient samples, a high false-negative rate, and an inability to distinguish between in situ and infiltrating lesions.[30,89] However, core-needle biopsy also has major shortcomings, including extensive tissue damage

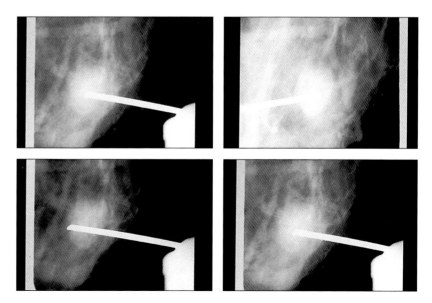

Figure 3.4
Demonstration of the positioning of the needle within the suspicious mammographic area (courtesy of Kambiz Dowlatshahi, MD).

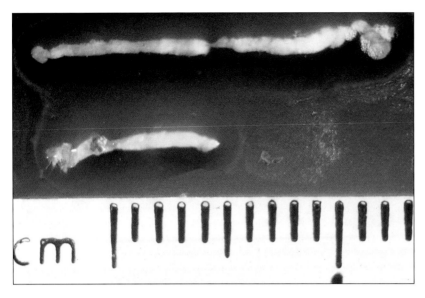

Figure 3.5
Macroscopic appearance of fragments of tissue obtained by core biopsy (courtesy of Kambiz Dowlatshahi, MD).

caused by the recommended multiple passes and the use of a 14-gauge needle. The long-throw mechanized core biopsy needle also has a practical limitation: it cannot be used in relatively small-breasted women with a compressed thickness less than approximately 4 centimeters, because the needle will hit the opposite skin and film holder and will bend. In addition, the core-needle biopsy is unlikely to facilitate confirmation of an in situ lesion. In situ lesions diagnosed by means of core-needle biopsy may show invasion on follow-up lumpectomy. Furthermore, malignant seeding from the needle track and epithelial displacement of breast tissue outside the targeted lesion has been associated with stereotaxic core biopsy of nonpalpable breast lesions.[93,94]

In summary, additional well-designed, controlled studies are required to assess the diagnostic value of FNAB and stereotactic core biopsy of nonpalpable breast lesions. The participation of pathologists in multidisciplinary investigations is the key to FNAB's success as a diagnostic technique. It is important that pathologists play an active role in fostering the merits of FNAB. This can be accomplished only by increasing technical skill and diagnostic ability. Pathologists also need to be aware of medicolegal issues

Table 3.7
Correlation of Results of FNAB Cytologic Assessment, Needle-Core Biopsy, and Both Techniques in 250 Mammographically Suspicious Breast Lesions[*]

Technique	Inadequate Sample (%)	Sensitivity (%)	Specificity (%)
Stereotaxic FNAB	24	86	72
Stereotaxic Core Biopsy	17	71	96
Combination	7	89	75

*Modified from: Dowlatshahi et al: Nonpalpable breast lesions: findings of stereotaxic needle-core biopsy and fine needle aspiration cytology. *Radiology*. 181:745–750, 1991.

relating to the choice of diagnostic method and the marketing power behind automated stereotactic core biopsy, because both law and financial considerations influence the practice of medicine in the United States.[89]

To avoid the demise of FNAB as a means of evaluating nonpalpable breast lesions, pathologists must make a concerted effort to enhance the clinical usefulness of FNAB. Combining the techniques of FNAB and core-needle biopsy may be an alternative means of increasing the overall sensitivity of these procedures and eliminating the need for surgical biopsy.[89]

Reporting and Management

Like reports on FNABs of palpable breast lesions, the results of fine needle aspirates of nonpalpable breast lesions are reported as insufficient, negative, inconclusive (suspicious), or positive for malignancy. The use of these terms, which go beyond the simple distinctions of benignity and malignancy, has been shown to improve diagnostic accuracy and reduce false-negative rates.[95] In situations where there is no or minimal cellular material, repeat aspiration or excisional biopsy is recommended. As has been previously mentioned, the criteria for adequacy of cytologic specimens varies in different institutions. Dowlatshahi et al[42] consider the presence of more than six epithelial clusters of more than 10 cells each a sufficient sample. Layfield et al[43] consider aspirates insufficient when less than 25 epithelial cells are present per slide.

Smears containing an adequate number of well-preserved benign cells are reported as negative. Follow-up of a patient with a nonpalpable breast lesion and negative FNAB depends on the extent of the mammographic abnormality seen in the patient. Abnormal mammograms depicting either soft-tissue masses or microcalcifications may be classified as having a high, intermediate, or low index of suspicion for malignancy. A highly suspicious lesion is usually seen as a solid soft-tissue mass with highly irregular or stellate borders or with fine, needle-like, linear branching microcalcifications, either clustered or scattered; as extremely polymorphic, clustered microcalcifications; or as a solid mass with irregular margins and suspicious or indeterminate microcalcifications. A solid soft-tissue mass with partially irregular or obscured borders or indeterminate microcalcifications is regarded as an intermediate lesion. A lesion with a low index of suspicion for malignancy is characterized by a 0.5- to 1.5-cm, well-defined mass; a 1- to 2-cm, asymmetric opacity; and regular, uniform, clustered microcalcifications.[76]

Considering the current increase in liability exposure in the United States, it is advisable to perform needle localization and open biopsy on lesions that have a high or intermediate risk of malignancy on mammography, even if the FNAB result is negative. An asymptomatic woman whose screening mammogram reveals a low-risk lesion and whose fine needle aspiration cytology reveals a negative result should undergo interval mammography within 6 to 12 months. This strategy is based on the likelihood of malignancy, which ranges from 10% for asymmetric, parenchymal densities and moderately suspicious microcalcifications to 50% to 70% for stellate masses and branching microcalcifications. Based on a well-conducted study performed in 1991, Sickles[96] reported that patients whose mammograms reveal a low degree of abnormality may be safely followed with interval mammography. Similarly, Hann et al[68] showed that the predictive value of negative cytologic findings in a lesion with a low index of suspicion on mammography was 100%.

Breast fine needle aspirates that show cells with significant cytologic atypia but that are not conclusive for malignancy are reported as inconclusive or suspicious. These cases require excisional biopsy and an intraoperative frozen section consultation to establish the final diagnosis. Aspirates that show conclusive evidence of malignancy are reported as positive. This diagnosis justifies proceeding directly to definitive therapy without frozen section confirmation unless the mammographic findings or other clinical factors do not agree with the positive FNAB result. In such cases, confirmation of malignancy by an intraoperative consultation diagnosis is recommended prior to definitive treatment (Figure 3.6). In the management of patients with nonpalpable breast lesions, FNAB results should always be complemented by mammographic findings.

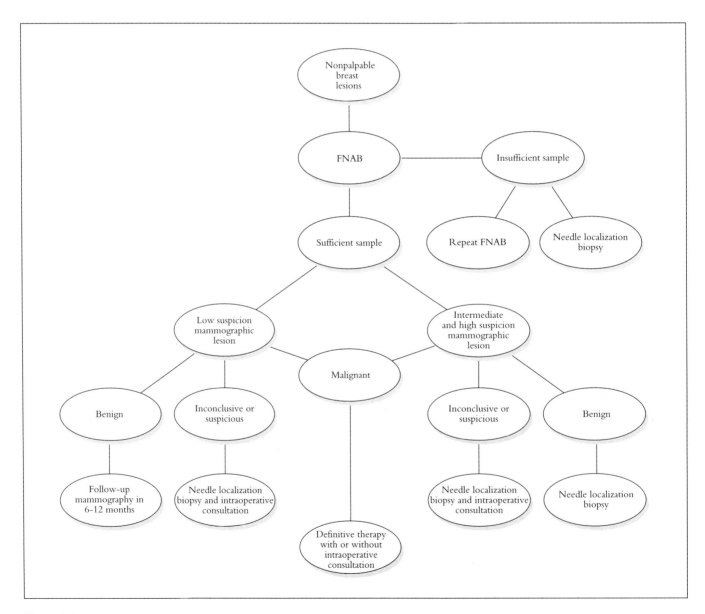

Figure 3.6
Management of patients with nonpalpable breast lesions.

Image 3.1
Microscopic section of the core tissue fragment shown in Figure 3.5 demonstrates the histologic features of fibroadenoma (H&E, 200X) (courtesy of Kambiz Dowlatshahi, MD).

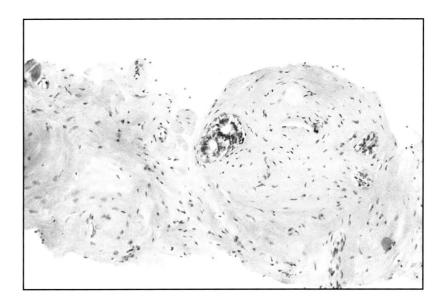

References

1. Zajdela A, Ghossein NA, Pilleron JP, et al: The value of aspiration cytology in the diagnosis of breast cancer: experience at the Fondation Curie. *Cancer* 35:499–506, 1975.

2. Zajicek J: Aspiration biopsy cytology, I. Cytology of supradiaphragmatic organs. In: Wied GL, ed. *Monographs in Clinical Cytology,* vol 4. Basel, Switzerland, S Karger, 1974, pp. 170–193.

3. Kline TS, Joshi LP, Neal HS: Fine needle aspiration of the breast: diagnosis and pitfalls. A review of 3545 cases. *Cancer* 44:1458–1464, 1979.

4. Wanebo HJ, Feldman PS, Wilhelm MC, et al: Fine needle aspiration biopsy in lieu of open biopsy in management of primary breast cancer. *Am Surg* 5:569–577, 1989.

5. Eisenberg AJ, Hajdu SI, Wihelmns J, et al: Preoperative aspiration cytology of breast tumors. *Acta Cytol* 30:135–145, 1986.

6. Griffith CN, Kern WH, Mikkelson WP: Needle cytologic examination in the management of suspicious lesions of the breast. *Surg Gynecol Obstet* 162:142–144, 1986.

7. Fessia L, Botta G, Arisio R, et al: Fine needle aspiration of breast lesions: role and accuracy in a review of 7495 cases. *Diagn Cytopathol* 3:121–125, 1987.

8. Gupta RK, Naran S, Buchanan A, et al: Fine needle aspiration cytology of breast: its impact on surgical practice with an emphasis on the diagnosis of breast abnormalities in young women. *Diagn Cytopathol* 4:206–209, 1988.

9. Gdabert HA, Hsiu I-G, Mullen JJ, et al: Prospective evaluation of the role of fine needle aspiration biopsy in the diagnosis and management of patients with palpable solid breast lesions. *Ann Surg* 56:263–267, 1990.

10. Silverman JF, Lannin DR, O'Brian K, et al: The triage role of fine needle aspiration biopsy of palpable breast masses. Diagnostic accuracy and cost-effectiveness. *Acta Cytol* 31:731–736, 1987.

11. Layfield LJ, Glasgow BJ, Cramer H: Fine needle aspiration in the management of breast masses. *Pathol Annu* 2:23–62, 1990.

12. Langmuir VK, Cramer SF, Hood ME: Fine needle aspiration cytology in the management of palpable, benign, and malignant breast disease. Correlation with clinical and mammographic findings. *Acta Cytol* 33:93–98, 1989.

13. Bell DA, Hajdu SI, Urban JR, et al: Role of aspiration cytology in the diagnosis and management of mammary lesions in office practice. *Cancer* 51:1182–1189, 1983.

14. Cohen MB, Rodgers C, Hales MS, et al: Influence of training and experience in fine needle aspiration biopsy of breast. Receiver operating characteristics curve analysis. *Arch Pathol Lab Med* 111: 518–520, 1987.

15. Lee KR, Foster RS, Papillo JL: Fine needle aspiration of the breast. Importance of the aspirator. *Acta Cytol* 31:281–284, 1987.

16. Barrows GH, Anderson TJ, Lamb JL, et al: Fine needle aspiration of breast cancer. Relationship of clinical factors to cytology results in 689 primary malignancies. *Cancer* 58:1493–1498, 1986.

17. Frable WJ: Needle aspiration of the breast. *Cancer* 53:671–676, 1984.

18. Bottles K, Miller JR, Cohen MB, et al: Fine needle aspiration biopsy: has its time come? *Am J Med* 81:525–531, 1986.

19. Elston CW, Cotton ER, Davies CJ, et al: A comparison of the use of "tru-cut" needle and fine needle aspiration cytology in the preoperative diagnosis of carcinoma of the breast. *Histopathology* 2:239–254, 1978.

20. Hajdu SI, Melamed MR: The diagnostic value of aspiration smears. *Am J Clin Pathol* 59:350–356, 1973.

21. Kern WH: The diagnosis of breast cancer by fine needle aspiration smears. *JAMA* 241:1125–1127, 1979.

22. Kline TS: Breast lesions: diagnosis by fine needle aspiration biopsy. *Am J Diagn Gynecol Obstet* 1:11–16, 1979.

23. Kline TS, Joshi LP, Neal HS: Fine needle aspiration of the breast. Diagnosis and pitfalls: a review of 3,545 cases. *Cancer* 44:1458–1464, 1979.

24. Naylor B: Fine needle aspiration cytology of the breast: an overview. *Am J Surg Pathol* 12(suppl):54–61, 1988.

25. Ortel YE, Galblum LI: Fine needle aspiration of the breast. Diagnostic criteria. *Pathol Annu* 18:375–407, 1983.

26. Rosen PP, Hajdu SI, Robbins G, et al: Diagnosis of carcinoma of the breast by aspiration biopsy. *Surg Gynecol Obstet* 134:837–838, 1972.

27. Wilson SL, Ehrmann RL: The cytologic diagnosis of breast aspirations. *Acta Cytol* 22:470–475, 1978.

28. Zajicek J, Caspersson T, Jakobsson P, Kudynowski J, Linsk J, Us-Krasarec M: Cytologic diagnosis of mammary tumors from aspiration biopsy smears: comparison of cytologic and histologic findings in 2,111 lesions and diagnostic use of cytophotometry. *Acta Cytol* 14:370–376, 1970.

29. Silverman J: Breast. In: Bibbo M, ed. *Comprehensive Cytopathology.* Philadelphia, Pa, WB Saunders Co, 1991, pp. 703–770.

30. Masood S: Fine needle aspiration biopsy of nonpalpable breast lesions. In: Schmidt WA, ed. *Cytopathology Annual 1994,* Chicago, Ill, ASCP Press, 1994, pp. 33–63.

31. Frable WJ: Needle aspiration biopsy: past, present and future. *Hum Pathol* 20:504–517, 1989.

32. Hammond S, Keyhani-Rofagha S, O'Toole RV: Statistical analysis of fine needle aspiration cytology of the breast. A review of 678 cases plus 4265 cases from the literature. *Acta Cytol* 31:276–280, 1989.

33. Kruezer G, Zajicek J: Cytologic diagnosis of mammary tumors from aspiration biopsy smears, III. Studies on 200 carcinomas with false negative or doubtful cytologic reports. *Acta Cytol* 16:249–252, 1972.

34. Pennes DR, Naylor B, Rebner M: Fine needle aspiration biopsy of the breast: influence of the number of passes and the sample size of the diagnostic yield. *Acta Cytol* 34:673–676, 1990.

35. Patel TJ, Gartell PC, Smallwood JA, et al: Fine needle aspiration cytology of breast masses. An evaluation of its accuracy and reasons for diagnostic failure. *Ann R Coll Surg Engl* 69:156–159, 1987.

36. Giard RWM, Hermans J: Fine needle aspiration cytology of the breast with immediate reporting of the results. *Acta Cytol* 37: 358–360, 1993.

37. Kline TS: *Handbook of Fine Needle Aspiration Biopsy Cytology.* St Louis, Mo, CV Mosby, 1988.

38. Kline TS: Survey of aspiration biopsy cytology of the breast. *Diagn Cytopathol* 7:98–105, 1991.

39. Al-Kaisi N: The spectrum of the "gray zone" in breast cytology. A review of 186 cases of atypical and suspicious cases. *Acta Cytol* 38:898–908, 1994.

40. Zajdela A, Zillhardt P, Voillenmot N: Cytologic diagnosis by fine needle aspiration without aspiration. *Cancer* 59:1201–1205, 1987.

41. Sneige N: Fine needle aspiration of the breast: a review of 1995 cases with emphasis on diagnostic pitfalls. *Diagn Cytopathol* 9:106–112, 1993.

42. Dowlatshahi K, Gent HJ, Schmidt R, et al: Nonpalpable breast tumors: diagnosis with stereotaxic localization and fine needle aspiration. *Radiology* 170:427–433, 1989.

43. Layfield L, Parkinson B, Wong J, et al: Mammographically guided fine needle aspiration biopsy of nonpalpable breast lesions. Can it replace open biopsy? *Cancer* 68:2007–2011, 1991.

44. Kline TS, Kline IK: *Breast: Guides to Clinical Aspiration Biopsy.* New York, NY, Igaku-Shoin, 1989.

45. Feldman PS, Corell JL: *Fine Needle Aspiration Cytology and Its Clinical Application: Breast and Lung.* Chicago, Ill, ASCP Press, 1985.

46. Goodson WH, Mailan RM, Miler TR: Three-year follow-up of benign fine needle aspiration biopsies of the breast. *Am J Surg* 154:58–61, 1985.

47. Grant CS, Goellner JR, Welch JS, et al: Fine needle aspiration of the breast. *Mayo Clin Proc* 61:377–381, 1986.

48. Koss LG, Woyke J, Olszewski W: *Aspiration Biopsy: Cytologic Interpretation and Histologic Bases.* Tokyo, Japan, Igaku-Shoin, 1989.

49. Linsk JA, Franzen S: *Clinical Aspiration Cytology.* Philadelphia, Pa, JB Lippincott, 1983.

50. Ulanow R, Galblum L, Carter JW: Fine needle aspiration in the diagnoses and management of solid breast lesions. *Am J Surg* 148:653-657, 1984.

51. Kline TS: Masquerades of malignancy. A review of 4241 aspirates from the breast. *Acta Cytol* 25:263–266, 1981.

52. Mazzara PF, Flint A, Naylor B: Adenoma of the nipple. Cytopathologic features. *Acta Cytol* 33:188–190, 1989.

53. Stanley MW, Tani EM, Skoog L: Fine needle aspiration of fibroadenomas of the breast with atypia. Spectrum including cases that cytologically mimic carcinoma. *Diagn Cytopathol* 6:375–382, 1990.

54. Whitlatch SP, Panke TW: Myoepithelial cells in needle aspirations of two cases of unusual breast lesions: an aid in differential diagnosis. *Diagn Cytopathol* 2:77–81, 1987.

55. Fanning TV, Sneige N, Staerkel G: Mucinous breast lesions. Fine needle aspiration findings. *Acta Cytol* 34:754, 1990.

56. Franzen S, Zajicek J: Aspiration biopsy in diagnosis of palpable lesions of the breast. Critical review of 3479 consecutive biopsies. *Acta Radiol [Ther](Stockh)* 7:241, 1968.

57. Linsk T, Kreuzer G, Zajicek J: Cytologic diagnosis of mammary tumors from aspiration biopsy smears, II. Studies on 210 fibroadenomas and 210 cases of benign dysplasia. *Acta Cytol* 16:130–138, 1972.

58. Peterse JL, Thunnissen FB, Van Heerde P: Fine needle aspiration cytology of radiation induced changes in non-neoplastic lesions. Possible pitfalls in fine needle aspiration biopsy. *Acta Cytol* 35: 229–233, 1991.

59. Holaday WF, Assor D: Ten thousand consecutive frozen sections. Retrospective study focusing on accuracy and quality control. *Am J Clin Pathol* 61:769–777, 1974.

60. Rosen PP: Frozen section diagnosis of breast lesions. Recent experience with 556 consecutive biopsies. *Ann Surg* 187:17–19, 1978.

61. Adye B, Jolly PC, Bauermeister DE: The role of fine needle aspiration in management of solid breast masses. *Arch Surg* 123:37–39, 1988.

62. Hermansen C, Paulsen HS, Jensen J, et al: Diagnostic reliability of combined physical examinations, mammography, and fine needle puncture ("triple-test") in breast tumors. *Cancer* 60:1866–1871, 1987.

63. Lamb J, Anderson TJ, Dixon MJ, et al: Role of fine needle aspiration cytology in breast cancer screening. *J Clin Pathol* 40:705–709, 1987.

64. Gupta RK, Dowle CS, Simpson JS: The value of needle aspiration cytology of the breast, with an emphasis on the diagnosis of breast disease in young women below the age of 30. *Acta Cytol* 34: 165–168, 1990.

65. Maygarden SJ, McCall JB, Frable WJ: Fine needle aspiration of breast lesions in women aged 30 and under. *Acta Cytol* 35:687–694, 1991.

66. Arishita GI, Cruz BK, Harding CL, et al: Mammogram-directed fine needle aspiration of nonpalpable breast lesions: *J Surg Oncol* 48:153–157, 1991.

67. Evans WP, Cade SH: Needle localization and fine needle aspiration biopsy of nonpalpable breast lesions with use of standard and stereotactic equipment. *Radiology* 173:53–56, 1989.

68. Hann L, Ducatman BS, Wang HH, et al: Nonpalpable breast lesions: evaluation by means of fine needle aspiration cytology. *Radiology* 171:373–376, 1989.

69. Helvie MA, Baker DE, Adler DD, et al: Radiographically guided fine needle aspiration of nonpalpable breast lesions. *Radiology* 174: 657–661, 1990.

70. Kehler M, Albrechtsson O: Mammographic fine needle biopsy of nonpalpable breast lesions. *Acta Radiol [Diagn] (Stockh)* 984:273–276, 1966.

71. Lofgren M, Andersson I, Bondeson L, et al: X-ray guided fine needle aspiration for the cytologic diagnosis of nonpalpable breast lesions. *Cancer* 61:1032–1037, 1988.

72. Masood S, Frykberg ER, McLellan GL, et al: Prospective evaluation of radiologically directed aspiration biopsy of nonpalpable breast lesions. *Cancer* 66:1480–1487, 1990.

73. Azavedo E, Svane G, Auer G: Stereotaxic fine needle biopsy in 2594 mammography detected nonpalpable lesions. *Lancet* 1:1033-1036, 1989.

74. Bibbo M, Scheiber M, Cajuhs R, et al: Stereotaxic fine needle aspiration cytology of clinically occult malignant and premalignant breast lesions. *Acta Cytol* 32:193–201, 1988.

75. Ciatto S, Cataliotti L, Distante V: Nonpalpable lesions detected with mammography: review of 512 consecutive cases. *Radiology* 165:99–102, 1987.

76. Dent DM, Kirkpatrick AE, McGoogan E, et al: Stereotaxic localization and aspiration cytology in nonpalpable breast lesions. *Clin Radiol* 40:380–382, 1989.

77. Dowlatshahi K, Jokich PM, Schmidt R, et al: Cytologic diagnosis of occult breast lesions using stereotaxic needle aspiration. *Arch Surg* 122:1343–1346, 1987.

78. Fajardo LL, Davis JR, Weins JL, et al: Mammography guided stereotactic fine needle aspiration cytology of nonpalpable breast lesions: prospective comparison with surgical biopsy results. *Am J Roentgenol* 155:977–981, 1990.

79. Gent HJ, Sprenger E, Dowlatshahi K: Stereotaxic needle localization and cytological diagnosis of occult breast lesions. *Ann Surg* 204:580–584, 1986.

80. Lofgren M, Anderson J, Lindholm K: Stereotaxic fine needle aspiration for cytologic diagnosis of nonpalpable breast lesions. *Am J Roentgenol* 154:1191–1195, 1990.

81. Mitnick J, Vazquez MF, Roses DF, et al: Stereotaxic localization for fine needle aspiration breast biopsy. Initial experience with 300 patients. *Arch Surg* 126:1137–1140, 1991.

82. Fornage B: Percutaneous biopsies of the breast: state of the art. *Cardiovasc Intervent Radiol* 14:29–39, 1991.

83. Fornage BD, Sneige N, Faroux MJ, et al: Sonographic appearance and ultrasound-guided fine needle aspiration biopsy of breast carcinomas smaller than 1 cm. *J Ultrasound Med* 9:559–568, 1990.

84. Sneige N, Fornage B, Saleh G: Ultrasound guided fine needle aspiration of nonpalpable breast lesions. Cytologic and histologic findings. *Am J Clin Pathol* 102:98–101, 1994.

85. Schwartz GF, Feig SA, Patchefsky AS: Significance and staging of nonpalpable carcinomas of the breast. *Surg Gynecol Obstet* 166:6–10, 1988.

86. Fisher ER, Fisher B: Lobular carcinoma of the breast: an overview. *Am Surg* 185:377–385, 1988.

87. Svane G, Silfversward C: Stereotaxic needle biopsy of nonpalpable breast lesions: cytologic and histologic findings. *Acta Radiol [Diagn] (Stockh)* 24:283–288, 1983.

88. Hall FM, Storella JM, Silverstone DZ, et al: Nonpalpable breast lesions: recommendation for biopsy based on suspicion of carcinoma at mammography. *Radiology* 167:353–358, 1988.

89. Masood S: Nonpalpable breast lesions and aspiration biopsy: a new challenge. *Diagn Cytopathol* 9:613–614, 1993.

90. Jackson VP, Reynolds HE: Stereotaxic needle-core biopsy and fine needle aspiration cytologic evaluation of nonpalpable breast lesions. *Radiology* 188:633–634, 1991.

91. Parker SH, Lovin JDF, Jobe WE, et al: Nonpalpable breast lesions: stereotactic automated large core biopsies. *Radiology* 180:403–407, 1991.

92. Dowlatshahi K, Yaremko NL, Kluskens LF, et al: Nonpalpable breast lesions: findings of stereotaxic needle core biopsy and fine needle aspiration cytology. *Radiology* 181:745–750, 1991.

93. Harter LP, Curtis JS, Ponto G, et al: Malignant seeding of the needle track during stereotaxic core needle biopsy. *Radiology* 185:713–717, 1992.

94. Youngson BJ, Liberman L, Rosen PP: Epithelial displacement in surgical breast specimens following stereotaxic core biopsy. *Mod Pathol* 8:29, 1995. Abstract.

95. Casey TT, Rodgers WH, Baxter WJ, et al: Stratified diagnostic approach to fine needle aspiration of the breast. *Am J Surg* 163:305–311, 1992.

96. Sickles EA: Periodic mammographic follow-up of probably benign lesion results in 3,784 consecutive cases. *Radiology* 179:463–468, 1991.

CHAPTER FOUR

Inflammatory Breast Lesions

The breast consists of major lactiferous ducts, branched ducts, lobules, and connective tissue stroma. In benign conditions, adipose tissue, epithelial cells, and stromal components are often seen. Cellularity is generally low or moderate, and the epithelial cells are arranged in clusters and small groups with myoepithelial cells present. Cytologic atypia and nuclear changes are minimal (Images 4.1 through 4.4). In aspirates of malignant breast disease, cellularity is usually high, with isolated single cells and clusters of discohesive epithelial cells present. Anisonucleosis, chromatin clumping, nuclear membrane abnormality, and necrosis are common cellular features in fine needle aspirates of malignant breast tissue (Images 4.5 through 4.10). The specific cellular characteristics of benign and malignant breast disease are summarized in Table 4.1. Although there are rare exceptions, such as high cellularity in lactating adenoma and insignificant atypia in well-differentiated primary breast carcinoma, these cellular characteristics are, in general, reliable indicators of most benign and malignant breast diseases.

Fine needle aspiration biopsy (FNAB) interpretation should be based on multiple parameters and not on a single criterion. Attempts have already been made to utilize new technologies, such as stereologic technique, cytometry, ploidy study, and molecular testing, to rapidly distinguish between benign and malignant breast disease. However, it has not been demonstrated that any of these techniques assist in differentiating between benign and malignant breast lesions. Cytomorphology remains the most effective approach.

Mastitis and Abscess

Mastitis is an inflammation of the breast that results from lactation, infection, or trauma. Acute suppurative mastitis is typically seen in the early

51

Table 4.1
General Cytomorphologic Features of Benign and Malignant Breast Disease

Cellular Characteristics	Benign	Malignant
Cell yield	Low to moderate	High tumor cellularity
Cellular arrangement	Cohesive, monolayer sheets of two cell population; scattered, bipolar, stripped nuclei	Discohesive, loosely arranged, one cell population Solid, multilayered clusters of cells with nuclear overlapping
Myoepithelial cells	Present	Frequently absent
Isolated, intact single cells	Inconspicuous	Conspicuous
Cellular pleomorphism	Inconspicuous	Conspicuous
Anisonucleosis	Inconspicuous	Conspicuous
Nucleoli	Inconspicuous	Conspicuous
Chromatin clumping	Inconspicuous	Conspicuous
Accompanying cells	Apocrine cells or macrophages	Lymphocytes and plasma cells
Cellular background	Clean background, fat and epithelial cells are separated	Necrotic, "dirty" background with degenerated red blood cells, fat, and epithelial cells intermingled

postpartum period and occurs in 1% to 3% of all lactating women. Staphylococci or, less commonly, streptococci are the microorganisms responsible for acute mastitis.[1] When inflammation localizes, it forms an abscess. Cytologically, an abundant number of inflammatory cells and a few reactive epithelial cells are present (Images 4.11 through 4.16). Epithelial atypia in inflammatory conditions presents a potential diagnostic dilemma, because occasionally the degree of cytologic atypia due to inflammation may approximate the changes seen in malignancy. An inflammatory background and a limited number of epithelial cells are features that militate against a diagnosis of carcinoma.

Chronic mastitis may evolve from an acute process and present as periductal inflammation and duct ectasia with cyst formation and fibrosis. The aspirate may be cellular and show scattered atypical epithelial cells, lymphocytes, plasma cells, fibroblasts, and histiocytes. The histiocytes are discrete, large, oval cells with distinctly delineated, pale, granular cytoplasm. The nuclei are bland and are either single and eccentric or multiple and peripheral (Images 4.17 through 4.21).

Cytomorphology of Mastitis and Abscess
Neutrophils
Foamy macrophages
Cytophagocytosis
Cell debris in background
Epithelial cells with nuclear enlargement and prominent nucleoli
Occasional multinucleated cells

Subareolar Abscess
Subareolar abscess of the breast is a specific clinicopathologic entity well known to surgeons but not readily recognized by pathologists.[2] It was first described in 1951 by Zuka et al.[3] Subareolar abscess is caused by a low-grade infection believed to originate in the lactiferous duct or sinus,

which can lead to abscess formation following rupture of the duct into the surrounding breast parenchyma. Abscess formation is followed by sinus tract formation, chronic recurrent infection, and fistula formation from the underlying subareolar abscess to the base of the nipple.[4,5]

A number of theories have been proposed regarding the pathogenesis of subareolar abscess of the breast. Zuka et al[3] have considered comedomastitis. Others suggest that squamous metaplasia of either normally occurring columnar epithelium of the large lactiferous ducts or congenital anomalies of the ductal system is the cause of this lesion.[4,5] This theory is supported by the demonstration of dilated ducts lined by squamous epithelium and surrounded by inflammatory cells. On histologic examination of the lesion, the ducts often contain macrophages, debris, and keratinous material.

Fine needle aspiration biopsy smears show similar features. The aspirate is cellular, with an inflammatory background containing abundant neutrophils, foreign body–type giant cells, and macrophages. The defining cytologic features of subareolar abscess are anucleated squamous cells, keratinous debris, cholesterol crystals, and numerous metaplastic and parakeratotic-type squamous cells (Images 4.22 and 4.23). Epithelial atypia secondary to infection may create diagnostic difficulty. However, the presence of keratinous debris or squamous cells associated with acute inflammation distinguish this lesion from a neoplastic process or other lesion occurring beneath the nipple.[2,6,7] The precise diagnosis of this lesion has major clinical implications, since the most effective treatment of chronic subareolar abscess is believed to be surgical excision of the abscess and the associated sinus tract and ducts (Figure 4.1 and Image 4.24).[5,8]

Cytomorphology of Subareolar Abscess
Cellular aspirate
Abundant acute inflammatory cells
Foreign body–type giant cells
Anucleated squamous cells
Keratinous material
Macrophages

Granulomatous Mastitis

Granulomatous mastitis, an inflammatory lesion of unknown etiology, was described by Kessler and Wallach in 1972.[9] It usually occurs in patients in their reproductive years with a history of a rapidly growing mass mimicking cancer. Morphologically, the disease is characterized by the presence of multiple, noncaseating granulomas and a giant cell reaction (Images 4.25 through 4.28). The diagnosis of granulomatous mastitis requires exclusion of other granulomatous lesions in the breast. The differential diagnosis of granulomatous lesions of the breast includes duct ectasia; fat necrosis; sarcoidosis; tuberculosis; fungal infection; epidermal inclusion cyst; and foreign bodies, such as suture, silicone, or paraffin leakage from cosmetic implants.[10] The value of FNAB in differentiating between granulomatous lesions of the breast and carcinoma cannot be overemphasized.

Duct ectasia, also called plasma cell mastitis or chemical mastitis, is characterized by a predominant population of plasma cells, granulomas, and

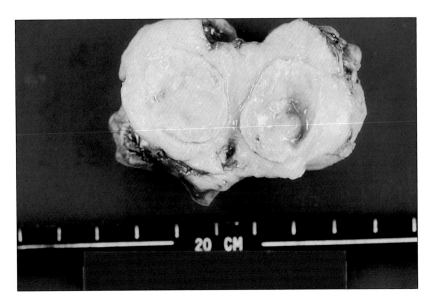

Figure 4.1
Gross photomicrograph of a resected subareolar abscess.

the absence of acid-fast bacilli. Fat necrosis is seen as a collection of lipophages with multinucleated giant cells and epithelioid cells. Foreign bodies produce multinucleated foreign body giant cells and histiocytes containing ingested foreign material. Epidermal inclusion cysts may rupture and cause secondary changes in the breast that clinically simulate carcinoma. In aspirate smears, keratinous material, squamous cells, and abundant inflammatory cells are seen (Images 4.29 through 4.32); however, in contrast to subareolar abscess, the location of the epidermal inclusion cyst may not be subareolar.

Sarcoidosis may also present as granulomatous mastitis but often shows no evidence of necrosis[11] (Images 4.33 through 4.35). If an inflammatory background and purulent material are present, the aspirated material should be sent for appropriate cultures and stains, such as Ziehl-Neelsen, which demonstrates acid-fast bacilli (Images 4.36 through 4.38).[12] It is also important to examine the cellular material for the presence of fungi. *Aspergillus* infection has been reported as a primary localized infection diagnosed by FNAB.[13] This fungus has also been associated with bilateral silicone implants.[14] Similarly, cases of fungal infection presenting as palpable breast lesions have been reported. In these cases, diagnoses of blastomycosis and histoplasmosis were substantiated by demonstration of the causative agents on silver stain.[15,16]

Actinomycosis of the breast can also induce chronic inflammatory changes and granulomatous reaction. It may involve the breast primarily, or it may be a secondary extension of thoracopleural disease.[17,18] The clinical appearance of actinomycosis is such that it has been mistaken for inflammatory breast carcinoma, with the actual diagnosis established following mastectomy or biopsy.[17,18] Diagnosis of actinomycosis of the breast is possible via FNAB by demonstration of polymorphonuclear leukocytes surrounding a typical sulphur granule composed of branching filaments.[19] Cat scratch disease can also involve the breast and present as a granulomatous inflammation. In a case of cat scratch disease reported by Chess et al[20] in 1990, a 21-year-old woman presented with a firm, tender, well-circumscribed lesion. The FNAB smears were highly cellular and consisted mainly of small, round lymphocytes; a few epithelial cells; histiocytes; and leukocytoclastic debris with microabscesses.

Parasitic infections rarely involve the breast.[21,22] We have seen only one case of a hydatid cyst presenting as a mass and diagnosed by FNAB. Associated with constitutional symptoms and a history of feline contact, hydatid cysts can be diagnosed cytologically by finding hooklets of *Echinococcus granulosus* in direct smears and in cytospin preparations (Image 4.39).

Filarial infection of the breast is an extremely rare cause of granulomatous mastitis. The first case diagnosed by FNAB was from a 35-year-old woman residing in an area in which *Wuchereria bancrofti* is endemic. She presented with a tender, cystic lump measuring 2 × 2 cm. The smear was characteristic of filariasis, showing numerous intact microfilariae and embryonated eggs, as well as a few inflammatory cells.[22]

Occasionally, it is difficult to distinguish the atypical, mononuclear, epithelioid histiocytes seen in granulomatous mastitis from neoplastic, mammary epithelial cells. Close attention to the inflammatory background and to the characteristic cytologic features of the histiocytes should help to avoid false-positive diagnosis by FNAB. Immunocytochemical staining is occasionally needed to establish the histiocytic origin of the atypical mononuclear cells. Histiocytes are positive for α_1-antitrypsin, α_1-antichymotrypsin, and lysozyme and are negative for epithelial markers. Awareness of the unusual and distinctive features of granulomatous mastitis and the use of special stains are key factors in substantiating the diagnosis.

Cytomorphology of Granulomatous Mastitis
Cellular aspirate
Lymphocytes and plasma cells
Granulomas with epithelioid and multinucleated giant cells
Reactive ductal epithelial cells with enlarged nuclei
Clusters of fibroblasts

Fat Necrosis and Organized Hematoma

Fat necrosis and organizing hematoma are inflammatory conditions that occur following trauma to the breast. They frequently imitate tumor, often presenting as firm, irregular masses in the breast. In a typical case, the diagnosis is not difficult. The cytologic specimen reveals a predominance of foamy or hemosiderin-laden macrophages, lymphocytes, plasma cells, fibroblasts, and fragments of fibrous tissue and small vessels (Images 4.40 through 4.44). However, groups of reactive epithelial ductal cells may cause great concern. Overinterpretation of epithelial atypia and the misinterpretation of histiocytes in fat necrosis have been reported to result in false-positive diagnoses of cancer.[24,25] The cells in fat necrosis and organizing hematomas are usually present in cohesive sheets, rarely display the degree of pleomorphism that cancer does, and rarely represent the majority of cellular elements, as they do in carcinoma (Images 4.45 and 4.46). Loose, isolated, highly atypical epithelial cells are not usually seen in reactive inflammatory conditions (Images 4.47 through 4.49). Fat necrosis may also coexist with cancer. Thus, lesions displaying fat necrosis should be carefully sampled, and patients with such lesions should receive follow-up.

Cytomorphology of Fat Necrosis and Organized Hematoma
Foamy or hemosiderin-containing macrophages
Inflammatory cells
Multinucleated cells
Fibroblasts
Small, newly formed vessels
Cholesterol crystals
Reactive epithelial cells
Necrotic background

Myospherulosis

Myospherulosis, a disease originally described by McClatchie et al in 1968,[26] results from an alteration of red blood cells after exposure to fats, such as petrolatum, lanolin, or human fats. These altered red blood cells, or spherules, have been produced in vivo and in vitro.[27,28] The spherules stain for antihemoglobin antibody, hemoglobin, peroxidase, and lipofuscin.[28-30] Myospherulosis is an inflammatory condition that results from iatrogenic exposure via intramuscular injections or following surgical impaction with petrolatum-covered gauze. It has been reported in soft tissue of the buttocks, in the brain, and in breast lesions.[31-33]

In 1991 Shabb et al[34] reported that myospherulosis is associated with both benign and malignant breast lesions, including breast carcinomas, fat necrosis, and mesenchymal repair. In their retrospective analysis of fine needle aspirates, Shabb et al suggested that myospherulosis is best seen in Papanicolaou-stained preparations. Spherulosis appears as many round spherules dispersed or in aggregates, with smooth, distinct borders and varied internal morphology. Some spherules of myospherulosis contain a single large, central body surrounded by a halo, while others have multiple bodies occasionally attached to the periphery. However, most spherules have a refractile or oily appearance (Images 4.50 and 4.51). Spherules can be confused with pollen grains, vegetable matter, algae, and fungi.[26,30] The fungal diseases most easily confused with myospherulosis are coccidioidomycosis and rhinosporidiosis. The absence of positive staining with periodic acid–Schiff and Gomori methenamine silver stains clearly substantiates a diagnosis of myospherulosis.[35] The presence of myospherulosis in an FNAB sample of a clinically suspicious breast lesion does not exclude the possibility of an underlying malignancy. Myospherulosis can also be caused by repeat aspirations of fatty tissue and the consequent release of endogenous fat in contact with blood.

Malakoplakia

Malakoplakia is a proliferation of benign histiocytes that phagocytize Michaelis-Gutmann bodies. The pathogenesis of malakoplakia is not yet well established.[36] Breast localization of this lesion is very infrequent.[36,37] In 1993 Perez-Guillermo et al[37] described the cytomorphology of malakoplakia in a patient who presented with a palpable lesion. Fine needle aspiration biopsy of the lesion yielded a cellular aspirate with numerous histiocytes showing round, eccentric nuclei and conspicuous nuclear pyknosis. The cytoplasm was microvacuolated and contained one or several inclusions with features characteristic of Michaelis-Gutmann bodies. Based on the diagnosis of malakoplakia by FNAB, the patient was placed on trimethoprimsulfamethoxazole; the mammographic follow-up performed after 2 months showed that the lesion had disappeared.

Cytologically, malakoplakia must be distinguished from fat necrosis and comedocarcinoma. The presence of Michaelis-Gutmann bodies is an important differentiating feature. Attention should always be paid to histiocytes, since they may lead one to diagnosis of malakoplakia.[38] A diagnosis of malakoplakia should alert the clinician to the possibility of other organ involvement.[36] The cytologic pattern of malakoplakia is distinct, which facilitates diagnosis. Fine needle aspiration biopsy can also be used to monitor the patient's response to therapy and may eliminate the need for surgical biopsy.[37]

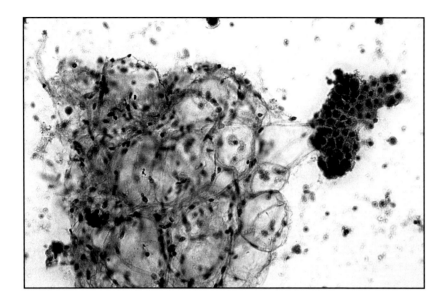

Image 4.1
Cytomorphology of benign breast disease: scant cellular yield with a fragment of adipose tissue and a cluster of epithelial cells (Papanicolaou, 200X).

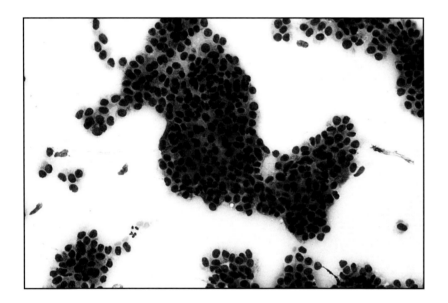

Image 4.2
Cytomorphology of benign breast disease: monolayer clustering of benign-appearing epithelial cells (Diff-Quik®, 200X).

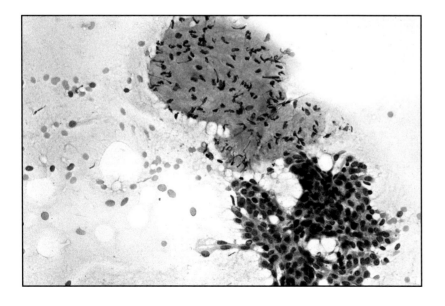

Image 4.3
Cytomorphology of benign breast disease: stromal elements and clusters of epithelial cells (Papanicolaou, 200X).

Image 4.4
Cytomorphology of benign breast disease: spindle cells of myoepithelial origin admixed with an epithelial component (Papanicolaou, 400X).

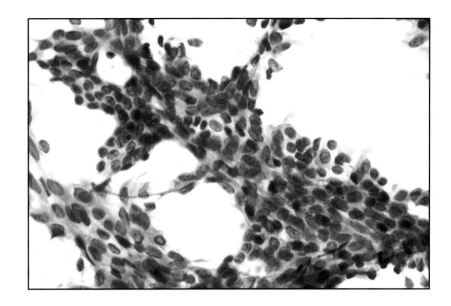

Image 4.5
Cytomorphology of malignant breast disease: cellular aspirate demonstrating loss of cellular cohesion (Diff-Quik, 400X).

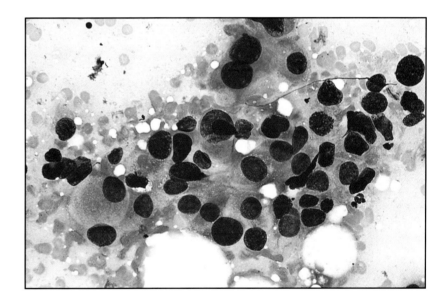

Image 4.6
Cytomorphology of malignant breast disease: cellular smear showing isolated atypical epithelial cells with conspicuous anisonucleosis (Papanicolaou, 400X).

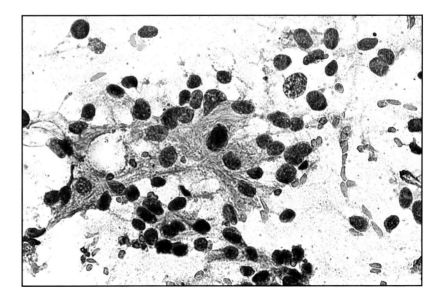

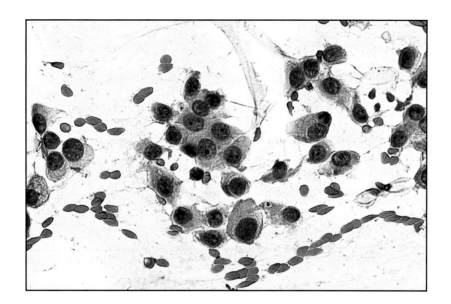

Image 4.7
Cytomorphology of malignant breast disease: scattered, dispersed cell pattern with hyperchromasia of the nuclei (Papanicolaou, 400X).

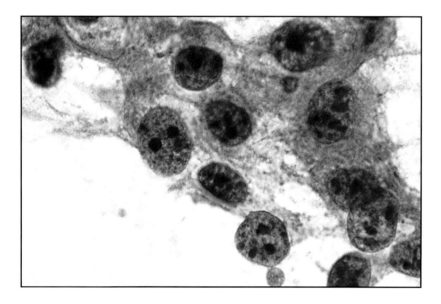

Image 4.8
Cytomorphology of malignant breast disease: hyperchromasia, coarse chromatin pattern, and presence of nucleoli (Papanicolaou, 1000X).

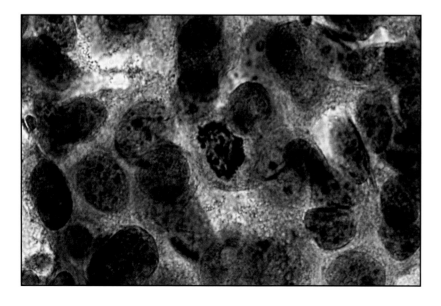

Image 4.9
Cytomorphology of malignant breast disease: prominent nucleoli and mitosis (Papanicolaou, 1000X).

Image 4.10
Cytomorphology of malignant breast disease: extensive necrosis. Cell block preparation (H&E, 200X).

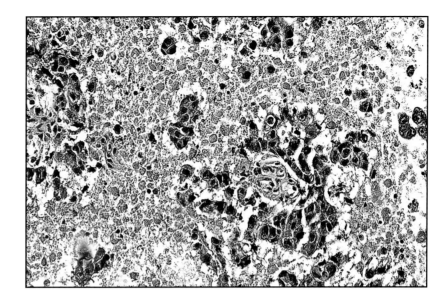

Image 4.11
Direct smear obtained via FNAB of a breast abscess shows necrotic debris, neutrophils, a cluster of epithelial cells, and histiocytes (Papanicolaou, 200X).

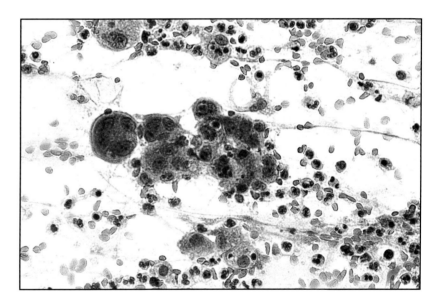

Image 4.12
Cluster of reactive epithelial cells surrounded by neutrophils in aspirate of a breast abscess (Papanicolaou, 200X).

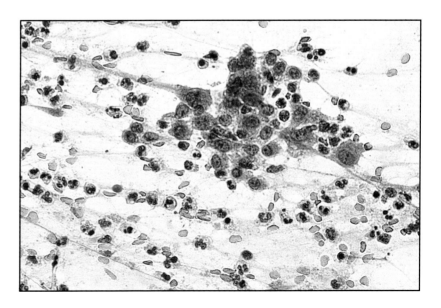

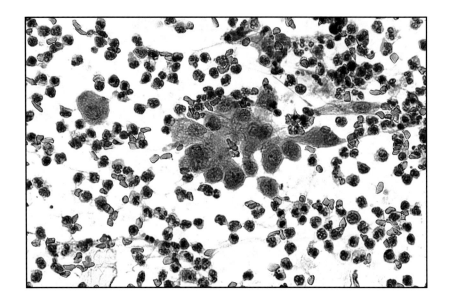

Image 4.13
Nuclear atypia and prominent nucleoli seen in epithelial cells as a response to inflammation. Note the inflammatory background and the lack of cellular discohesion (Papanicolaou, 400X).

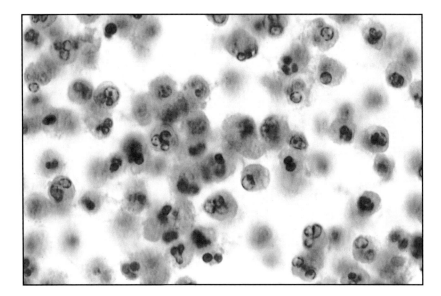

Image 4.14
Cytospin preparation of acute mastitis demonstrating abundant neutrophils (Papanicolaou, 400X).

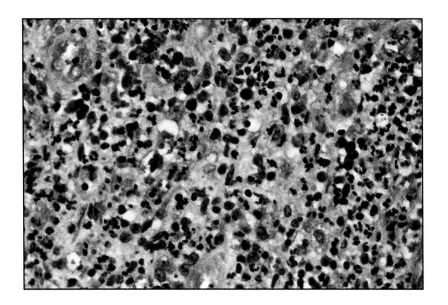

Image 4.15
Corresponding tissue section of an organized breast abscess showing infiltration of acute inflammatory cells (H&E, 200X).

Image 4.16
Higher magnification of the same case
demonstrates necrotic debris, acute
inflammatory cells, and binucleated histiocytes (H&E, 400X).

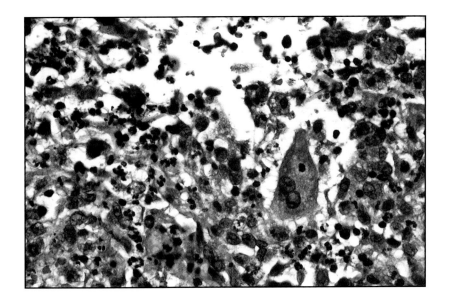

Image 4.17
Cellular smear from FNAB of a patient
with chronic mastitis demonstrates
lymphocytes, plasma cells, fibroblasts,
and histiocytes (Papanicolaou, 100X).

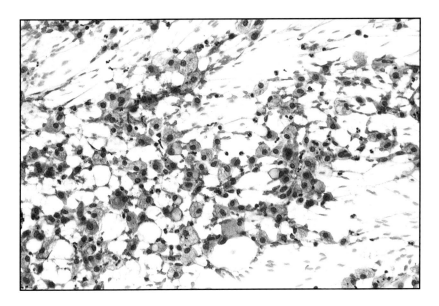

Image 4.18
Collection of histiocytes in the same
case. The histiocytes are discrete and
oval, with distinct cell borders and vacuolated cytoplasm. The nuclei are
peripherally located (Papanicolaou,
1000X).

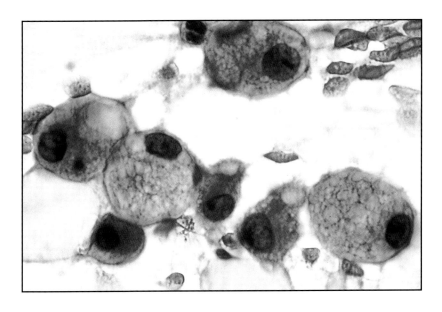

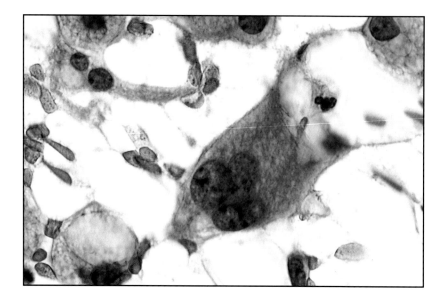

Image 4.19
Histiocytes in a case of chronic mastitis. One shows peripherally located, multiple nuclei (Papanicolaou, 1000X).

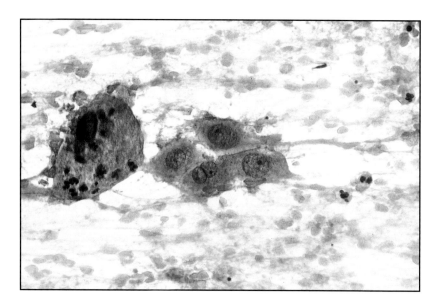

Image 4.20
Histiocytes in the same case show evidence of phagocytosis adjacent to a reactive cluster of epithelial cells (Papanicolaou, 400X).

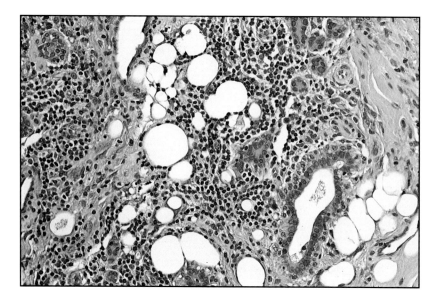

Image 4.21
Tissue section of the same case demonstrates chronic inflammation (H&E, 200X).

Image 4.22
Direct smear from a subareolar abscess: cellular smear with numerous acute inflammatory cells and necrotic debris (Papanicolaou, 200X).

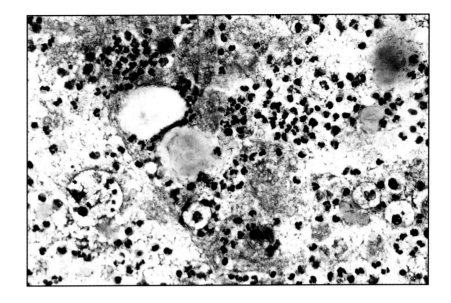

Image 4.23
Higher magnification of the same case demonstrates the presence of squamous and denucleated cells (Papanicolaou, 400X).

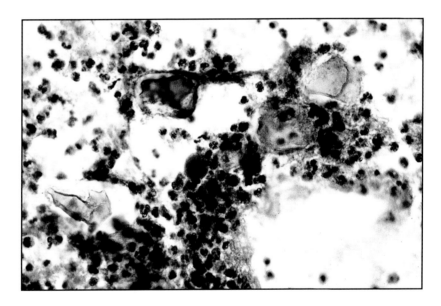

Image 4.24
Tissue section of a subareolar abscess with inflammatory cell infiltrate (H&E, 200X).

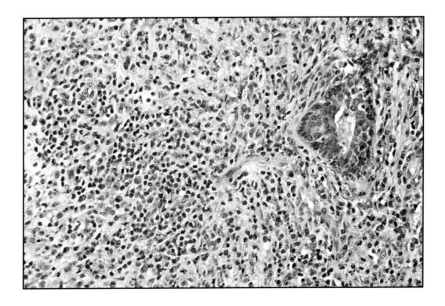

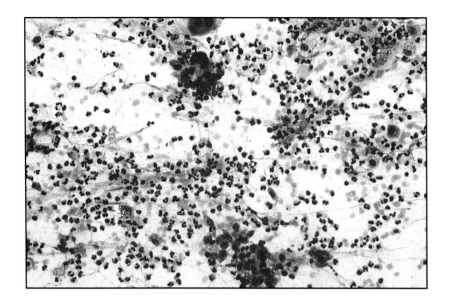

Image 4.25
Direct smear from an FNAB of a patient with granulomatous mastitis. The cellular aspirate consists of lymphocytes, plasma cells, and histiocytes (Diff-Quik, 200X).

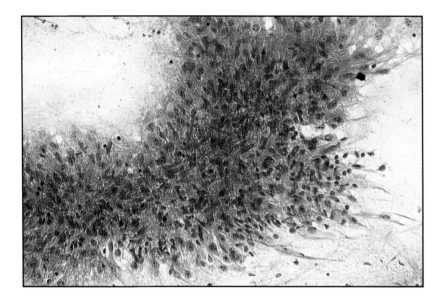

Image 4.26
Direct smear from the same case shows the presence of noncaseating granulomas surrounded by chronic inflammatory cells (Papanicolaou, 200X).

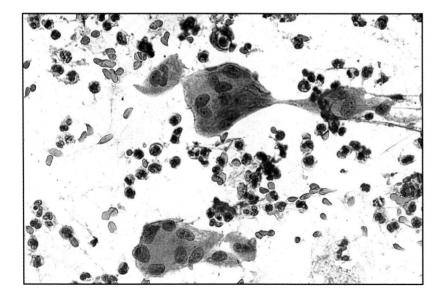

Image 4.27
Higher magnification of other areas of the same case reveals the presence of multinucleated giant cells (Papanicolaou, 400X).

Image 4.28
Cell block preparation of the same case demonstrates a granuloma and many histiocytes (H&E, 200X).

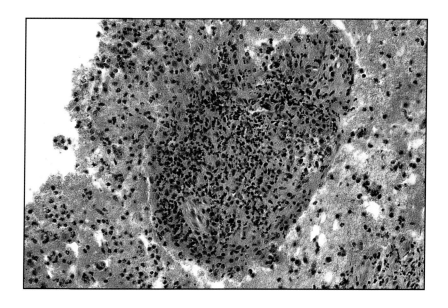

Image 4.29
Photomicrograph of FNAB smear from a patient with a ruptured epidermal inclusion cyst. Note the presence of numerous acute and chronic inflammatory cells and foreign body–type giant cells (H&E, 200X).

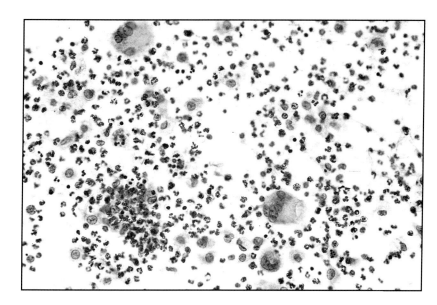

Image 4.30
Higher magnification of the same case demonstrates giant cells and inflammatory cells (H&E, 400X).

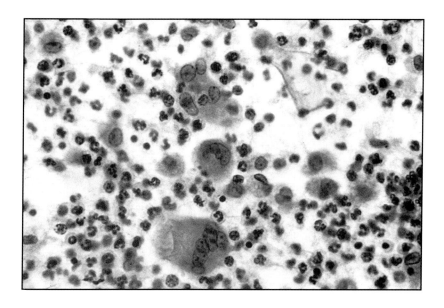

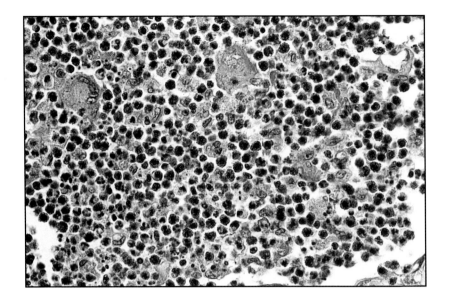

Image 4.31
Cell block preparation of the same case shows inflammatory exudate and giant cells (H&E, 200X).

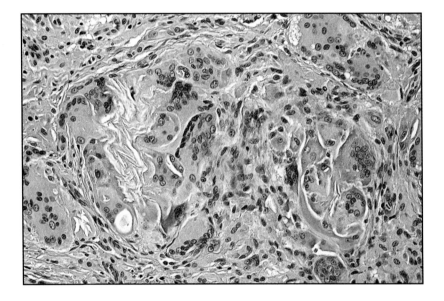

Image 4.32
Surgically excised lesion of the same case with foreign body giant cell reaction to keratin and inflammatory cells (H&E, 400X).

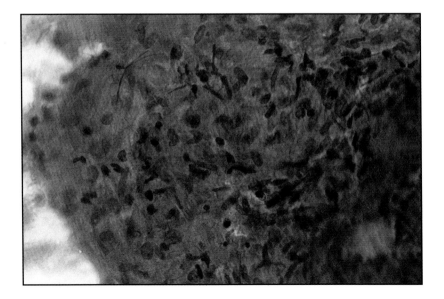

Image 4.33
Direct smear from a diffuse lesion in a breast of a woman with history of sarcoidosis. Note the presence of epithelioid cells embedded in dense, fibrous tissue (Papanicolaou, 400X).

Image 4.34
Direct smear from the same case demonstrates epithelial cells forming a granuloma (Diff-Quik, 1000X).

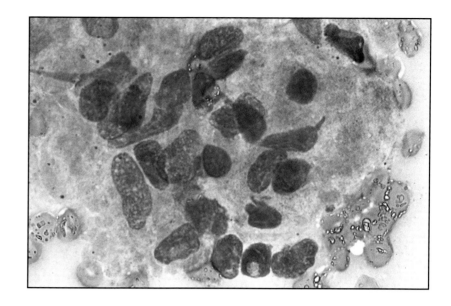

Image 4.35
Previously biopsied lymph node of the same patient demonstrates the presence of a noncaseating granuloma and the absence of acid-fast bacilli, features consistent with sarcoidosis (H&E, 400X).

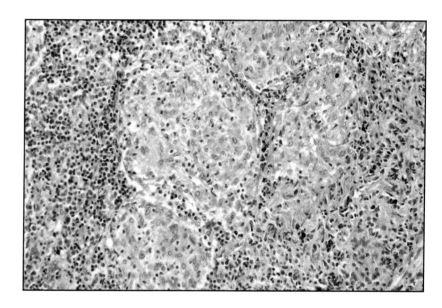

Image 4.36
Granuloma formation seen in direct smear obtained from FNAB of patient with advanced tuberculosis (Papanicolaou, 1000X).

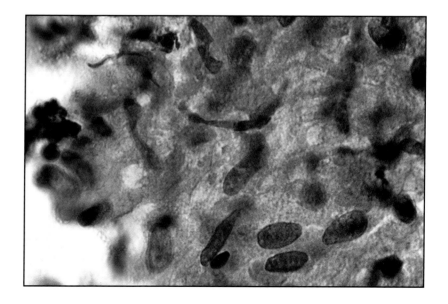

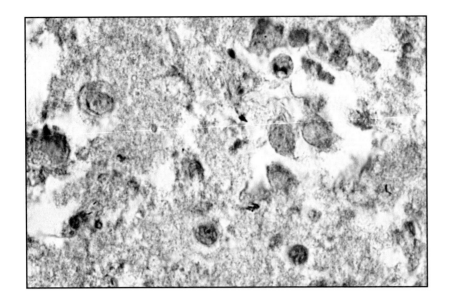

Image 4.37
Direct smear of the same case demonstrates the presence of acid-fast bacilli (Ziehl–Neelsen stain, 1000X).

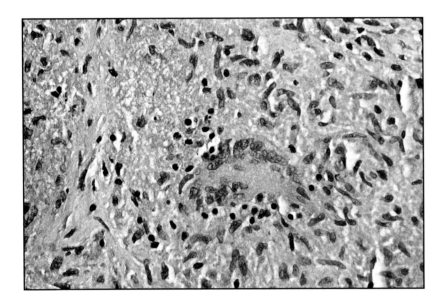

Image 4.38
Tissue section of previously biopsied lesion from the lymph node of the same patient, who was diagnosed with advanced tuberculosis, shows granulomatous inflammation (H&E, 400X)

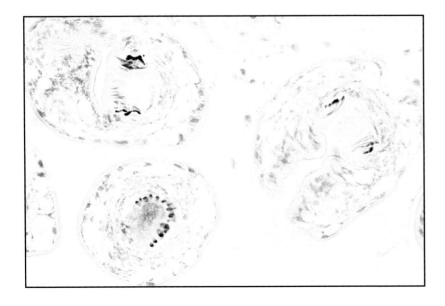

Image 4.39
Cytospin preparation from a patient with a localized breast lesion demonstrates scolices of *Echinococcus granulosus*, diagnosed as a hydatid cyst by FNAB (Papanicolaou, 400X).

Image 4.40
Aspirate of fat necrosis. Cellular smear demonstrates amorphous debris, inflammatory cells, and lipid-laden macrophages (Diff-Quik, 200X).

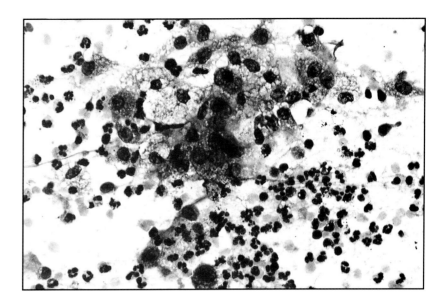

Image 4.41
Papanicolaou-stained smear of the same case shows similar features (100X).

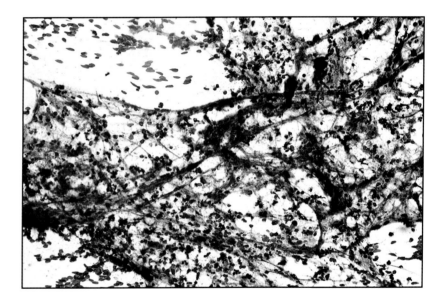

Image 4.42
Cellular debris, inflammatory cells, and small vessels in aspirate of fat necrosis (Papanicolaou, 200X).

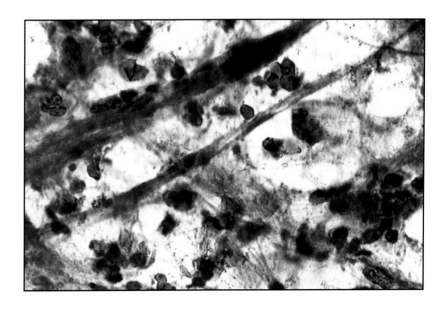

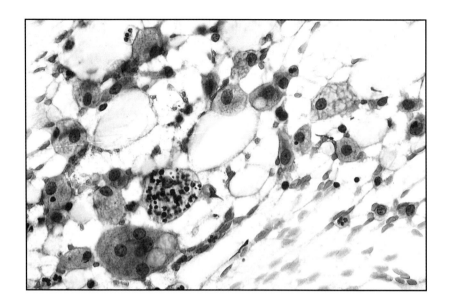

Image 4.43
Aspirate of fat necrosis consisting of lipid-laden macrophages with abundant, vacuolated cytoplasm in an inflammatory background (Papanicolaou, 200X).

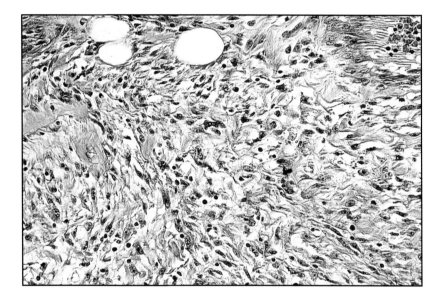

Image 4.44
Fat necrosis in corresponding excisional biopsy of the same case depicted in Images 4.42 and 4.43 (H&E, 200X).

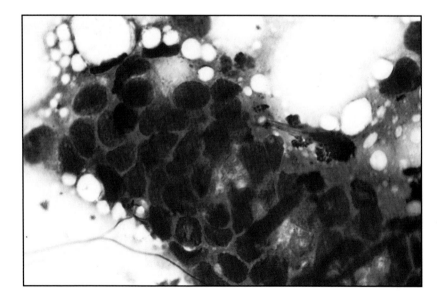

Image 4.45
Aspirate of fat necrosis displaying clusters of atypical epithelial cells with some loss of polarity (Diff-Quik, 400X).

Image 4.46
Papanicolaou-stained slide of the same case shows the presence of atypical cells. Single, isolated epithelial cells are rare in aspirates of fat necrosis (200X).

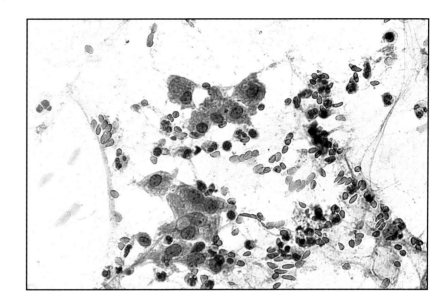

Image 4.47
Aspirate of an infiltrating duct cell carcinoma in a fatty background. In contrast to fat necrosis, the cells show loss of cellular cohesion and conspicuous anisonucleosis (Diff-Quik, 400X).

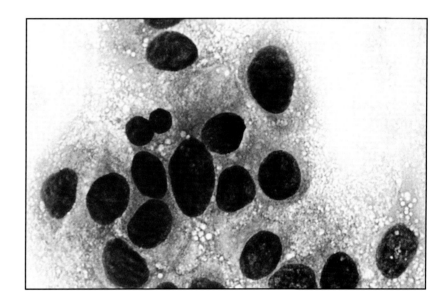

Image 4.48
Higher-power view of the same case shows isolated atypical epithelial cells (Diff-Quik, 1000X).

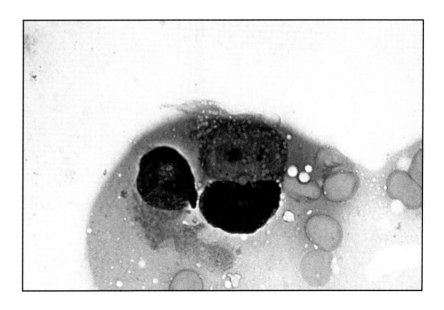

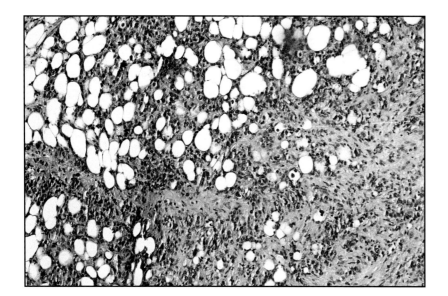

Image 4.49
Corresponding tissue section shows infiltration of neoplastic epithelial cells into the mammary adipose tissue (H&E, 200X).

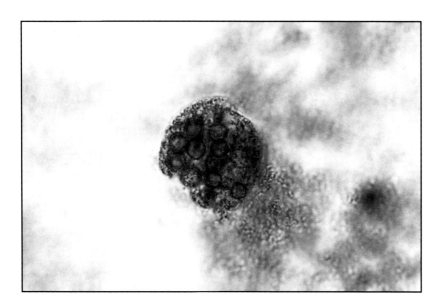

Image 4.50
Direct smear of an aspirate diagnosed as myospherulosis demonstrates many round spherules with smooth, distinct borders and varied internal morphology in a granular background (Papanicolaou, 200X).

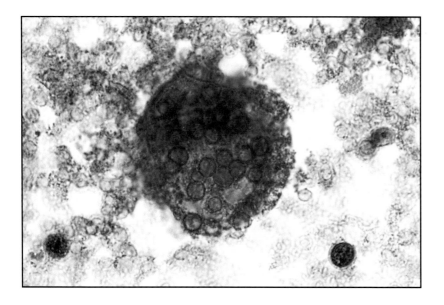

Image 4.51
Higher magnification of the same case (Papanicolaou, 400X).

References

1. Weiss RL, Matsen JM: Group B streptococcal breast abscess. *Arch Pathol Lab Med* 111:74–75, 1987.

2. Galblum LI, Oertel YC: Subareolar abscess of the breast: diagnosis by fine needle aspiration. *Am J Clin Pathol* 80:496–499, 1983.

3. Zuka JJ, Crite G Jr, Aryes WW: Fistulas of lactiferous ducts. *Am J Surg* 81:312–317, 1951.

4. Hahif DV, Persin KH, Lipton R, et al: Subareolar abscess associated with squamous metaplasia of lactiferous ducts. *Am J Surg* 119: 523–526, 1970.

5. Patey DH, Thackray AC: Pathology and treatment of mammary-duct fistula. *Lancet* 2:871–873, 1958.

6. Oertel YC, Galblum LI: Fine needle aspiration biopsy of the breast: diagnostic criteria. *Pathol Annu* 1:375–407, 1983.

7. Silverman JF, Lannin DR, Unverferth M, et al: Fine needle aspiration cytology of subareolar abscess of the breast. Spectrum of cytomorphologic findings and potential diagnostic pitfalls. *Acta Cytol* 30:413–419, 1986.

8. Rosenthal LJ, Greenfield DS, Lesnick GJ: Breast abscess: management in subareolar and peripheral disease. *N Y State J Med* 81:182–183, 1981.

9. Kessler E, Wallach Y: Granulomatous mastitis: a lesion clinically simulating carcinoma. *Am J Clin Pathol* 58:642–646, 1972.

10. Macansh S, Greenberg M, Barraclough B, et al: Fine needle aspiration cytology of granulomatous mastitis. Report of a case and review of the literature. *Acta Cytol* 34:38–42, 1990.

11. Gansler TS, Wheeler JE: Mammary sarcoidosis. *Arch Pathol Lab Med* 108:673–675, 1984.

12. Jayaram G: Cytomorphology of tuberculosis mastitis. A report of nine cases with fine needle aspiration cytology. *Acta Cytol* 29:974–978, 1985.

13. Govindarajan M, Verghese S, Kurutilla S: Primary aspergillosis of the breast: report of a case with fine needle aspiration cytology diagnosis. *Acta Cytol* 37:234–236, 1993.

14. Williams K, Walton RL, Bunkis I: *Aspergillus* colonization associated with bilateral silicone mammary implants. *J Surg Pathol* 71:260–261, 1982.

15. Farmer C, Bardales R, Bradshaw R, et al: Mycoses of the breast: diagnosis by fine needle aspiration. *Acta Cytol* 37:809, 1993. Abstract.

16. Houn HYD, Granger J: Granulomatous mastitis secondary to histoplasmosis: Report of a case diagnosed by fine needle aspiration biopsy. *Diagn Cytopathol* 7:282–285, 1991.

17. Gogas J, Sechas M, Diamantis S, et al: Actinomycosis of the breast. *Int Surg* 57:664–665, 1972.

18. Schouten A: A case of primary actinomycosis of the breast. *Arch Chir Neerl* 25:319–323, 1973.

19. Pinto MM, Longstreth GB, Khoury GM: Fine needle aspiration of actinomycosis, infection of the breast. A novel presentation of thoracopleural actinomycosis. *Acta Cytol* 35:409–416, 1991.

20. Chess G, Santarseieri V, Kostroff K: Aspiration cytology of cat scratch disease of the breast. *Acta Cytol* 34:761, 1990.

21. Quedrazgo E-G: Lekysle hydatique du sein: etude de 20 observations. *J Gynecol Obstet Biol Reprod (Paris)* 14:187–194, 1985.

22. Sagin HB, Kiroglu Y, Aksoy F: Hydatid cyst of the breast diagnosed by fine needle aspiration biopsy. A case report. *Acta Cytol* 38: 965–967, 1994.

23. Bapat KC, Pandit AA: Filarial infection of the breast. Report of case with diagnosis by fine needle aspiration cytology. *Acta Cytol* 36: 505–506, 1992.

24. Biedrzycki T, Dabska M, Sikorowa L, et al: On cytologic vagaries in the diagnosis of breast tumor. *Tumori* 66:191–196, 1980.

25. Layfield LJ, Glasgow BJ, Cramer H: Fine needle aspiration in the management of breast masses. *Pathol Annu* 24:23–62, 1989.

26. McClatchie S, Warambo MW, Bremmer AD: Myospherulosis: a previously unreported disease. *Am J Clin Pathol* 57:699–704, 1969.

27. Rosai J: The nature of myospherulosis. *Am J Clin Pathol* 69: 475–481, 1978.

28. Wheeler TM, McGavarn MH: Myospherulosis: future observations. *Am J Clin Pathol* 73:685–686, 1980.

29. DeSchryrer-Kecskemeti K, Kyriakos M: Myospherulosis: an electron microscopic study of a human case. *Am J Clin Pathol* 67: 555–561, 1977.

30. Travis WD, Li CY, Weiland LH: Immunostaining for hemoglobin in two cases of myospherulosis. *Arch Pathol Lab Med* 110:263–265, 1986.

31. Shimada K, Kobayashi S, Yamadori I, et al: Myospherulosis in Japan: a report of two cases and an immunohistochemical investigation. *Am J Surg Pathol* 129:427–432, 1988.

32. Mills SE, Lininger JR: Intracranial myospherulosis. *Hum Pathol* 13:596–597, 1982.

33. Ferrell LD: Myospherulosis of the breast: diagnosis by fine needle aspiration. *Acta Cytol* 28:726–728, 1984.

34. Shabb N, Sneige N, Dekmezian RH: Myospherulosis. Fine needle aspiration cytologic findings in 19 cases. *Acta Cytol* 35:225–228, 1991.

35. Kyriakos M: Myospherulosis of the paranasal sinuses, nose and middle ear. *Am J Clin Pathol* 67:118–130, 1977.

36. McClaure J. Malakoplakia. *J Pathol* 140:275–330, 1983.

37. Perez-Guillermo M, Sola-Perez J, Rodriguez-Bermejo M: Malakoplakia and Rosai-Dorfman disease: two entities of histiocytic origin infrequently localized in the female breast. The cytologic aspect in aspirates obtained via fine needle aspiration cytology. *Diagn Cytopathol* 9:698–704, 1993.

38. Stanton MJ, Maxted W: Malakoplakia: a study of the literature and current concepts of pathogenesis, diagnosis and treatment. *J Urol* 125:139–146, 1981.

CHAPTER FIVE

Noninflammatory Breast Lesions

Cysts

Cysts are the most common lesion of the female breast and are frequently subject to fine needle aspiration biopsy (FNAB). In recent years, the practice of combining sonography and FNAB has become popular in breast clinics and in gynecologic offices.[1] In 1988 Gupta et al[2] reported that in their review of 3,226 cases of breast FNAB, cysts constituted 17.2% of lesions in women over age 30.

Cysts produce fluid that varies in appearance from clear to opaque dark brown or yellow-green to bloody. Benign cysts are acellular and only occasionally contain foamy cells, epithelial cells, or apocrine cells (Images 5.1 and 5.2). Aspirates from apocrine cysts and chronic cystic mastitis may be more cellular than those from duct ectasia (Images 5.3 through 5.6). Occasionally, intracytoplasmic, eosinophilic inclusion bodies can be seen in benign cyst fluids. These inclusions are morphologically similar to the well-known intracytoplasmic, eosinophilic inclusion bodies seen in urine specimens (Images 5.7 and 5.8). Ultrastructural studies have shown that these inclusions represent giant lysosomes within the macrophages and indicate a degenerative process.[3,4]

The question of how to evaluate breast cyst fluids is somewhat controversial, since more than 99% of them are derived from benign cysts. Reports in the literature and our own experience suggest that cytologic examination of cyst fluids should be limited to fluids that are bloody in nature.[5] Cysts that form due to tumors are virtually always bloody, with some residual thickening. If a residual mass persists after a cyst is aspirated, the mass should be reaspirated and examined.

The presence of a clinically and radiologically occult intracystic lesion, such as a papilloma or carcinoma, may be suspected when the cyst fluid is bloody (Images 5.9 through 5.14).[6–9] However, since such lesions have been found even in the absence of blood in the cyst fluid, some authors have recommended performing routine pneumocystography[10] and/or cytologic studies[11,12] on all breast cysts. Cystic lesions with a clear fluid and no residual mass rarely harbor malignant lesions. Rarely, medullary carcinomas become cystic, and the aspirated samples consist of clear fluid. The smears show a mixture of inflammatory cells and tumor cells (Images 5.15 through 5.18). If tumor cells are sparse in an aspirated smear of cystic medullary carcinoma, accurate diagnosis may become difficult.[13,14] In fluid specimens with many inflammatory cells, the possibility of tumor must be anticipated. A mammogram should be performed following a cyst aspiration.

In a review of 6,782 cases, Ciatto et al[5] assessed the cost-effectiveness and diagnostic value of breast cyst fluid aspiration cytology in detecting occult breast cancer. They found five clinically and radiologically inapparent intracystic papillomas (1%). Each of the five cases produced a blood-stained fluid and showed an intracystic mass on pneumocystography. One incidental case of occult in situ lobular carcinoma was also detected. No true occult intracystic cancer was observed. Based on these observations, Ciatto et al concluded that routine examination of all breast cyst fluids is not cost-effective. Although the cytologic examination of simple cysts with clear fluid has limited diagnostic value, such specimens are occasionally sent to the laboratory for cytologic evaluation—mainly because the patient is apprehensive or the clinician fears legal liability.

Fibroadenoma

Fibroadenomas are the most commonly observed neoplasm in women under age 25 and appear to be more prevalent in the black population.[15–17] These slow-growing tumors are believed to occur as the result of unopposed estrogenic influence on susceptible tissue.[18,19] Fibroadenomas often present as small, solitary, painless nodules. Radiologically they appear as well-defined lesions (Figure 5.1). The incidence of multiplicity in reported series varies from 7% to 16% of cases.[19,20] Rapidly growing tumors, referred to as giant, juvenile, or fetal fibroadenomas, occur in adolescent females and may become as large as 19 cm.[19] Carcinoma arising in a fibroadenoma is very rare and constitutes only 0.1% of all cases.[16] In situ and infiltrating lobular carcinomas are reportedly the most common malignant lesions associated with fibroadenoma.[21]

Fibroadenomas can be diagnosed by FNAB. The aspirates are typically cellular and demonstrate a biphasic pattern consisting of epithelial and stromal elements (Images 5.19 and 5.20). The cell population consists of two different cell types. Large cells form sheets of monolayered epithelial clusters with finger-like projections in an antler-horn pattern (Image 5.21). The second cell type, small cells with naked nuclei, may be bipolar or spindle shaped, admixed with epithelial cells, and/or lie freely in the background (Images 5.22 and 5.23). The origin of these cells is controversial.[22,23] Immunostains for muscle specific actin (MSA) can be applied to identify myoepithelial cells in the aspirate smear.[24] Scattered histiocytes,

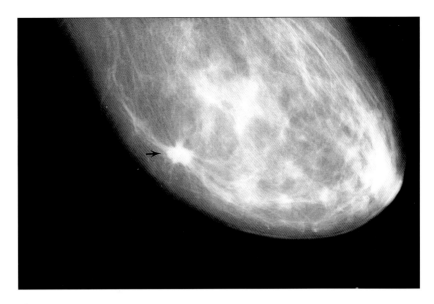

Figure 5.1
Mammographic appearance of a fibroadenoma appearing as a well-defined mass.

apocrine cells, and occasional multinucleated giant cells may also be present in cellular aspirates of fibroadenoma (Images 5.24 and 5.25).[22,25,26]

Juvenile fibroadenomas are typically large lesions with distinct cytomorphology.[27] The characteristic feature of juvenile fibroadenoma is an almost monomorphic cellular aspirate consisting of a conspicuous number of monolayered sheets of cells and papillae, which are composed of uniform, bland, columnar cells surrounded by a few foam cells and histiocytes (Figure 5.2 and Images 5.26 through 5.28). The age of the patient substantiates the correct diagnosis.

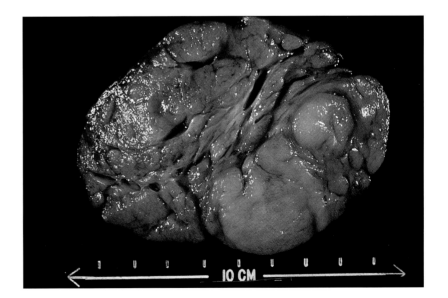

Figure 5.2
Gross appearance of a giant fibroadenoma. The lesion is large and well demarcated, with a whorled surface.

Fibroadenomas have many faces and can display a variety of architectural patterns and cellular features. The cytologic differential diagnosis includes the spectrum of fibrocystic change, including atypical hyperplasia and papillary lesions. Fibroadenomas can also mimic phyllodes tumors and low-grade carcinomas, including tubular carcinoma. Cytologic differentiation between fibroadenoma and the spectrum of fibrocystic change may be difficult. Linsk et al[22] and Bottles et al[25] found that the two conditions have overlapping cytologic features, including cellularity, fronds, naked nuclei, and stromal fragments. However, Bottles et al[25] concluded that the presence of well-demarcated stroma containing fibrillary clusters of spindle cells is the most important differentiating feature. This feature was present in 97% of fibroadenomas and was not seen in any of the cases of fibrocystic change. In a similar study, Butler et al,[28] using the same criteria of cellularity, fronds, naked nuclei, and stromal fragments, found that the combination of a honeycomb pattern; antler horn–like projections; and numerous, bipolar, naked nuclei is the most important factor in making the diagnosis of fibroadenoma. Linsk et al,[22] on the other hand, believe that the defined cytologic criteria should be analyzed quantitatively to distinguish between fibroadenoma and fibrocystic change.

Fibroadenomas may be associated with significant cytologic atypia, resulting in a false-positive diagnosis (Image 5.29).[28-35] The potential pathogenetic mechanisms for atypia in fibroadenoma include response to hormonal stimulation, focal secretory activity, response to inflammation, squamous and apocrine metaplasia, and preneoplastic atypia. We have seen many cases in which the cytologic features of atypical hyperplasia coexisted with histologically proven fibroadenomas (Images 5.30 through 5.37). Fibroadenomas may also be characterized by the presence of cell balls and distended cords, simulating lobular neoplasia (Images 5.38 and 5.39). Pregnancy and lactational changes increase the cellularity of fibroadenoma and produce moderate nuclear atypia and conspicuous nucleoli (Images 5.40 and 5.41). In these circumstances, the cellularity of the aspirate, loose cohesion, occasional papillary structures, anisonucleosis, and macronuclei can simulate carcinoma. The presence of naked nuclei, stromal fragments, and finger-like projections should suggest the benign nature of the lesion. The absence of a necrotic background and isolated, single, pleomorphic epithelial cells are also helpful in separating fibroadenoma from carcinoma.[10,20,21,25,33,36]

In elderly patients, fibroadenomas may be clinically suspicious for malignancy. The high cellularity of the aspirate may also cause concern. However, a diagnosis of carcinoma by FNAB in a patient with a clinical impression of fibroadenoma should be based on all the cytologic criteria of malignancy in a well-preserved cellular preparation.[35] A fibroadenoma with mucous degeneration may be misdiagnosed as mucinous carcinoma. The presence of mucus in the background of a breast smear should not be regarded as sufficient to render a diagnosis of mucinous carcinoma. The presence of stromal fragments and numerous bare nuclei and the absence of cells with eccentric nuclei can distinguish fibroadenoma from mucinous carcinoma (Images 5.42 and 5.43).[28]

Low-grade carcinoma of the breast can simulate fibroadenoma.[37] Cytologically, low-grade carcinomas are characterized by bland-appearing epithelial cells in clusters and in a dispersed cellular pattern, mimicking atypical fibroadenomas that show loss of cellular cohesion. Morphologic distinction between these lesions may be difficult. Immunostaining for MSA to detect myoepithelial cells is most helpful (Images 5.44 through 5.47). The presence or absence of immunoreactivity for MSA in the smears may also be of great help in differentiating between fibroadenoma and tubular carcinoma.[38] Tubular carcinoma is characterized by tightly cohesive clusters of cells and minimal atypia. In contrast to fibroadenoma, tubular carcinoma is marked by impressive monomorphism due to a lack of myoepithelial differentiation (Images 5.48 through 5.51). Rigid, sometimes bent, tubular structures, along with fragments of elastic material and isolated cells that retain their cytoplasm, are among the most useful diagnostic features.[39]

Carcinoma arising in or adjacent to a breast fibroadenoma presents another diagnostic difficulty.[40] The cytologic presentation may differ depending on how the lesion is sampled and where the needle is placed. Naturally, if only a malignant lesion is sampled, the smear may show a population of one cell type exhibiting cytologic evidence of malignancy. Simpson et al[41] reported a case in which the aspirate contained many epithelial cells with a variable amount of cytoplasm, irregular nuclei, and large nucleoli. A few vacuoles were seen in the cytoplasm, and there was no myoepithelial or stromal component. Histologic examination of the excised lesion showed the presence of ductal carcinoma in situ in a fibroadenoma.

Ductal adenoma, a rare benign tumor of the breast, also shares some cytologic features with fibroadenoma. However, in contrast to fibroadenoma, in which there is distinct separation between the stroma and the epithelial cells, ductal adenoma shows an intimate association between the two components. In addition, the stroma in ductal adenoma is acellular.[42]

The cytologic distinction between fibroadenoma and phyllodes tumors is based primarily on the pattern and cellularity of the stromal fragments and may present a diagnostic challenge (Images 5.52 and 5.53). Stromal fragments in phyllodes tumor are conspicuously cellular. Also, the spindle cells in phyllodes tumor are embedded in pink-staining, acid mucopolysaccharide of the stroma, which is best demonstrated by metachromatic stains.[26,43–45] Stromal overgrowth, atypical stromal cells, and mitoses favor a diagnosis of high-grade phyllodes tumor.[46] Morphologically, the distinction between fibroadenoma and benign phyllodes tumor is somewhat difficult. Clinically, however, phyllodes tumor presents as a large, rapidly growing lesion. In contrast to fibroadenoma, phyllodes tumor occurs in older age groups. An excisional biopsy can confirm a diagnosis of phyllodes tumor and distinguish between benign and malignant types.

Cytomorphology of Fibroadenoma

Cellular aspirate
Stromal fragments
Sheets of monolayered, ductal epithelial cells forming antler horns
Bipolar, naked nuclei
Occasional apocrine cells
Rare multinucleated giant cells

Papilloma

Papillomas are generally solitary lesions of the major ducts, commonly located in the subareolar region. They occur most frequently in women over 50. Papillomas also occur in men.[47–49] Presenting symptoms include nipple discharge; a central, subareolar mass; or nipple retraction.[50] Intraductal papillomas are not associated with significant risk for subsequent development of cancer.[51] Papillomas are characterized by the formation of epithelial fronds supported by a fibrovascular stroma. Papillomas are lined by two layers of uniform, columnar or cuboidal cells and myoepithelial cells.[52] Metaplastic apocrine cells are not uncommon.[50] The epithelial cells rarely undergo oncocytic changes.[53] Thrombosis and hemorrhagic infarction occur occasionally.[45] Mucinous, clear, sebaceous, and squamous metaplasia also occur in papilloma.[53,54]

Cytologic diagnosis of intraductal papilloma can be made either by examining the serous or bloody nipple secretion or by FNAB of a palpable lesion. The smears are relatively cellular and show a striking, proteinaceous background with a large number of foamy macrophages. The epithelial cells are arranged in three-dimensional papillary clusters. Occasionally, tall columnar cells representing hyperplastic duct and epithelial cells of the cyst wall are also present. These cells characteristically have eccentric nuclei and cytoplasm that narrows at one end, where the nucleus is located, giving the cell a conical appearance. The tall columnar cells resemble bronchial and endocervical epithelial cells but lack cilia and mucous vacuoles. Cell balls are common. Occasionally, loosely cohesive groups of cells, isolated cells, and naked nuclei may be seen. Some degree of anisonucleosis and a few macronucleoli may be observed (Images 5.54 through 5.58). Some of these features may also be seen in other papillary lesions of the breast. Clinical presentation, location, age, and the presence of more than one lesion of the same type may assist in precise classification of papillary lesions of the breast.

Morphologic distinction between papilloma and well-differentiated papillary carcinoma can be difficult. Among various histologic features, the single most important finding is the presence of a relatively uniform layer of myoepithelial cells in the proliferating, papillary, intraluminal component of the lesion (Images 5.59 through 5.61). The importance of this finding explains the wisdom of avoiding frozen-section diagnosis of papillary lesions. The recommended approach for correct diagnosis of papillary lesions of the breast is total excision of the mass along with a rim of uninvolved breast tissue.

Cytologic findings that suggest a diagnosis of intraductal papilloma include the presence of sheets of hyperplastic ductal cells blending imperceptibly with apocrine metaplastic cells and the characteristic polymorphous cell population (Image 5.62). Immunostaining for MSA can also be performed to detect myoepithelial cells in destained Papanicolaou direct smear preparations or in cell block preparations.[24] Papillary carcinomas are often characterized by a monomorphic cell population with mild to moderate pleomorphism and isolated, atypical columnar cells (Image 5.63).[55,56]

Another lesion that should be differentiated from papilloma is fibroadenoma. Cellularity, tissue fragments, and occasional naked nuclei are overlapping cytologic features. However, the presence of cell balls, red blood cells, foamy macrophages, and cellular polymorphism are features that favor a diagnosis of papilloma (Images 5.64 and 5.65).

Cytomorphology of Papilloma
Cellular aspirate
Proteinaceous or bloody background

Foamy or hemosiderin-containing macrophages
Tall columnar cells
Three-dimensional papillary clusters
Presence of myoepithelial cells
Cell balls

Nipple Adenoma (Papillomatosis)

Nipple adenoma is a rare tumor that occurs beneath the nipple and subareolar region. Patients with nipple adenoma often present with nipple discharge and/or ulceration and crusting of the nipple. The tumor can simulate Paget's disease clinically and adenocarcinoma histologically.[57]

Nipple adenoma is a benign tumor with a potential for local recurrence.[58] Rarely, carcinoma has been associated with nipple adenoma.[59] Nipple adenoma is also known as florid papillomatosis, subareolar duct papillomatosis, erosive adenomatosis, and papillary adenoma of the nipple.[60–62] Nipple adenoma results from the proliferation of epithelial cells within the lactiferous ducts. Morphologically, the cells have a papillary pattern and contain a core of connective tissue. The epithelial cells are columnar in nature and are admixed with myoepithelial cells (Image 5.66).

Fine needle aspiration biopsy of this lesion yields a cellular aspirate composed of a large number of epithelial cells, which may be present both singly and in clusters. The epithelial cell nuclei are uniform with a fine chromatin pattern and inconspicuous nucleoli (Images 5.67 and 5.68). A few cells may show anisonucleosis and hyperchromasia. Naked nuclei and papillary clusters with or without a vascular core may be present. The cellular background may display cellular debris, inflammatory cells, and hemosiderin-containing macrophages.[63,64] When combined with the typical clinical presentation, the cytologic features of nipple adenoma, although not particularly distinctive, are sufficiently characteristic to render a correct diagnosis.

Paget's disease, infiltrating carcinoma, fibrocystic change, mammary duct ectasia, fibroadenoma, intraductal papilloma, and chronic subareolar abscess may also involve the nipple. Paget's disease is characterized by a pleomorphic, hyperchromatic population of cells that contain multiple, variably sized nucleoli and are mucin positive. Infiltrating carcinoma involving the nipple is often poorly differentiated and is associated with significant cytologic abnormalities not commonly observed in nipple adenoma. Furthermore, carcinomas are associated with a significant lack of cohesion and the presence of many single cells. The cytologic features of nipple adenoma and other benign lesions can overlap. However, there are a few features that may assist in a correct distinction. These include the presence of white blood cells in duct ectasia, cell balls in intraductal papilloma, monolayering and fronds in fibroadenoma, and apocrine cells and foam cells in lesions associated with fibrocystic change (Table 5.1).

Cytomorphology of Nipple Adenoma
Cellular aspirate
Inflammatory background
Hemosiderin-containing macrophages

Table 5.1
Cytologic Differential Diagnosis of Nipple Adenoma*

	Nipple Adenoma	Duct Ectasia	Intraductal Papilloma	Fibroadenoma
Cytoplasm	Moderate amount	Scant to moderate	Scant, clear	Scant
Nuclear features	Regular shape, slight hyperchromasia	Regular shape, pyknotic	Hyperchromatic	Small, naked nuclei
Nucleoli	1–2, small	Inconspicuous	Small	Small
Other features	Few naked nuclei	White blood cells	Spheres of cells	Fronds, monolayer sheets

	Fibrocystic Change	Invasive Carcinoma	Paget's Disease	Subareolar Abscess
Cytoplasm	Scant	Moderate, possibly vacuolated	Moderate, possibly vacuolated	Moderate
Nuclear features	Hyperchromatic	Irregular, pleomorphic	Hyperchromatic, pleomorphic	Slight pleomorphism
Nucleoli	Inconspicuous	Multiple, large	Multiple, variable size	Small
Other features	Apocrine cells, foam cells	Single cells, loose clusters	Mucin positive	Anucleated squames, neutrophils, histiocytes

*Modified from: Mazzara PF, Flint A, Naylor B: Adenoma of the nipple. *Acta Cytol* 33:189–190, 1989.

Papillary clusters
Naked nuclei

Juvenile Papillomatosis

Juvenile papillomatosis (Swiss-cheese disease) is a proliferative breast disorder that affects young women (age range, 10–40; average, 21 years). The lesions associated with juvenile papillomatosis are discrete, well-defined, and characterized by cystically dilated ducts and various degrees of intraductal hyperplasia.[65] The cysts are lined by flat epithelium or metaplastic apocrine cells and show areas of papillary hyperplasia with or without atypia. Fine needle aspiration biopsy of this lesion often obtains cyst fluid. The cytologic features of juvenile papillomatosis include rich cellularity, well-ordered fragments of ductal epithelial cells with a papillary configuration, apocrine cells, naked nuclei, macrophages, and fragments of fibrous connective tissue in the background (Images 5.69 through 5.71).[66,67]

Depending on the degree of hyperplastic change, the cytologic differential diagnosis of juvenile papillomatosis includes fibroadenoma, proliferative breast disease with or without atypia, sclerosing adenosis, papillomatosis, carcinoma in situ, and an invasive lesion. Due to the multicystic nature of juvenile papillomatosis, even when cytologic and clinical findings, including the presence of fluid and a residual lump, are combined, one can only suggest a diagnosis and recommend a confirmatory open biopsy.[67] Also, because of the associated increased risk of breast cancer, long-term follow-up of patients with juvenile papillomatosis is highly recommended.[68] Intraductal lobular carcinoma in situ and secretory carcinoma have been associated with juvenile papillomatosis.[69,70]

Cytomorphology of Juvenile Papillomatosis
Cyst fluid and highly cellular aspirate
Well-ordered fragments of epithelial cells forming papillae
Apocrine cells
Naked nuclei

Microglandular Adenosis

Originally described by McDivitt et al[71] in 1968, microglandular adenosis (MGA) is a peculiar benign proliferative lesion of the breast. Clinically, patients with MGA present with a localized mass, which often recurs in middle-aged women. Microscopically, microglandular adenosis is characterized by a poorly circumscribed, organoid proliferation of glands within loose, fibrous or fat stroma. The glands have a round shape and regular size and are delineated by uniform, cuboid, epithelial cells with vacuolated, glycogen-containing, clear cytoplasm. In contrast to other types of adenosis, MGA lacks a distinct layer of myoepithelial cells. The features of MGA can be easily confused with those of invasive carcinoma.[71–73]

Description of the cytomorphologic features of MGA is based on FNABs of two cases reported by Gherardi et al[74] in 1993. In both cases, the diagnosis was inconclusive and excisional biopsies were performed. The smears showed striking similarities. Cellularity was sparse, and the background was rich in red blood cells, with a few fibroblasts present. No myoepithelial cells were identified. The predominant feature in both aspirates was a monotonous population of medium-sized, round to oval cells with clear cytoplasm containing small vacuoles or granules. The cells had no definite borders due to fragmentation of the cytoplasm. The nuclei were uniform, with a fine chromatin pattern and small nucleoli. The clear cells formed gland-like clusters with empty lumens. In contrast to other benign breast lesions, the smears showed a lack of various ancillary cells, such as foam cells.

The presence of clear cells in a solid, noncystic breast lesion poses diagnostic difficulty. The cytologic differential diagnosis summarized in Table 5.2 includes fibrocystic change, fat necrosis, organized hematoma, secretory carcinoma, colloid carcinoma, lobular carcinoma, and metastatic renal cell carcinoma. Secretory changes can also occur in benign breast lesions, so that even in the absence of pregnancy or hormonal manipulation, cells can appear vacuolated.[75,76] However, the lack of myoepithelial cells in MGA is a contrasting feature that helps substantiate the diagnosis. The absence of necrotic debris and inflammatory cells in the background can easily exclude a diagnosis of fat necrosis or organized hematoma. Secretory carcinoma can be distinguished from MGA by its higher cellularity, different cell arrangements, and more pronounced nuclear atypia.[77] In contrast to colloid carcinoma, in MGA there is no mucin in the background. Similarly, unlike lobular carcinoma, there are no mucin-producing cells or signet ring cells in MGA.[78,79]

Metastatic renal cell carcinoma is a possibility that should be excluded by clinical investigation. We have seen three cases of unexpected renal cell carcinoma in which the patient presented with a superficial breast lesion.

Cytomorphology of Microglandular Adenosis
Sparse cellularity
Bloody background
Monotonous population of epithelial cells with clear cytoplasm
Lack of definite cell borders
Uniform nuclei with small nucleoli
Absence of myoepithelial cells

Pregnancy and Lactational Changes

Pregnancy is associated with significant hormonal alterations in the breast, which result in an increase in the number of acini per lobule and the accumulation of secretory material in the lobular epithelial cells (Images 5.72 and 5.73). Pregnancy-associated lesions in the breast occur de novo or due to the enlargement of preexisting small breast tumors. Lactating adenoma and tubular adenoma are strongly associated with pregnancy and lactational influences.[80,81]

Similarly, preexisting fibroadenoma undergoes significant morphologic changes during pregnancy.[82] Although unusual, breast cancer does occur in pregnant women; it is second only to cervical carcinoma as the most frequent newly diagnosed cancer in pregnant women.[83,84] It is estimated that the incidence of breast cancer in pregnant women is 3 cases per 10,000 pregnancies.[85] Breast cancer in pregnancy is associated with poor prognosis.[86–88] Youth, breast enlargement, increased vascularity, and lymphatic permeability due to pregnancy are thought to be responsible for the rapid growth and early metastasis of breast carcinoma in these patients.

Table 5.2
Differential Diagnosis of Clear Cells in Breast Fine Needle Aspiration Biopsy[*]

Cytologic Findings	Microglandular Adenosis	Fibrocystic Change	Fat Necrosis	Organized Hematoma
Cellularity	Sparse	Cellular	Sparse	Sparse
Cellular pattern	Clustered	Singly	Singly	Singly
Nuclear features	Bland chromatin	Hyperchromasia with nucleoli	Bland chromatin	Bland chromatin
Bare nuclei	Absent	Present	Absent	Absent
Background	Red blood cells and fibroblasts	Cytoplasmic debris	Inflammatory cells, necrotic debris	Inflammatory cells, fibroblasts, fibrin, necrotic debris

Cytologic Findings	Secretory Carcinoma	Colloid Carcinoma	Lobular Carcinoma with Mucinous Changes
Cellularity	Cellular	Variable	Variable
Cellular pattern	Clustered	Clustered	Singly
Nuclear features	Slight pleomorphism	Minimal atypia	Minimal atypia, indented or lobulated shape
Bare nuclei	Absent	Absent	Absent
Background	Necrotic debris	Cell balls, mucinous background	Signet ring cells and necrotic debris

[*]Modified from: Gherardi G, Bernardi C, Marveggio C: Microglandular adenosis of the breast: fine needle aspiration biopsy of two cases. *Diagn Cytopathol* 9:72–76, 1993.

It is important to distinguish between pregnancy-associated lesions and carcinoma in the lactating breast. Breast aspirates from pregnancy-associated lesions may present worrisome cytologic features. However, if one is alerted to the possibility of pregnancy, these changes are rather specific and are not difficult to recognize. Frequently, masses in lactating breasts are tender and show a high cellular yield.[89–93] The main cytologic feature seen in all pregnancy-associated lesions is the presence of proteinaceous, bubbly vacuoles in the background of the smear. Unlike signet ring cells in cancer, several vacuoles are usually present in the cytoplasm. Cytoplasmic vacuolization, with fraying of the cytoplasmic borders, is characteristic of cytoplasmic secretion, which may facilitate the distinction between cancer and pregnancy-associated changes (Images 5.74 through 5.77).

In addition to the spectrum of cytologic findings seen in pregnancy-associated lesions, there are characteristic clinical and cytologic features that can be used to reliably differentiate between galactocele, lactating adenoma, and fibroadenoma on FNAB.[94] Aspirates from galactocele lesions in the postpartum period contain cloudy fluid and are associated with immediate regression of the mass following FNAB. The smears show low to moderate cellularity and numerous foam cells. The background is granular, foamy, and replete with lipid micelles admixed with proteinaceous material. The epithelial cells are few and are seen in monolayers, with vacuolated cytoplasm and lipid droplets. Occasional dispersed cells are seen (Image 5.78).

The clinical history of patients with fibroadenoma and lactational change often reveals that the breast nodule was present prior to pregnancy. Women with lactating adenomas, on the other hand, usually notice the mass initially during pregnancy. Aspirates from lactating adenomas are cellular and typically have several large, grape-like clusters of epithelial cells representing lobular units composed of uniform, expanded acini attached to terminal ductules (Images 5.79 and 5.80). The acini have smooth, rounded borders, giving the tissue fragments a scalloped appearance. In contrast to fibroadenoma, naked nuclei and epithelial clusters in an antler-horn pattern are not commonly seen.[92] Similarly, fibroadenomas with lactational changes rarely demonstrate the grape-like clusters of expanded lobular units, and the background is replete with bipolar, oval, stripped nuclei. Compared to lactational adenoma, the fragments of fibrous stroma in fibroadenoma tend to be larger in size and present more frequently. The background also has fewer proteinaceous secretions and lipid droplets and may contain giant cells (Images 5.81 and 5.82).

O'Hara and Page[81] have reported that tubular and lactating adenomas and lesions caused by lactational changes in fibroadenoma have overlapping histomorphologic features. The same observation has been made cytologically as well. After studying FNABs of 11 pregnant women with breast lesions, Finley et al[90] reported a wide spectrum of cytomorphologic features. Some lesions had cytomorphologic features similar to those of fibroadenoma or proliferative breast disease with minor lactational changes, while others yielded markedly cellular aspirates containing predominantly dissociated cells with microtissue fragments showing lobular hyperplasia. The dispersed cells displayed anisonucleosis with prominent nucleoli. Naturally, this range of cytomorphologic features makes diagnosing breast lesions in pregnant women a significant challenge for an inexperienced pathologist, particularly since some pregnancy-associated changes have also been described in nonlactating breast.[82,94,95]

Most ductal carcinomas show more discohesion, loss of polarity, necrosis, hyperchromasia, and nuclear atypia than pregnancy-associated lesions[86] (Images 5.83 through 5.90). However, adenoma with lactational changes and lobular hyperplasia can be misdiagnosed as lobular carcinoma if the presence of myoepithelial cells is not appreciated. In addition, lobular carcinomas are often sparsely cellular and show no evidence of the foamy or chicken-wire background seen in most lactating adenomas. Lobular carcinomas present as groups of small cells in a signet ring pattern with eccentric nuclei and inconspicuous nucleoli. Lactating adenomas also share cytologic features with malignant lymphoma and granulocytic sarcoma of the breast. The overlapping features are a proteinaceous background, the presence of intact lobules of benign breast tissue, and a dispersed cellular pattern. In addition to the hyperchromasia seen in malignant lymphoma, eosinophilic, cytoplasmic granules with intranuclear and cytoplasmic vacuoles are common in granulocytic sarcoma. Clinical history remains an important factor in the correct diagnosis of lactational adenoma. Attempts have also been made to use cytomorphometric analysis to distinguish lactating adenoma from well-differentiated ductal carcinoma and lobular carcinoma. However, no statistically significant differences in the nuclear areas of these lesions have been found.[92]

Cytologic study remains an effective tool in distinguishing between benign and malignant processes and in reducing the delay in the diagnosis of breast cancer in pregnant and lactating women. Naturally, suspicious lesions or those that persist after pregnancy should be further biopsied. A team approach involving both the clinician and the pathologist is mandatory. Fine needle aspiration biopsy also reduces the number of unnecessary open biopsies in pregnant women.

Cytomorphology of Pregnancy-Associated Lesions
High cell yield
Granular, proteinaceous background
Dispersed cells and loosely arranged cell clusters
Large epithelial cells with uniform nuclei and prominent nucleoli
Abundant, foamy, vacuolated cytoplasm with fraying of cytoplasmic borders
Bipolar, naked nuclei
Foamy macrophages
Occasional multinucleated giant cells

Treatment-Induced Changes

With more widespread acceptance of conservative therapy, lumpectomy and axillary dissection combined with irradiation are now frequently the treatment of choice for breast cancer. This means that pathologists may be confronted with another diagnostic challenge: distinguishing recurrent carcinoma from radiation atypia. Radiation treatment results in the formation of dense, fibrous tissue and scattered epithelial and stromal cells, which may appear extremely atypical. Clinically, patients present with thickening at the site of previous operation or radiation therapy. Relatively low cellularity, with a paucity of malignant epithelial cells and the presence of reactive, atypical histiocytes and giant cells, compounds the diagnostic problem.

Radiation is known to cause epithelial atypia in the terminal duct lobular unit of the breast. The cells are enlarged, with hyperchromatic nuclei and occasional prominent nucleoli. The cytoplasm is pale and eosinophilic, and evidence of vacuolization is present. Atrophy and fibrosis of the lobules are also observed.[94] Although the value of FNAB in distinguishing radiation-induced changes from carcinoma has occasionally been questioned,[94] the FNAB procedure can play a significant role in the evaluation of an irradiated breast.[95–97]

Peterse et al[95] suggest that radiation-induced changes in the breast exhibit three different patterns in the FNAB smear: epithelial atypia, fat necrosis, or poor cellularity. They did not see evidence of cellular discohesion or necrotic cell debris in FNAB smears from radiated, nonneoplastic breast lesions. Cytologically, aspirates obtained from irradiated breasts are poorly cellular. The epithelial cells are atypical, with pleomorphic, hyperchromatic nuclei. Anisonucleosis, reticular chromatin patterns, and prominent nucleoli are often seen (Images 5.91 through 5.93) and may be indistinguishable from malignant changes. False-positive diagnoses of malignancy have been reported by several investigators.[94–97]

Peterse et al[96] described features of malignancy in an irradiated breast as including loss of cellular cohesion; arrangement of cells in small clusters; nuclei with multiple nucleoli, anisonucleosis, and irregular nuclear membrane; and necrosis.[95] In our experience, the most important feature in distinguishing between a recent radiation-induced change and a recurrent cancer is the rich cellularity of the aspirate (Images 5.94 through 5.99).

In a recent study, Filomena et al[98] assessed the diagnostic accuracy of FNABs performed on 60 patients with a history of radiation therapy for breast carcinoma. They found that FNAB had a sensitivity of 86%, a specificity of 98%, a positive predictive value of 86%, a negative predictive value of 98%, and an efficiency of 97%. They suggested that aspirator experience is the key to obtaining an adequate sample. Lack of cellularity in a smear was considered evidence against local recurrent carcinoma. Filomena et al believe that an unequivocal diagnosis of recurrent carcinoma in an irradiated breast should be made only if there is an abundance of epithelial cells, both singly and in clusters. Cellular characteristics are less helpful, since nuclear enlargement, increased N/C ratio, and prominent nucleoli are present in both radiated nonneoplastic and radiated neoplastic breast lesions.[98] Therefore, epithelial atypia in a sparsely cellular aspirate from an irradiated breast lesion should be interpreted with great caution to avoid a false-positive diagnosis.

According to Schnitt et al,[99] epithelial changes in irradiated breast are not related to the presence or absence of carcinoma or to radiation dosage, patient age, time interval between the radiation and the biopsy, or the use of adjuvant chemotherapy. Peterse et al[96] did not find any induction of epithelial atypia in breast cancer patients who underwent adjuvant chemotherapy. However, extensive granulomatous reaction has been observed in FNAB smears of a breast cancer patient with locally advanced disease who showed complete response to preoperative chemotherapy.[100] In another study, Soyage-Rabie et al[101] reviewed the cytology of 100 breast lesions following lumpectomy and irradiation. The authors concluded that FNAB is a valuable tool, with a sensitivity of 100%, a specificity of 94%, a positive predictive value of 69%, a negative predictive value of 100%, and an efficiency of 93%.

Suture granulomas and surgery-induced fibrosis may also exhibit worrisome cytologic features that result in a false-positive diagnosis.[102,103] The differential diagnosis of postsurgical lesions in breast cancer includes benign, surgery-associated lesions; recurrent tumor; and new, unrelated breast or soft tissue lesions. The classic suture granuloma is characterized by the presence of granulation tissue and granulomatous inflammation, along with leukocytes, histiocytes, fibroblasts, blood vessels and multinucleated giant cells (Images 5.100 through 5.104).[55,104,105] Refractile suture material may occasionally be seen in the giant cells and/or free in the background.[55,104,105] However, occasionally suture granulomas exhibit atypical features that may suggest malignancy, such as abundant granulation tissue; fat necrosis; or atypical, immature fibroblasts.[55,104,106,107] A cellular, cicatricial nodule around suture granulomas may be the only component sampled by aspiration biopsy and may exhibit atypical spindle cells (Images 5.105 and 5.106). Brifford et al[105] reported that of 135 subcutaneous nodules sampled in patients with a history of surgical treatment for breast cancer, the presence of these reactive fibroblasts resulted in erroneous suspicion of malignancy in one case.

Similarly, Maygarden et al[108] reported three FNABs of suture granulomas of the breast that were either interpreted as suspicious for or conclusively diagnosed as recurrent cancer. On review, each smear contained a variable number of spindle cells and fragments of cellular stroma. However, the multinucleated giant cells characteristic of suture granuloma were not seen in the aspirated material. To avoid a false-positive diagnosis, it is best to adhere to the usual cytologic characteristics of suture granuloma, which include low to moderate cellularity, heterogeneity of the cytologic sample, and inflammation admixed with histiocytes.[66,106,109–123]

Other remote and yet important differential diagnoses of atypical suture granuloma, which is characterized by absence of multinucleated cells, suture material, and abundance of spindle cells, are breast tumors with prominent spindle cell components, such as pseudosarcomatous metaplastic carcinoma, sarcoma, phyllodes tumor, salivary gland–type primary breast carcinomas, pleomorphic adenoma of the breast, myoepithelioma, myofibroblastoma, fibromatosis, nodular fasciitis, and other mesenchymal tumors of the breast.[43,107,109–122] Lack of cytologic similarity to the primary tumor and predominance of spindle cells are important diagnostic clues in excluding the presence of a recurrent tumor. Ancillary studies, such as a panel of immunostains or electron microscopic studies, are most helpful in distinguishing a reactive process from a recent tumor. Nevertheless, when associated with strong clinical suspicion, the presence of atypical cytologic features warrants surgical biopsy of the lesion.

Cytomorphology of Treatment-Induced Changes
Poor cellularity
Granulation tissue
Fat necrosis
Epithelial atypia
Granulomatous reaction
Fibroblastic reaction

Implants and Silicone-Induced Changes

In the past two decades, silicone has been used extensively in joint prostheses and in plastic surgical procedures, notably breast reconstruction or augmentation. The link between silicone and connective tissue diseases remains controversial. However, well-documented complications secondary to silicone use involving both joint prostheses and breast implants have been reported.[124–126]

It is well recognized that the presence of silicone in breast tissue, whether via direct injection into the chest wall or due to the rupture of a mammary prosthesis, will result in a local inflammatory tissue response.[125] This has been confirmed by animal studies.[127] The character of the tissue response varies with the physical form of the silicone.[128] Particles of elastomer (rubber) used in arthroplasty elicit a foreign-body giant cell reaction, while the gel and liquid forms used in gel-bag prostheses and direct injections of silicone into tissue induce migration of macrophages into the cystic space but are associated with relatively few multinucleated giant cells. The location of inflammatory response also influences the morphology of the lesion, with the foreign-body giant cell reaction more pronounced in lymph nodes than in connective tissue.

Silicone implants used in reconstructive surgery for breast cancer induce an inflammatory response that can produce a localized lesion or an area of induration. Distinguishing between a silicone-induced change and a recurrent cancer is a diagnostic challenge.[129] Our experience is limited to an FNAB of the chest wall of a woman with a history of primary breast cancer. The smears from this patient were moderately cellular and displayed scattered, tightly packed, vacuolated cells with fine droplets of refractile material that was assumed to be silicone. A few macrophages and chronic inflammatory cells were also present. No malignant cells were identified (Images 5.107 and 5.108).

Similar cytologic features have also been described in a fine needle aspirate from a 39-year-old woman with silicone lymphadenopathy.[130] The patient had an intact prosthesis and a mass in the right axilla. The smears revealed mononucleated and multinucleated giant cells intermingled with benign-appearing lymphoid cells. The most striking feature of the aspirate was the cytoplasmic vacuolization of the macrophages. The vacuoles contained refractile, homogeneous, faintly yellow material that was not birefringent. Asteroid bodies were occasionally seen. The surgically excised lymph node contained many spaces filled with a clear, mucoid material. Microscopically, the sinusoid was distended by a large amount of microglobular, refractile, nonpolarizing material. Scanning electron microscopic study confirmed the presence of material consistent with a silicone polymer implant.

In addition to silicone granulomas occurring in axillary lymph node and in breast tissue, breast carcinoma can occur in the presence of intact mammary prostheses.[129] In our experience, the cytology of malignant tumor in a patient with intact breast implants is similar to that of any primary breast carcinoma (Figure 5.3 and Images 5.109 through 5.112). When performing the aspiration, one must be particularly careful not to puncture the implant. A mass associated with an implant can be clinically misinterpreted as silicone granuloma and a cancer can be missed.

Cytomorphology of Silicone-Induced Changes
Moderate cellularity
Vacuolated macrophages containing refractile homogeneous material,
  dispersed and in clusters
Multinucleation

Collagenous Spherulosis

Collagenous spherulosis, a benign breast lesion, is often associated with intraductal papilloma, sclerosing adenosis, or radial scar. It is frequently an incidental finding and is characterized histologically by acellular, eosinophilic, fibrillar spherules surrounded by a proliferation of bland, round or oval, epithelial and myoepithelial cells. The fibrils are arranged in a concentric, star-shaped pattern. The spherules show a positive immunostaining reaction for type IV collagen. Ultrastructurally, the spherules demonstrate features similar to those of basement membrane material.[131,132]

Fine needle aspiration biopsy of collagenous spherulosis shows scattered, metachromatic hyaline globules surrounded by numerous groups of benign-appearing ductal epithelial cells, some of which form papillae. The globules exhibit a positive reaction with periodic acid–Schiff stain. The differential diagnosis includes adenoid cystic carcinoma, which, in contrast to collagenous spherulosis, presents as a palpable mass (Images 5.113 and 5.114).[133–136] Cytologically, the spherules in adenoid cystic carcinoma are surrounded by mildly atypical cells rather than the flattened myoepithelial cells typically seen in collagenous spherulosis. Another lesion considered in the differential diagnosis is intraductal signet ring carcinoma, which is characterized by an eccentric, atypical nucleus. In contrast to collagenous spherulosis, the spherules of intraductal signet ring carcinoma contain intracellular mucin.[133,134]

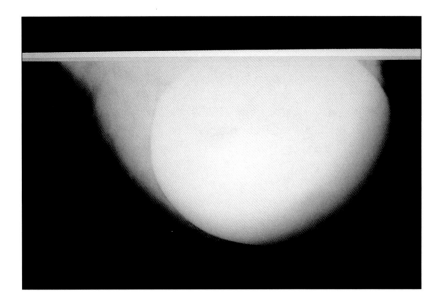

Figure 5.3
Mammogram of an implant with adjacent radiologic abnormality.

Cytomorphology of Collagenous Spherulosis
Sparse to moderate cellularity
Hyaline globules surrounded by uniform ductal epithelial cells
PAS positivity of the spherules

Amyloid Tumor

Amyloid tumor of the breast, a localized collection of amyloid, may occur as a primary tumor of the breast or as a manifestation of secondary amyloidosis. It may also be associated with multiple myeloma.[137] This lesion is found in elderly women and may simulate carcinoma clinically and mammographically.[138] Cytologically, amyloid tumor appears as an amorphous, eosinophilic, nonfibrillar mass, occasionally surrounded by foreign body giant cells. As in other sites, it stains positively with Congo red stain and has a greenish blue illumination under polarized light.[139,140] Electron microscopic study shows straight, nonbranching fibrils measuring 4 to 9 nm, a feature diagnostic of amyloid tumor. In conjunction with ancillary studies, FNAB can substantiate a diagnosis of amyloid tumor of the breast.[137]

Cytomorphology of Amyloid Tumor
Low cellularity
Amorphous, eosinophilic, nonfibrillar mass, positive with Congo red stain
Multinucleated cells

Adenosis Tumor

Adenosis tumor is an infrequent lesion of the breast that can be clinically and histologically confused with breast cancer, particularly in frozen section.[141–145] Even its mammographic pattern of calcification may mimic that of carcinoma.[146] This lesion occurs in a wide age range, from 20 to 67 years (mean, 37 years). The average size of the lesion is 2.4 cm. Treatment consists of local excision with close clinical follow-up.[143–145] Adenosis tumor may present as a well-delineated lesion or may be ill defined. Microscopically, adenosis tumor is characterized by an organoid, lobulated proliferation of a closely packed aggregate of tubules, many of which display open lumens. The tubules are lined by epithelial and myoepithelial cell layers (Image 5.115). The epithelial cells may show apocrine metaplasia and cellular atypia, creating diagnostic difficulty. Occasionally, perineural invasion may be demonstrated.[141,142]

The cytomorphology of adenosis tumor is rarely described.[145] Fine needle aspiration biopsy smears of adenosis tumor are highly cellular and contain numerous groups of uniform, benign ductal cells arranged in small groups and microtissue fragments. Some clusters may display a finger-like branching arrangement. Bipolar, naked nuclei are numerous, and fragments of localized, eosinophilic stroma are present (Images 5.116 through 5.119). The spindle cells show positive immunostaining for muscle specific actin, confirming the myoepithelial origin of some cells. Electron microscopic study of adenosis tumor demonstrates ductal cells surrounded by myoepithelial cells resting on a delicate basal lamina surrounded by bundles of collagen.[145,147]

Precise diagnosis of adenosis tumor by FNAB may not be possible. However, the benign nature of this unusual breast lesion can be ascertained. The cytologic features of adenosis tumor are essentially the same as those of sclerosing adenosis.[145,148] The cytologic differential diagnosis includes myoepithelioma, proliferative breast disease, juvenile papillomatosis, and cellular fibroadenoma.[145] The presence of cohesive groups of duct cells and naked nuclei clearly distinguishes adenosis tumor from carcinoma. In addition, immunostaining for muscle specific actin clearly demonstrates the myoepithelial origin of the tumor and confirms the benign nature of the lesion.

Cytomorphology of Adenosis Tumor
Cellular aspirate
Clusters of uniform epithelial cells
Numerous naked nuclei
Eosinophilic stroma

Radial Scar

Radial scar is best defined as a fibroelastic core surrounded by radiating ducts and lobules displaying various amounts of epithelial hyperplasia, adenosis, or ectasia. The central core often shows entrapped tubular structures.[149] Radial scar occurs in women ranging in age from 47 to 72, with a mean of 55 years. It is observed more frequently in women with fibrocystic change and is strongly associated with bilaterality and multicentricity.[150] Radial scars are often small, measuring no more than a few millimeters. Radiographically, they appear as small, spiculated structures that mimic invasive carcinoma. Grossly, the lesion's firmness and stellate or nodular appearance, with central puckering and creamy white streaks of elastica, make it easy to mistake for cancer.[151]

Microscopically, the radial pattern of the lesion is invariably evident. The appearance of the lesion depends on the degree of sclerosis and the nature of the proliferative changes (Image 5.120). Radial scar has been associated with both malignant and benign lesions.[152] It appears that women with biopsy-treated radial scar do not have an increased risk of subsequently developing breast cancer.[153] However, the presence of intraductal carcinoma or lobular neoplasia within the radial scar results in an unfavorable prognosis.[151]

Radial scar typically forms a nonpalpable but mammographically detectable mass and is difficult to diagnose by frozen section.[154] Similarly, its cytologic features, as seen in stereotaxic fine needle aspiration specimens, may simulate those of carcinoma.[155] Cytologic specimens of radial scar are frequently obtained via a stereotaxic FNAB. The smears are cellular and contain small, uniform cells arranged in small groups and round or angular clusters. There is a tendency for the cells to form tubules (Images 5.121 and 5.122). Branching sheets are uncommon, and single cells are frequent. The cells have distinct cytoplasmic borders and are evenly spaced. Nuclei are small and regular with inconspicuous nucleoli. Occasionally, cytoplasmic vacuoles are seen. The cytologic differential diagnosis includes low-grade neoplasms, such as noncomedo-type duct cell carcinoma in situ and lobular and tubular carcinoma. Familiarity with the cytomorphology of radial scar may prevent overdiagnosis of malignancy in stereotaxic FNAB specimens. The rare occurrence of carcinoma within a radial scar may justify confirmatory excisional biopsy when a diagnosis of carcinoma appears possible cytologically.

Cytomorphology of Radial Scar
Cellular aspirate
Small groups of uniform cells
Tendency for tubule formation
Frequent single cells
Small nuclei with inconspicuous nucleoli
Occasional cytoplasmic vacuoles

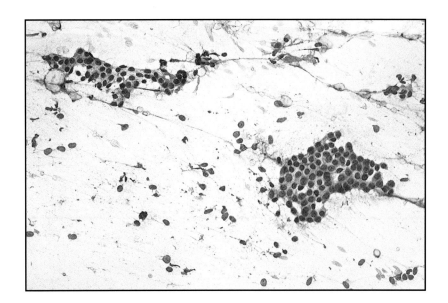

Image 5.1
Benign cyst demonstrating clusters of uniform, monolayered cells admixed with foamy cells (Papanicolaou, 100X).

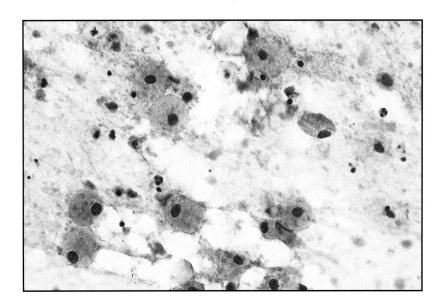

Image 5.2
Higher magnification of the same case shows bland, foamy macrophages (Papanicolaou, 200X).

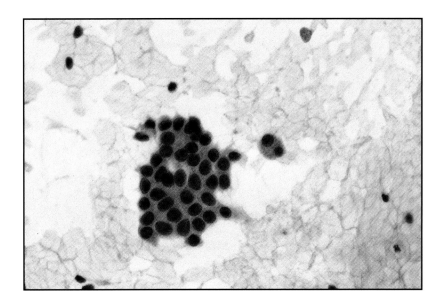

Image 5.3
A cluster of apocrine cells scattered in the background of cyst fluid (H&E, 200X).

Image 5.4
Corresponding tissue section diagnosed as an apocrine cyst (H&E, 200X).

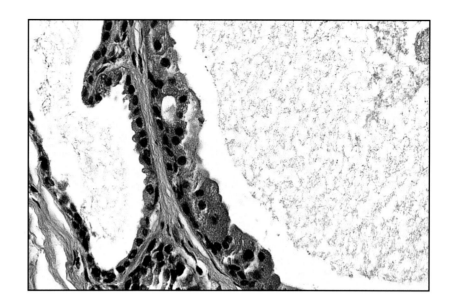

Image 5.5
Cytospin preparation obtained from an FNAB of chronic cystic mastitis demonstrates a cluster of reactive epithelial cells surrounded by inflammatory cells (H&E, 200X).

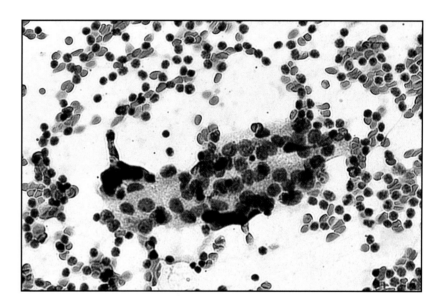

Image 5.6
Cell block preparation of the same case shows cellular debris, degenerated epithelial cells, and inflammatory cells (H&E, 400X).

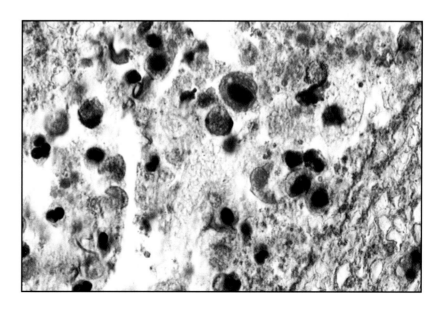

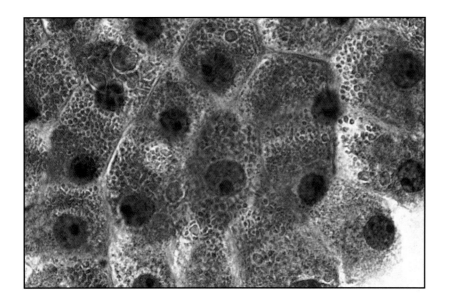

Image 5.7
A cluster of reactive apocrine cells with intracytoplasmic, eosinophilic inclusions seen in cytospin preparation of an apocrine cyst (Papanicolaou, 1000X).

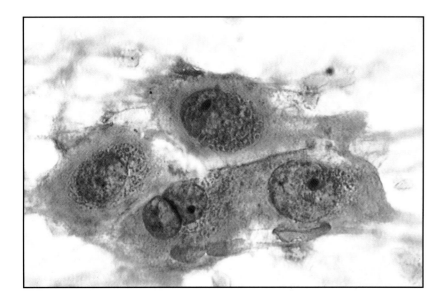

Image 5.8
Another view of the same case shows eosinophilic inclusions and binucleation (Papanicolaou, 1000X).

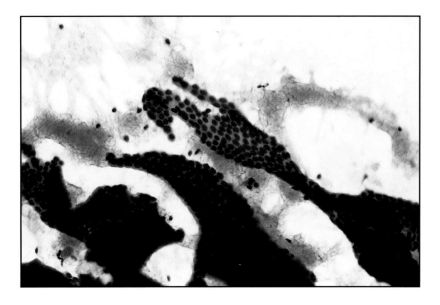

Image 5.9
Cytospin preparation from a cystic lesion demonstrates clusters of three-dimensional epithelial cells in a proteinaceous background (H&E, 200X).

Image 5.10
Tissue section of the corresponding surgically excised specimen, which was diagnosed as intraductal papilloma (H&E, 200X).

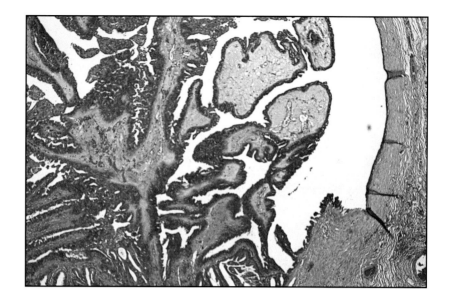

Image 5.11
Cytospin preparation from an intracystic carcinoma demonstrates a bloody background containing a few isolated epithelial cells and a cluster of loosely cohesive groups of epithelial cells (Papanicolaou, 200X).

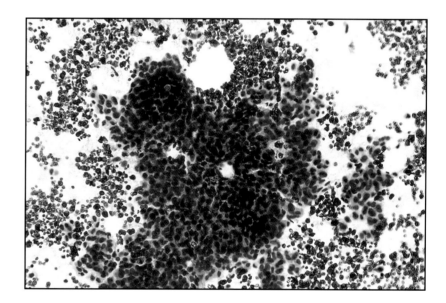

Image 5.12
Higher magnification of the same case shows crowding of the nuclei, loss of polarity, and anisonucleosis, with a few isolated atypical cells in the bloody background (Papanicolaou, 400X).

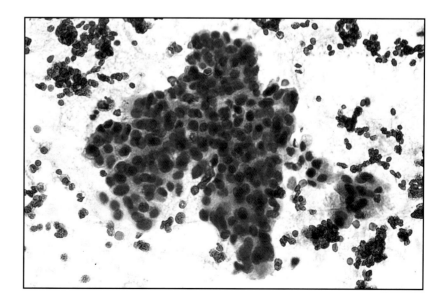

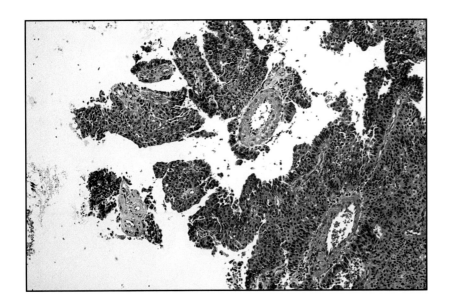

Image 5.13
Cell block preparation of the same case shows fragments of highly vascular tissue with a papillary configuration (H&E, 200X).

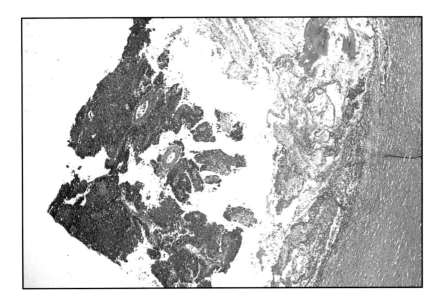

Image 5.14
Corresponding surgically excised lesion confirms the diagnosis of intracystic carcinoma with no evidence of invasion into the cyst wall (H&E, 200X).

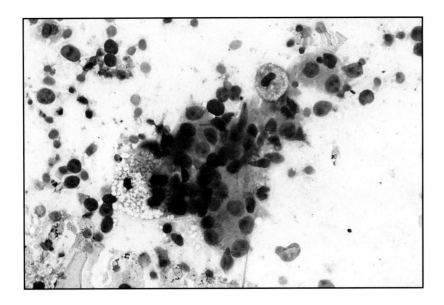

Image 5.15
Cystic medullary carcinoma. A cluster of atypical epithelial cells surrounded by inflammatory cells and histiocytes (Diff-Quik®, 200X).

Image 5.16
Cytospin preparation of a cystic medullary carcinoma demonstrates syncytial grouping of neoplastic epithelial cells in an inflammatory background (Papanicolaou, 200X).

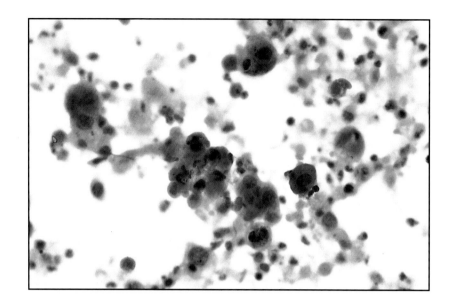

Image 5.17
Corresponding tissue section with characteristic histologic features in medullary carcinoma. Note that the neoplastic epithelial cells are surrounded by lymphocytes (H&E, 200X).

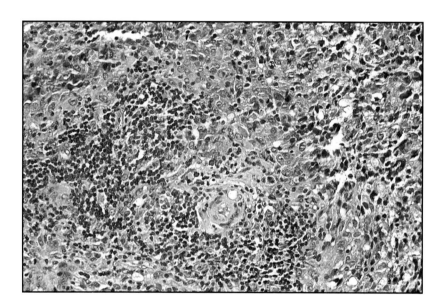

Image 5.18
Cystic degeneration seen in the same case (H&E, 200X).

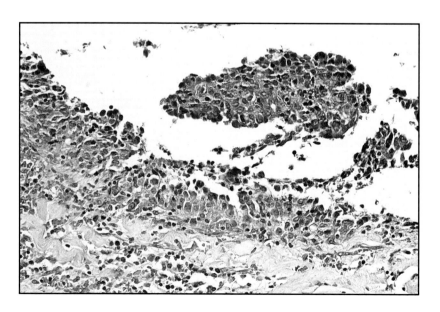

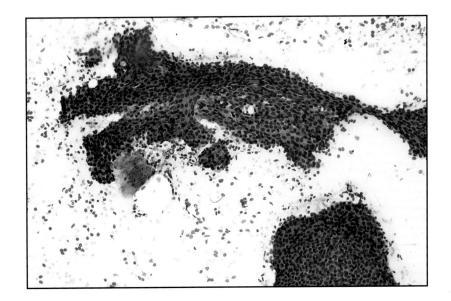

Image 5.19
Direct smear of an FNAB of fibro-adenoma. The aspirate is cellular, with a biphasic pattern consisting of epithelial and stromal elements (Diff-Quik, 200X).

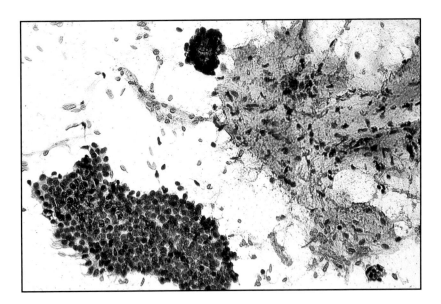

Image 5.20
Papanicolaou-stained smear of the same case shows the presence of stromal and epithelial components (200X).

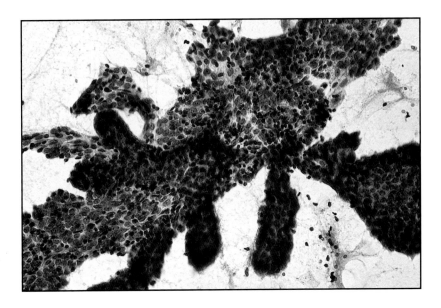

Image 5.21
Sheets of monolayered epithelial cells with finger-like projections forming an antler-horn pattern in a direct smear of fibroadenoma (Papanicolaou, 200X).

Image 5.22
Higher magnification of the same case demonstrating two cell populations: larger cells with round to oval nuclei of epithelial origin and smaller, spindle-shaped cells of myoepithelial origin (Papanicolaou, 400X).

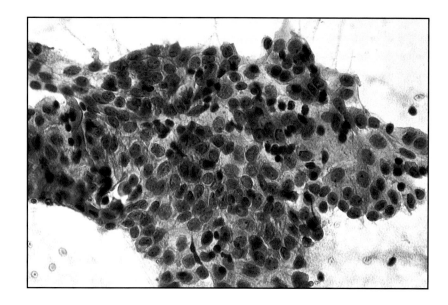

Image 5.23
Scattered, naked nuclei of myoepithelial origin seen in the background of a direct smear of an FNAB of a patient with fibroadenoma (Diff-Quik, 400X).

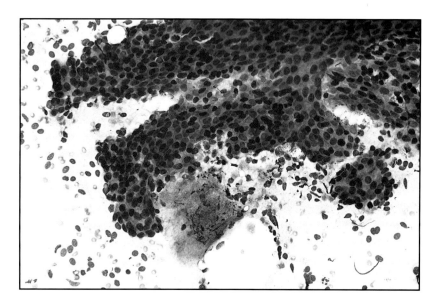

Image 5.24
Apocrine cells as accompanying cells in a fibroadenoma (Diff-Quik, 400X).

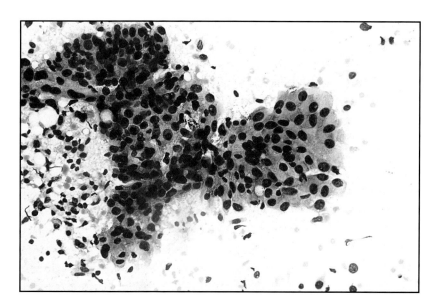

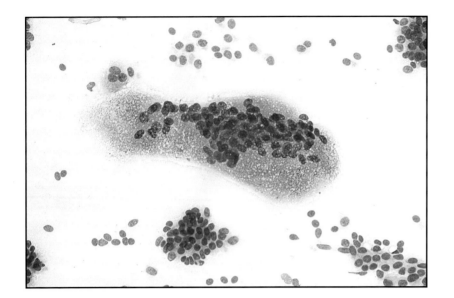

Image 5.25
Multinucleated cells occasionally seen in aspirates of fibroadenoma (Diff-Quik, 400X).

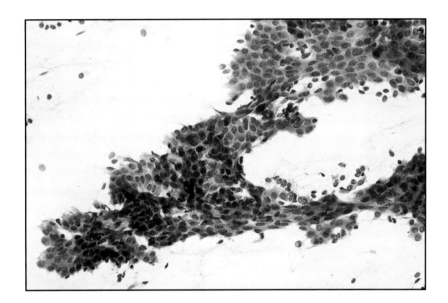

Image 5.26
Juvenile fibroadenoma. Branching sheet of epithelial cells with a few scattered, naked nuclei in the background (Papanicolaou, 200X).

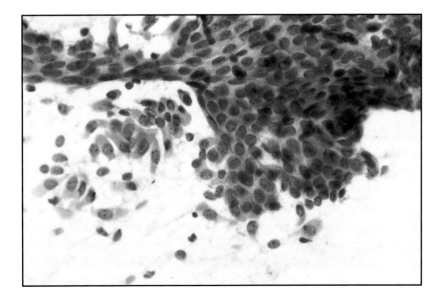

Image 5.27
Higher magnification of the same case demonstrates the presence of tall columnar cells (Papanicolaou, 400X).

Image 5.28
Clusters of epithelial cells with columnar differentiation surrounded by a few histiocytes (Papanicolaou, 400X).

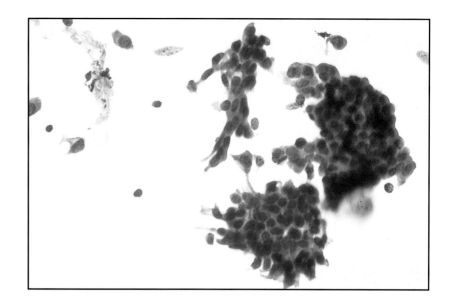

Image 5.29
Smear from fibroadenoma demonstrates atypical nuclei, including overlapping, mild hyperchromasia, prominent nucleoli, and rare mitoses, simulating carcinoma (Papanicolaou, 400X).

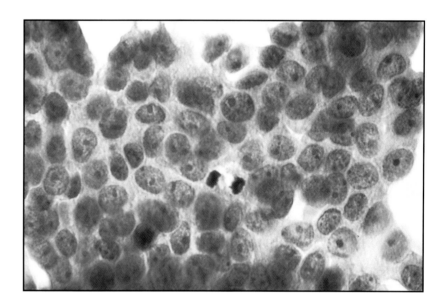

Image 5.30
Smear of fibroadenoma showing two clusters of epithelial cells. One is tightly cohesive and uniform, the other is loosely cohesive and atypical (Papanicolaou, 200X).

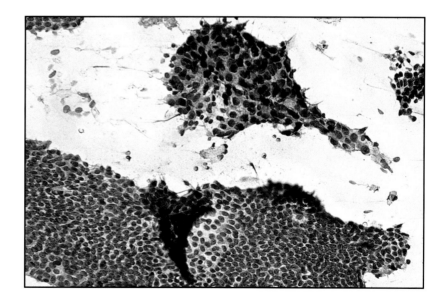

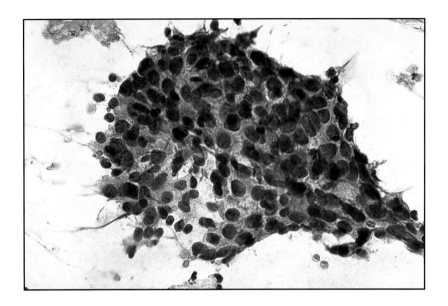

Image 5.31
Higher magnification of the atypical cluster from the same case demonstrates hyperchromasia, anisonucleosis, and the presence of nucleoli (Papanicolaou, 400X).

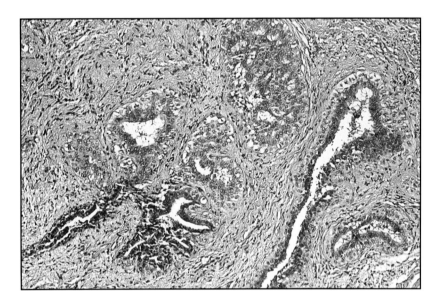

Image 5.32
Tissue section of the corresponding surgically excised lesion, which has the morphologic features of fibroadenoma (H&E, 200X).

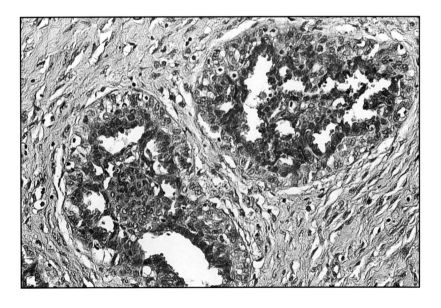

Image 5.33
High magnification of an area of atypical ductal hyperplasia in the same fibroadenoma (H&E, 400X).

Image 5.34
Cellular aspirate with atypical cells isolated and in clusters, simulating carcinoma (Papanicolaou, 200X).

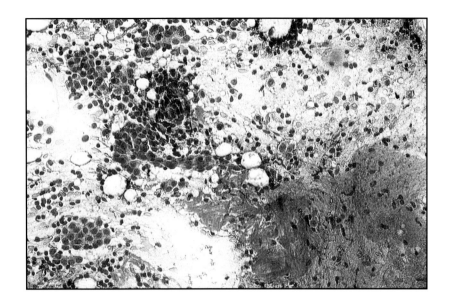

Image 5.35
Stromal elements in other areas of the same aspirate mixed with clusters of epithelial cells (Papanicolaou, 400X).

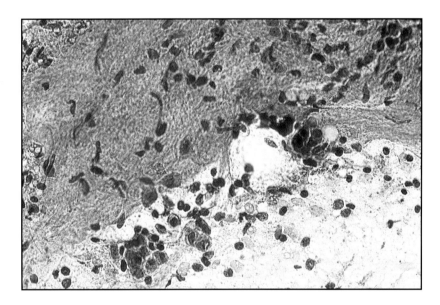

Image 5.36
Biphasic pattern of stromal and epithelial components in the same aspirate confirms a diagnosis of fibroadenoma with atypia (Papanicolaou, 400X).

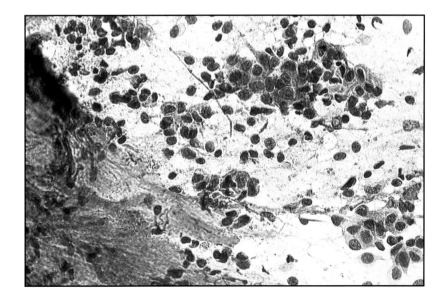

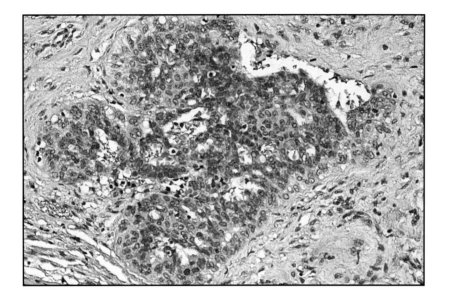

Image 5.37
Tissue section of the same case diagnosed as fibroadenoma with areas of atypical hyperplasia (H&E, 400X).

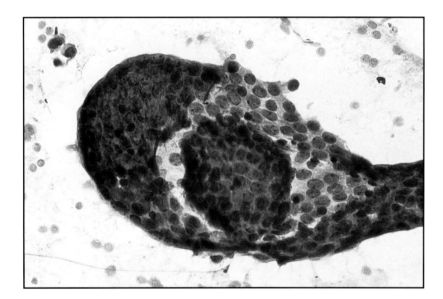

Image 5.38
FNAB of fibroadenoma demonstrates a cell ball within a distended cellular structure, resembling a tennis racket with a ball (Papanicolaou, 400X).

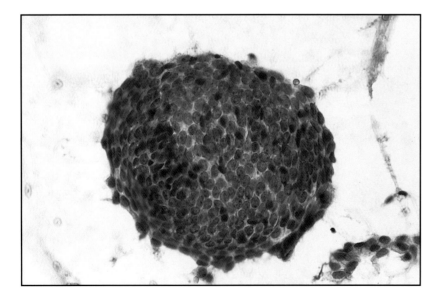

Image 5.39
A cell ball from the same case shows extreme crowding of the nuclei (Papanicolaou, 400X).

Image 5.40
FNAB of a fibroadenoma in a pregnant woman. Direct smear shows a loosely cohesive cluster of epithelial cells surrounded by naked nuclei in a proteinaceous background (Papanicolaou, 200X).

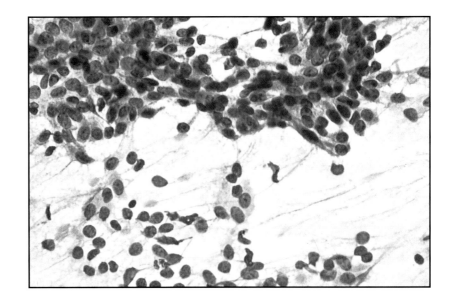

Image 5.41
Higher magnification of the same case shows a cluster of epithelial cells with prominent nucleoli and indistinct cytoplasmic borders (Papanicolaou, 400X).

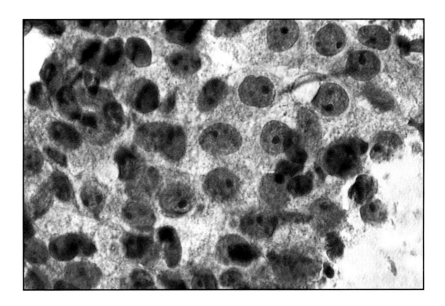

Image 5.42
Direct smear from an FNAB of fibroadenoma shows stromal elements with areas simulating mucoid change surrounded by naked nuclei (Papanicolaou, 200X).

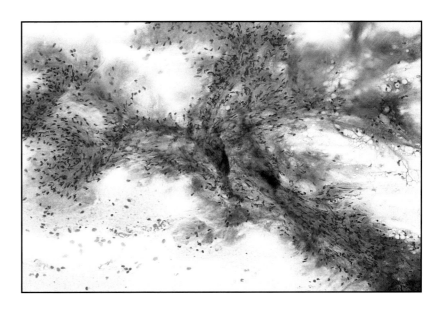

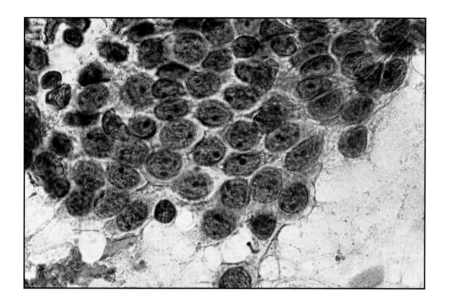

Image 5.43
A cluster of benign-appearing epithelial cells in a mucoid background. These features may be misinterpreted as colloid carcinoma (Papanicolaou, 200X).

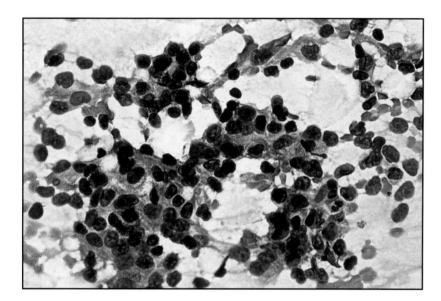

Image 5.44
FNAB of low-grade breast carcinoma. The direct smear demonstrates bland epithelial cells and a dispersed cellular pattern, simulating fibroadenoma (Papanicolaou, 200X).

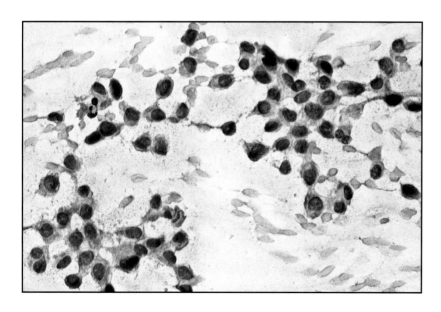

Image 5.45
Absence of the expression of muscle specific actin in direct smear of the same case (200X).

Image 5.46
Direct smear from an FNAB of atypical fibroadenoma with loss of cellular cohesion (Papanicolaou, 200X).

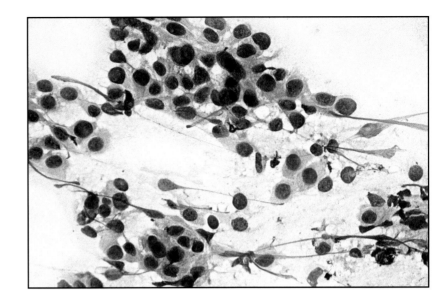

Image 5.47
Expression of muscle specific actin in a reticular pattern in the same case, evidence of myoepithelial cell differentiation (Immunostaining, 1000X).

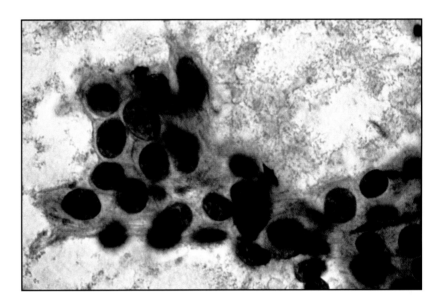

Image 5.48
Direct smear from FNAB of tubular carcinoma shows tubular structure with blunted end. Note the lack of myoepithelial cells (Diff-Quik, 200X).

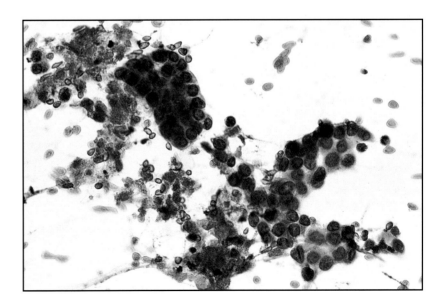

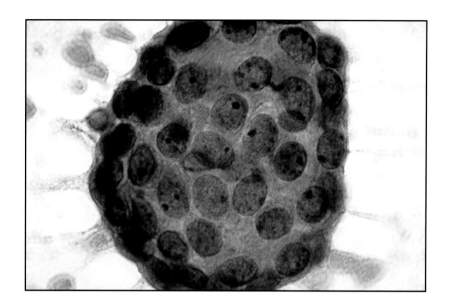

Image 5.49
Conspicuous monomorphism and absence of myoepithelial cells in the same case (Papanicolaou, 1000X).

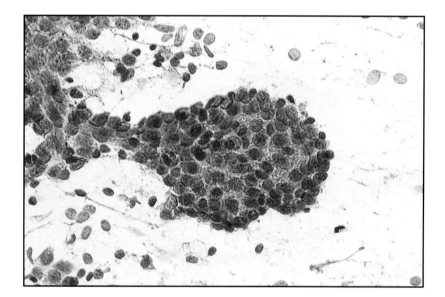

Image 5.50
Tubular structure in a fibroadenoma. Note the presence of scattered myo-epithelial cells in the background (Papanicolaou, 400X).

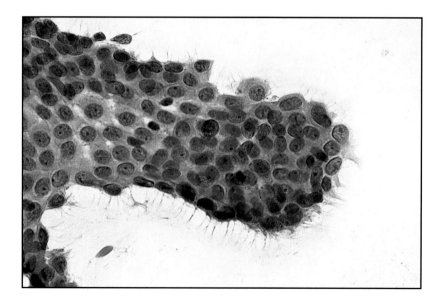

Image 5.51
Tubular structure in a fibroadenoma. The myoepithelial cells are small and admixed with the cluster of epithelial cells (Papanicolaou, 400X).

Image 5.52
Biphasic pattern in direct smear of an FNAB of phyllodes tumor. Note the similarity of these features to those of fibroadenoma (Papanicolaou, 200X).

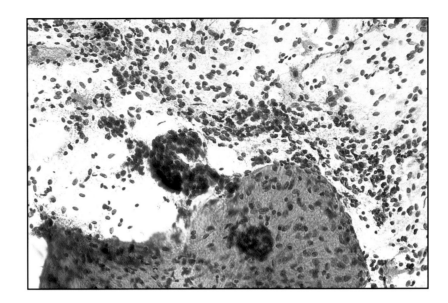

Image 5.53
A cellular stromal component commonly seen in phyllodes tumor (Papanicolaou, 400X).

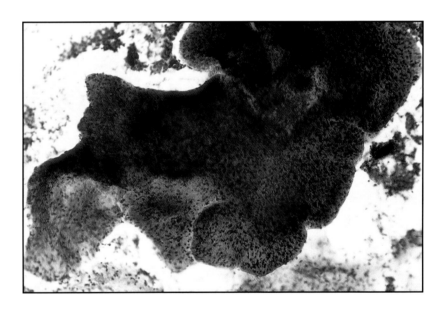

Image 5.54
Cellular aspirate demonstrating three-dimensional papillary fragments and tall columnar cells in a case of intraductal papilloma (Diff-Quik, 200X).

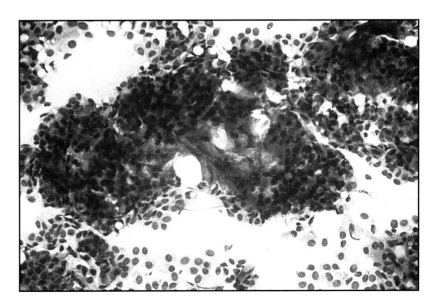

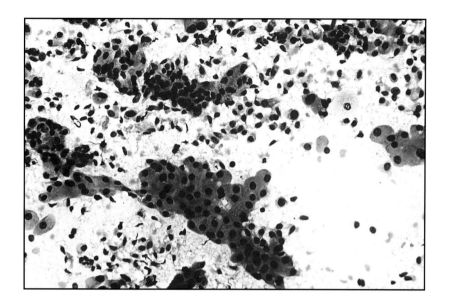

Image 5.55
Another view of the same case shows apocrine cells, histiocytes, a few tall columnar cells, and naked nuclei (Diff-Quik, 200X).

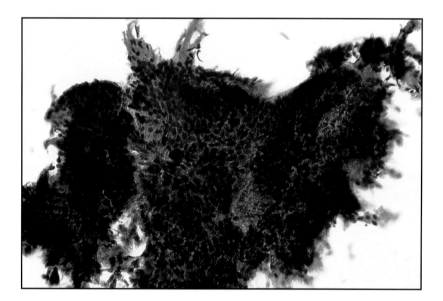

Image 5.56
Sheet of epithelial cells with conspicuous nuclear overlap forming a papilloma. Tall columnar cell differentiation is seen on the periphery (Papanicolaou, 400X).

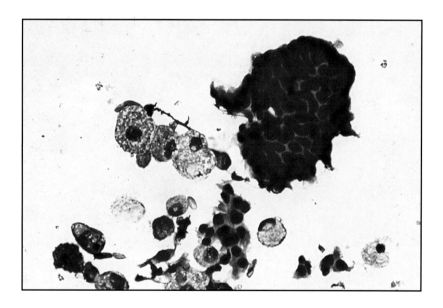

Image 5.57
Scattered histiocytes and cell ball seen in intraductal papilloma (Diff-Quik, 400X).

Image 5.58
Loosely cohesive cluster of atypical cells with some degree of anisonucleosis in FNAB smear of intraductal papilloma (Diff-Quik, 400X).

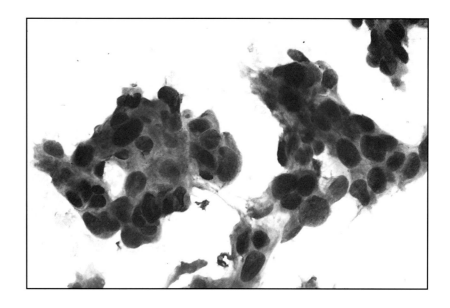

Image 5.59
Corresponding tissue section of surgically excised lesion diagnosed as intraductal papilloma (H&E, 400X).

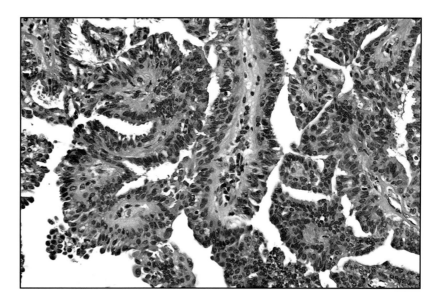

Image 5.60
Demonstration of a uniform layer of myoepithelial cells in the proliferating, papillary, intraluminal component of the corresponding tissue section (Immunostaining for MSA, 200X).

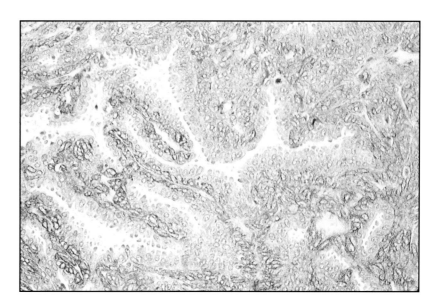

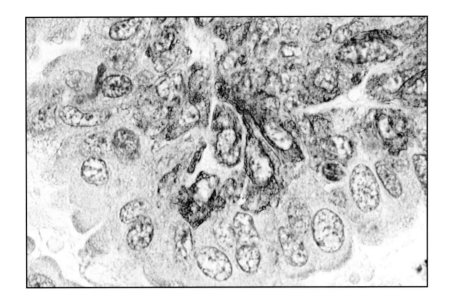

Image 5.61
Higher magnification of the same case shows differential immunoreactivity of myoepithelial cells (Immunostaining for MSA, 1000X).

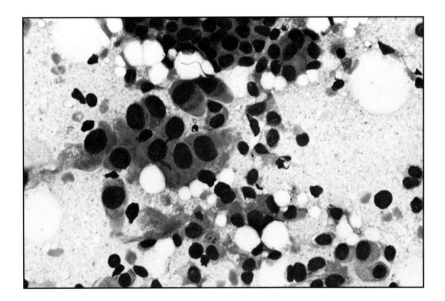

Image 5.62
Intraductal papilloma. Despite discohesiveness, the presence of a polymorphous population of epithelial cells with apocrine differentiation and columnar cells in a granular background distinguishes this lesion from a well-differentiated papillary carcinoma (Diff-Quik, 400X).

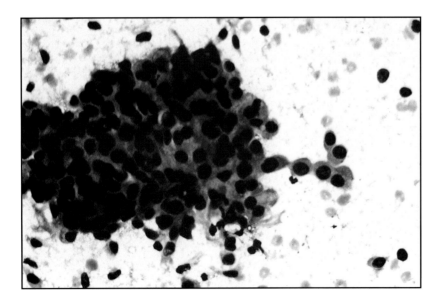

Image 5.63
Intracystic papillary carcinoma: a population of monomorphic epithelial cells isolated and in clusters with columnar differentiation (Diff-Quik, 400X).

Image 5.64

The overlapping cytologic features of fibroadenoma and intraductal papilloma include rich cellularity, tissue fragments, and occasional naked nuclei. Direct smear from an intraductal papilloma (Diff-Quik, 200X).

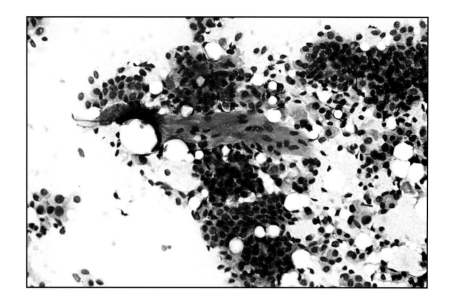

Image 5.65

The absence of polymorphism and the presence of a conspicuous number of naked nuclei in the background differentiates this fibroadenoma from intraductal papilloma (Diff-Quik, 200X).

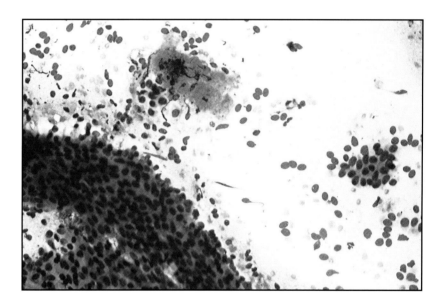

Image 5.66

Histologically, nipple adenoma is characterized by a proliferation of epithelial cells with a papillary pattern surrounding a core of connective tissue (H&E, 200X).

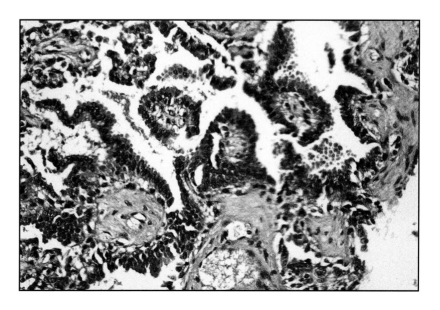

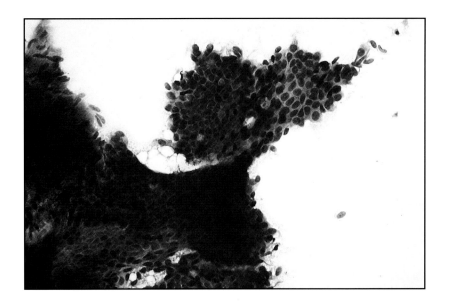

Image 5.67
Direct smear of nipple adenoma demonstrates clusters of epithelial cells in sheets and a three-dimensional pattern intertwined with dense connective tissue (Diff-Quik, 200X).

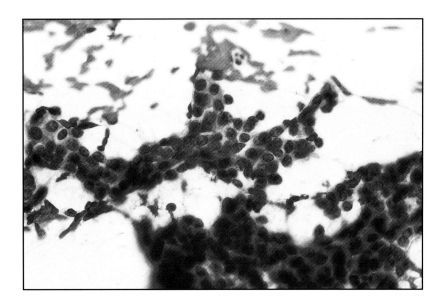

Image 5.68
Papanicolaou-stained smear of the same case demonstrating a few myoepithelial cells admixed with clusters of epithelial cells in sheets and a three-dimensional pattern. The cells have uniform nuclei and inconspicuous nucleoli (200X).

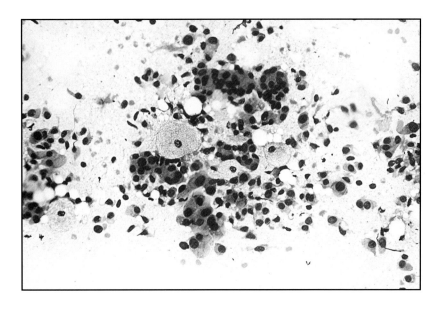

Image 5.69
Direct smear of juvenile papillomatosis demonstrates a polymorphous population of ductal epithelial cells, apocrine cells, histiocytes, and naked nuclei in a cystic fluid background (Diff-Quik, 200X).

Image 5.70
Another view of the same case of juvenile papillomatosis shows an orderly arrangement of ductal epithelial cells mixed with myoepithelial cells (Diff-Quik, 400X).

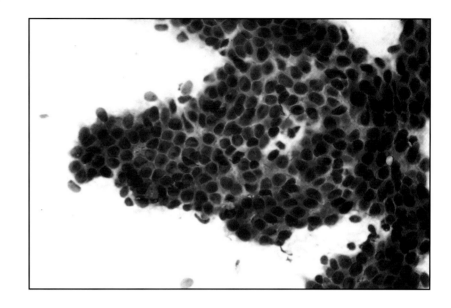

Image 5.71
Tissue section of the corresponding surgically excised lesion diagnosed as juvenile papillomatosis demonstrates many dilated cysts lined by flat epithelium (H&E, 400X).

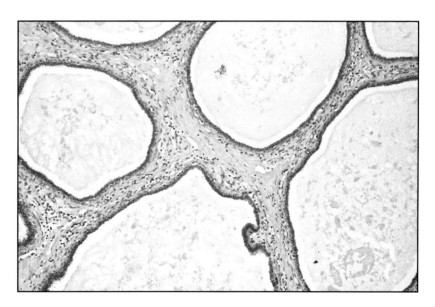

Image 5.72
Pregnancy-associated changes, including lobular hyperplasia and the presence of secretory vacuoles in the lobular epithelial cells (H&E, 400X).

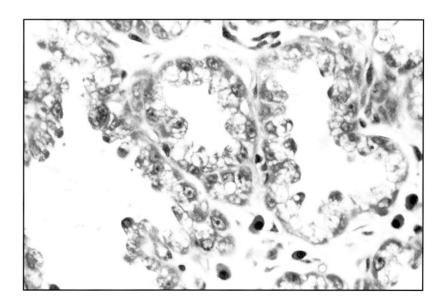

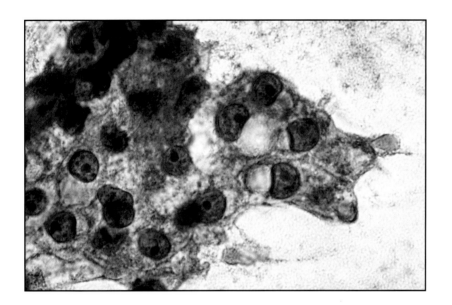

Image 5.73
Direct smear of pregnancy-associated change demonstrates uniform cells with granular, vacuolated cytoplasm; indistinct cell borders; and prominent nucleoli in a proteinaceous background (Papanicolaou, 1000X).

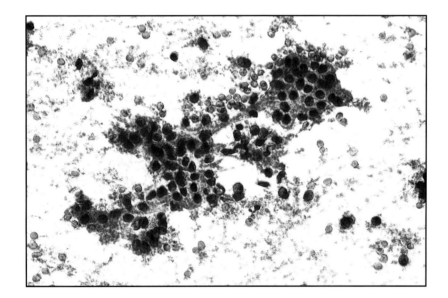

Image 5.74
Low magnification of pregnancy-associated change. The smear is cellular, with cells in loose clusters and a dispersed pattern, simulating carcinoma (Papanicolaou, 200X).

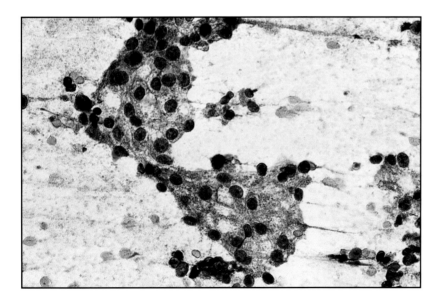

Image 5.75
Another view of the same case provides more convincing evidence that the morphologic features are those of pregnancy-associated change rather than carcinoma (Papanicolaou, 200X).

Image 5.76
Pregnancy-associated change. A cluster of loosely cohesive epithelial cells with frayed cytoplasm (Papanicolaou, 200X).

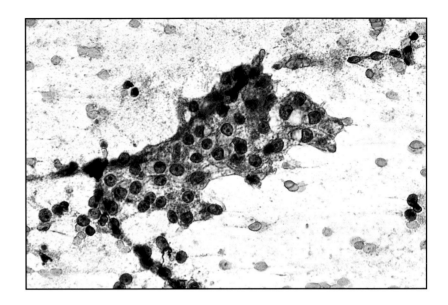

Image 5.77
Higher magnification of the same case shows a proteinaceous background and vacuolated cytoplasm (Papanicolaou, 400X).

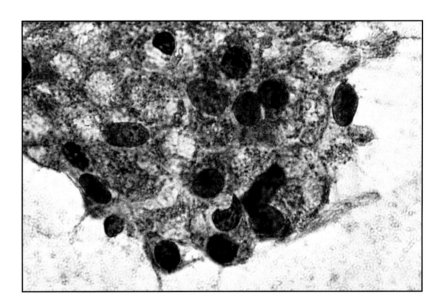

Image 5.78
Galactocele. Cytospin preparation depicts abundant, foamy macrophages and a cluster of epithelial cells (Papanicolaou, 200X).

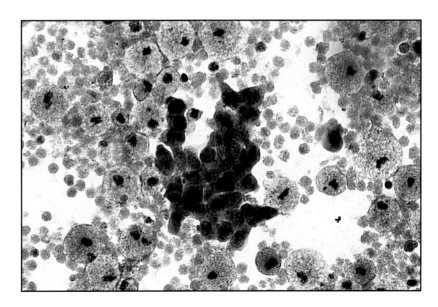

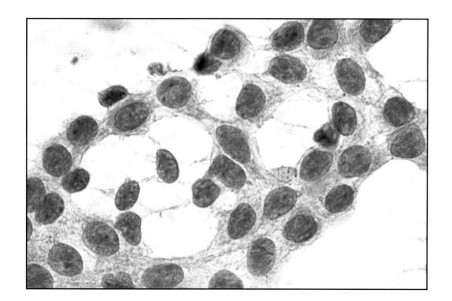

Image 5.79
Lactational adenoma. Slightly proteinaceous background contains epithelial cells with granular cytoplasm lining ill-defined, distended acini attached to terminal ductules (H&E, 200X).

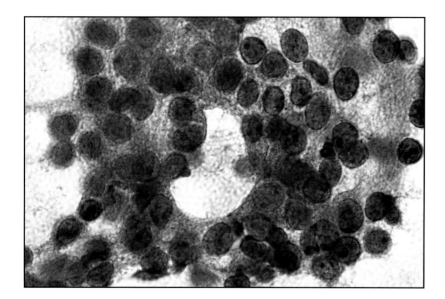

Image 5.80
Higher magnification of the same case demonstrates an acinus with uniform cells and frayed cytoplasm (Papanicolaou, 400X).

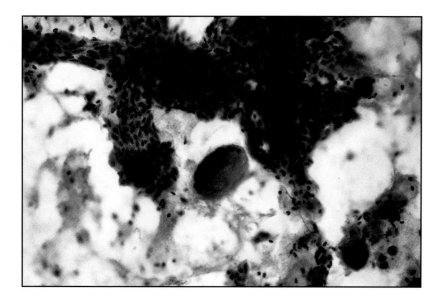

Image 5.81
Fibroadenoma in pregnancy. The proteinaceous background contains naked nuclei, multinucleated giant cells, and complex sheets of epithelial cells (H&E, 200X).

Image 5.82
Papanicolaou-stained smear of the same case demonstrates similar features (200X).

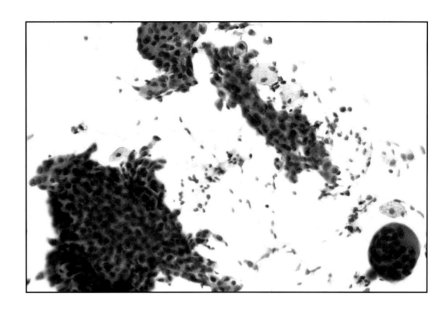

Image 5.83
Cancer in pregnancy. Smear shows a dispersed cell pattern with a mild degree of pleomorphism (Papanicolaou, 200X).

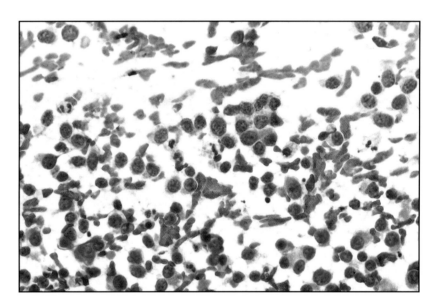

Image 5.84
High-power magnification of the same case demonstrating occasional isolated and clusters of highly atypical epithelial cells (Papanicolaou, 400X).

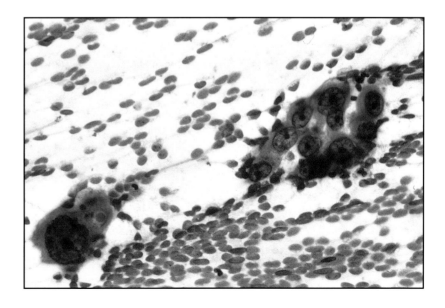

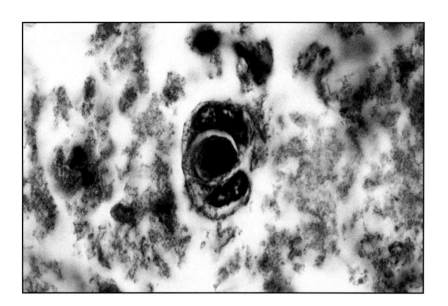

Image 5.85
Cell block preparation of the same case shows a cluster of malignant neoplastic cells with conspicuous nuclear molding diagnosed as ductal carcinoma (H&E, 400X).

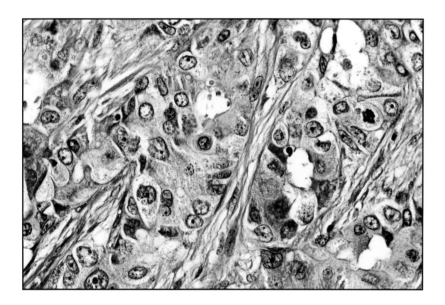

Image 5.86
Tissue section from a mastectomy specimen from a 26-year-old pregnant woman. The histologic features are those of infiltrating duct cell carcinoma (H&E, 400X).

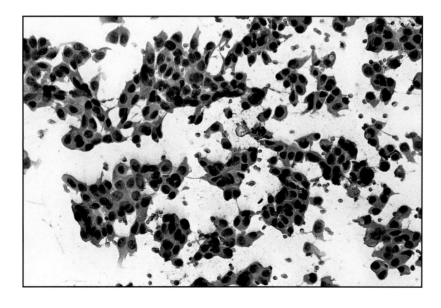

Image 5.87
Cancer in pregnancy. This direct smear from an FNAB of a breast lesion in a young pregnant woman is cellular, showing a dispersed, pleomorphic population of atypical epithelial cells (Papanicolaou, 200X).

Image 5.88
Higher magnification of the same case of breast cancer demonstrates marked hyperchromasia (Papanicolaou, 400X).

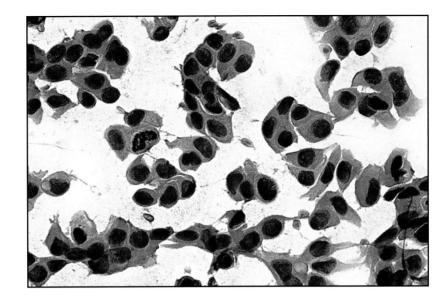

Image 5.89
Oil magnification of the same case shows abnormal nuclei and mitoses, features characteristically seen in breast carcinoma (Papanicolaou, 1000X).

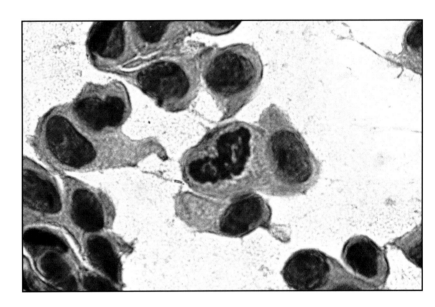

Image 5.90
Corresponding tissue section of mastectomy specimen diagnosed as high-grade infiltrating duct cell carcinoma (H&E, 400X).

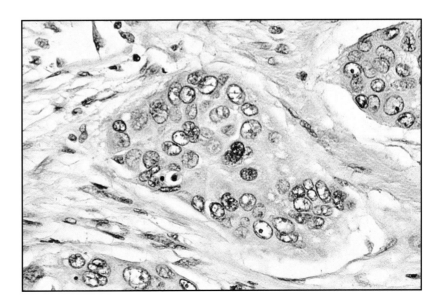

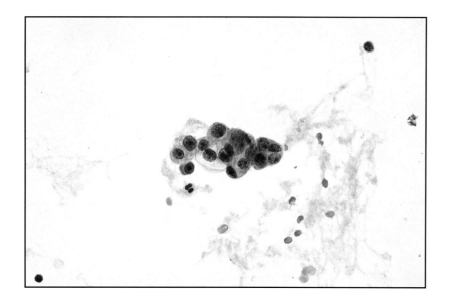

Image 5.91
This smear from an irradiated breast is poorly cellular, showing only a cluster of epithelial cells (Papanicolaou, 200X).

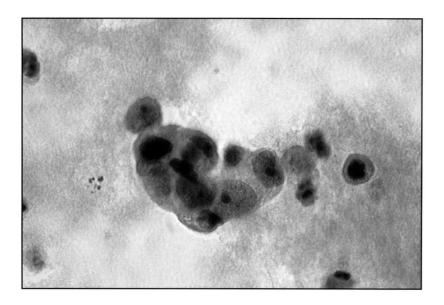

Image 5.92
Higher magnification of the same case demonstrates epithelial atypia characterized by pleomorphic, hyperchromatic nuclei; anisonucleosis; and prominent nucleoli; features that simulate recurrent carcinoma (Papanicolaou, 400X).

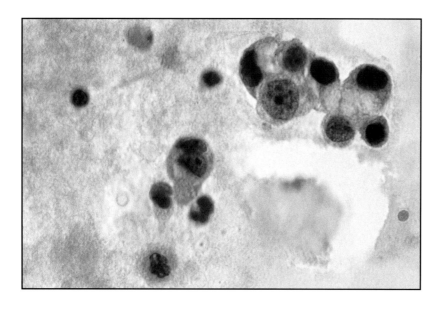

Image 5.93
Radiation changes, including degenerated cytoplasmic vacuoles and nuclear atypia (Papanicolaou, 400X).

Image 5.94
Recurrent carcinoma in an irradiated breast. This cellular aspirate shows a dispersed cell pattern (Papanicolaou, 100X).

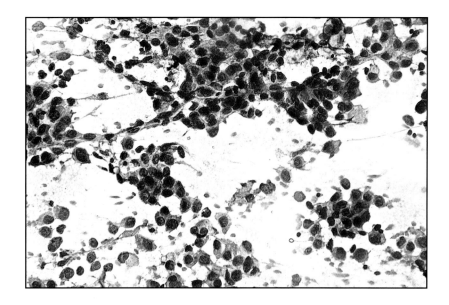

Image 5.95
Higher magnification of the same case demonstrates clusters of atypical epithelial cells and a few large mononuclear cells (Papanicolaou, 200X).

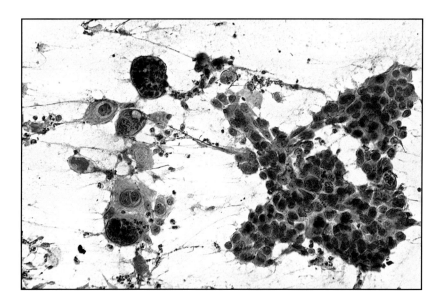

Image 5.96
Higher magnification of the same case shows the presence of atypical cells with conspicuous, enlarged nuclei and a few reactive fibroblasts (Papanicolaou, 400X).

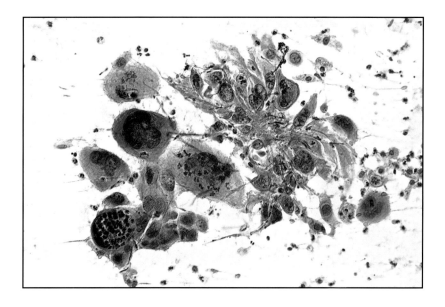

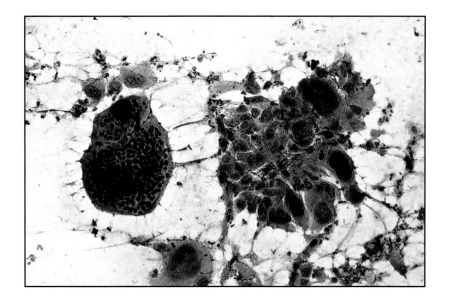

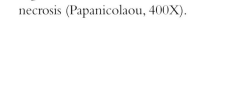

Image 5.97
Different view of the same case showing radiation-induced individual cell necrosis (Papanicolaou, 400X).

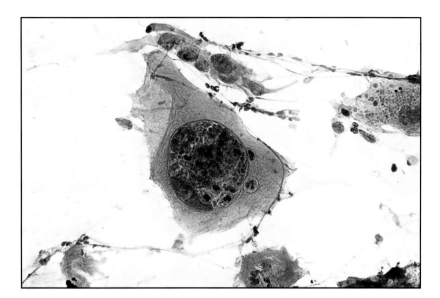

Image 5.98
Cytomorphology of radiation-induced change seen in malignant cells (Papanicolaou, 400X).

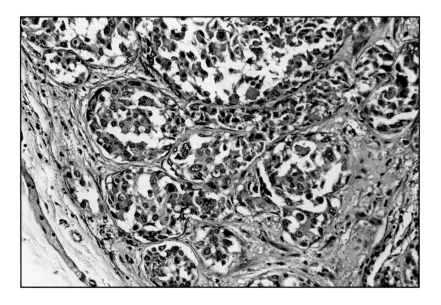

Image 5.99
Tissue section of the corresponding surgically excised lesion demonstrates a recurrent carcinoma (H&E, 200X).

Image 5.100
This cellular aspirate of suture granuloma shows mixed inflammatory cells,
histiocytes, and cellular debris (Diff-
Quik, 200X).

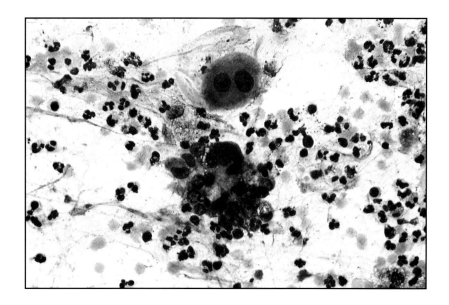

Image 5.101
Different view of the same case
demonstrating vacuolated histiocytes
(Papanicolaou, 200X).

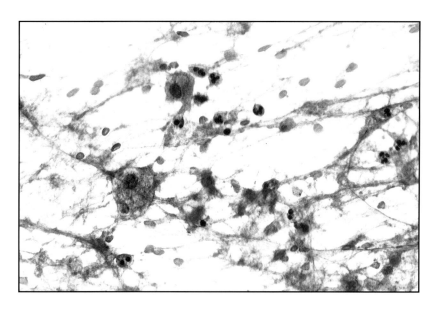

Image 5.102
Presence of atypical fibroblasts in the
same case (Papanicolaou, 200X).

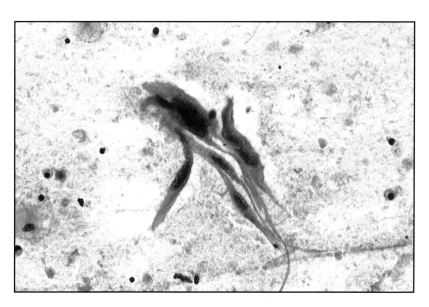

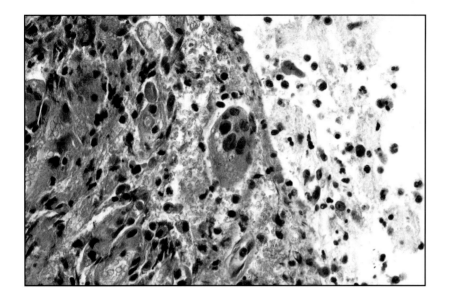

Image 5.103
Cell block preparation of the same case with fibrosis, inflammation, and foreign-body giant cell reaction (H&E, 200X).

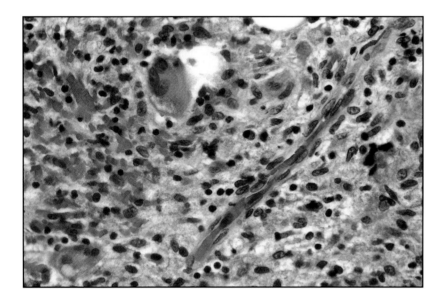

Image 5.104
Corresponding surgically excised lesion with similar features (H&E, 200X).

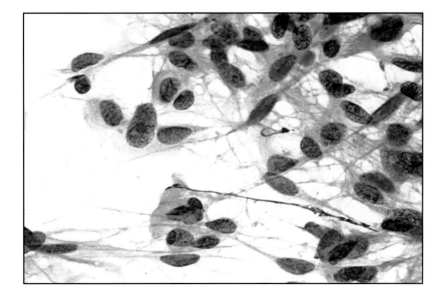

Image 5.105
Suture granuloma. In the absence of classic granulomatous inflammation in the aspirate, the predominance of atypical spindle cells simulates a variety of malignancies (H&E, 400X).

Image 5.106
Another view of the same atypical cells (H&E, 400X).

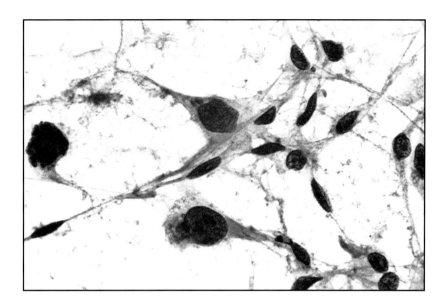

Image 5.107
Direct smear of silicone-induced change demonstrates a collection of vacuolated cells with foreign-body materials assumed to be silicone (Diff-Quik, 1000X).

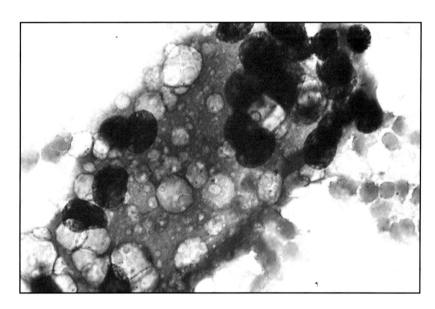

Image 5.108
Different view of the same case demonstrating multinucleated giant cells with refractile material (Papanicolaou, 1000X).

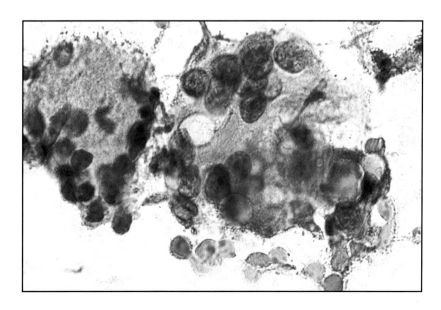

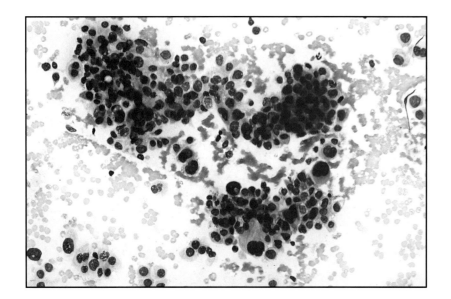

Image 5.109
Direct smear from FNAB of a malignant breast lesion adjacent to an implant demonstrates a dispersed cell pattern with significant pleomorphism and anisonucleosis (Diff-Quik, 200X).

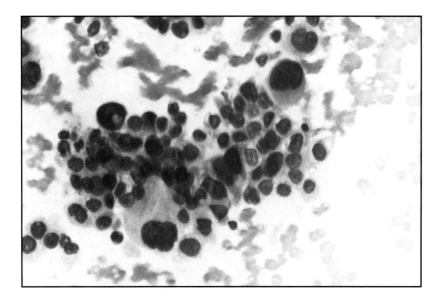

Image 5.110
Higher magnification of the same case shows similar features (Diff-Quik, 400X).

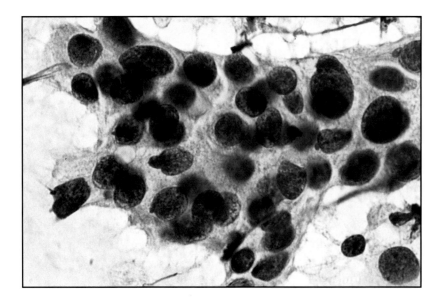

Image 5.111
Cellular pleomorphism, nuclear atypia, hyperchromasia, and anisonucleosis interpreted as a high-grade ductal carcinoma (Papanicolaou, 400X).

Image 5.112
Corresponding surgically excised lesion of the same case (H&E, 400X).

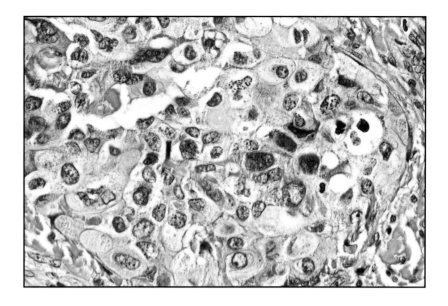

Image 5.113
Direct smear of collagenous spherulosis shows several blue globules, some surrounded by epithelial cells scattered among benign-appearing clusters of epithelial cells (Papanicolaou, 200X) (courtesy of Nour Sneige, MD).

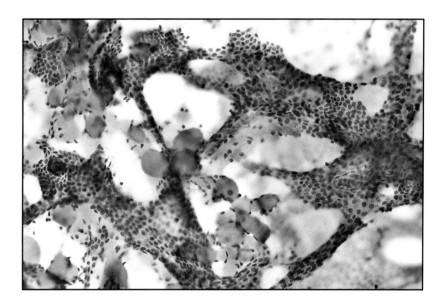

Image 5.114
Higher magnification of another example of collagenous spherulosis depicts bland-appearing ductal epithelial cells with hyaline globules (H&E, 400X).

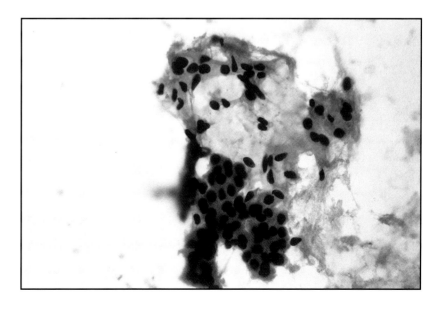

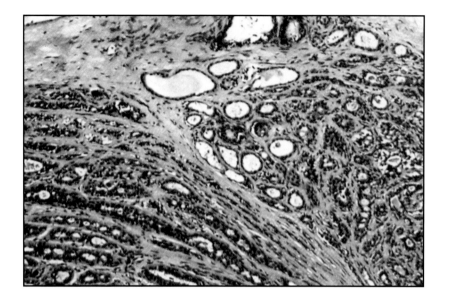

Image 5.115
Tissue section of an adenosis tumor shows an organized proliferation of closely packed tubules with open lumens (H&E, 200X).

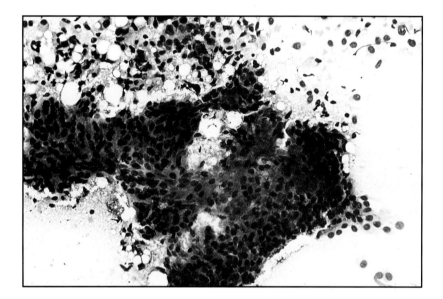

Image 5.116
Cellular aspirate of adenosis tumor shows a uniform population of ductal epithelial cells wih fragments of stroma surrounded by naked nuclei (Diff-Quik, 200X).

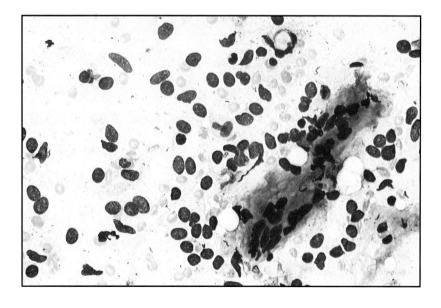

Image 5.117
Bipolar, naked nuclei appear to lie on top of localized, eosinophilic stroma (Diff-Quik, 400X).

Image 5.118
Papanicolaou-stained smear of adenosis tumor displays small groups of ductal epithelial cells intermixed with myoepithelial cells (200X).

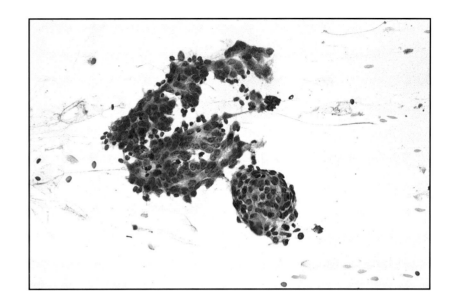

Image 5.119
Higher magnification of the same case shows similar features (Papanicolaou, 400X).

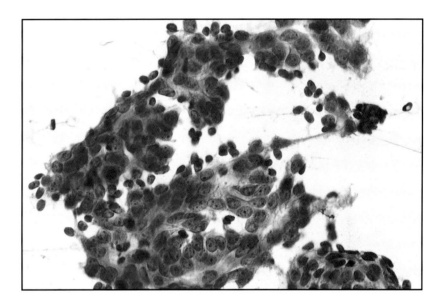

Image 5.120
Tissue section of a radial scar demonstrates a scleroelastic center with few tubular structures and adjacent dilated ducts (H&E, 200X).

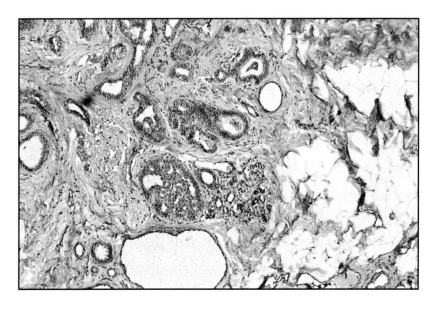

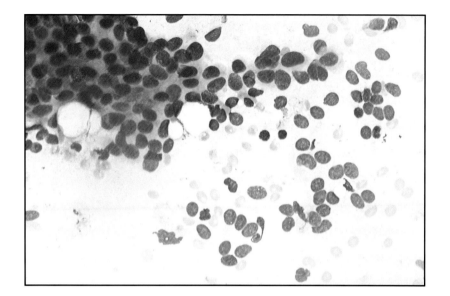

Image 5.121
Direct smear of radial scar showing a cluster of small, uniform cells with regular nuclei and a few scattered single cells in a clean background (Diff-Quik, 200X).

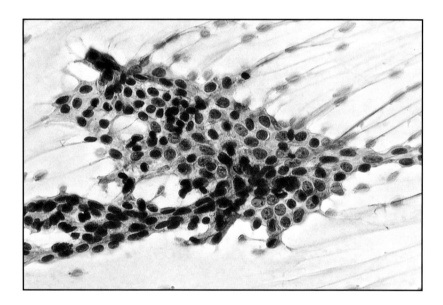

Image 5.122
Direct smear of radial scar shows tight clusters of epithelial cells forming a tubular structure (Papanicolaou, 200X).

References

1. Nyiryesy I, Billingsley FS: Management of breast problems in gynecologic office practice using sonography and fine needle aspiration. *Obstet Gynecol* 79:669–702, 1992.

2. Gupta RK, Naran S, Buchanan A, et al: Fine needle aspiration cytology of breast, its impact on surgical practice with an emphasis on the diagnosis of breast abnormalities in young women. *Diagn Cytopathol* 4:206–209, 1988.

3. Nagy GK, DeCiero JG, Pomerantz SN: Intracytoplasmic eosinophilic inclusion bodies in breast cyst fluids. *Acta Cytol* 30:45–47, 1986.

4. Nagy GK, Jacob JB, Mason-Saras A, et al: Intracytoplasmic eosinophilic inclusion bodies in breast cyst fluids are giant lysosomes. *Acta Cytol* 33:99–103, 1989.

5. Ciatto S, Cariaggi P, Bulgares P: The value of routine cytologic examination of breast cyst fluids. *Acta Cytol* 31:301–304, 1987.

6. Ciatto S, Roselli Del Turco M, Cariaggi P: Diagnostic and therapeutic role of breast pneumocystography. *Int J Breast Pathol* 2:27–29, 1983.

7. Cohen PN, Bensen GA: Cytological study of fluid from breast cysts. *Br J Surg* 106:209–211, 1976.

8. Dixon JM, Clarks PJ: Refilling of breast cysts as indicators of breast biopsy. *Lancet* 2:608, 1985.

9. Forrest APM, Kirkpatrick JR, Roberts MM: Needle aspiration of breast cyst. *Br Med J* 3:30–37, 1975.

10. Tabar L, Pentek Z, Dean PB: The diagnostic and therapeutic value of breast cyst puncture and pneumocystography. *Radiology* 141:659–663, 1981.

11. Abramson AS: A clinical evaluation of aspiration of cysts of the breast. *Surg Gynecol Obstet* 139:531–537, 1974.

12. Czernobilsky B: Intracystic carcinoma of the female breast. *Surg Gynecol Obstet* 124:93–98, 1967.

13. Kline TS, Kline IK: *Breast: Guides to Clinical Aspiration Biopsy.* New York, NY, Igaku-Shoin, 1989.

14. Kline TS, Kannan V: Appraisal and cytomorphologic analysis of common carcinomas of the breast. *Diagn Cytopathol* 1:188–193, 1985.

15. Hagensen CC: *Diseases of the Breast,* 3rd ed. Philadelphia, Pa, WB Saunders Co, 1986.

16. Rosai J: Breast. In: Rosai J, ed. *Ackerman's Surgical Pathology,* 6th ed. St. Louis, Mo, CV Mosby Co, 1981, pp. 1193–1267.

17. Funderburk WW, Rosero G, Leffall LD: Breast lesions in blacks. *Surg Gynecol Obstet* 135:58–60, 1972.

18. Lewis D, Hartman CG: Tumors of the breast related to the oestrin hormone. *Am J Cancer* 21:828–859, 1934.

19. Oliver RL, Major RC: Cyclomastopathy: a physio-pathological conception of benign breast tumors, with an analysis of four hundred cases. *Am J Cancer* 21:1–85, 1934.

20. Geschickter CF: *Diseases of the Breast: Pathology, Treatment,* 2nd ed. Philadelphia, Pa, JB Lippincott Co, 1945, pp. 291–324.

21. McDivitt RW, Stewart FW, Farrow JH: Breast carcinoma arising in solitary fibroadenoma. *Surg Gynecol Obstet* 125:572–576, 1967.

22. Linsk JA, Kreuzer G, Zajicek J: Cytologic diagnosis of mammary tumors from aspiration biopsy smears, II. Studies on 210 fibroadenomas and 210 cases of benign dysplasia. *Acta Cytol* 16:130–138, 1972.

23. Tsuchiya S, Maruyama Y, Koike Y, et al: Cytologic characteristics and origin of naked nuclei in breast aspirate smears. *Acta Cytol* 31:285–290, 1987.

24. Masood S, Lu L, Assaf-Munasifi N, et al: Application of immunostaining for muscle specific actin in detection of myoepithelial cells in breast fine needle aspirates. *Diagn Cytopathol* 13:71–74, 1995.

25. Bottles K, Chan JS, Holly EA, et al: Cytologic criteria for fibroadenoma: a stepwise logistic regression analysis. *Am J Clin Pathol* 89:707–713, 1988.

26. Simi U, Moretti D, Iaccom P, et al: Fine needle aspiration cytopathology of phyllodes tumor, differential diagnostic with fibroadenoma. *Acta Cytol* 32:63–66, 1988.

27. Degrell I: Histological and needle biopsy studies of juvenile mastopathy. *Acta Morphol Hung* 29:365–376, 1981.

28. Butler KR, Cason Z, Nick TG, et al: Fibroadenoma versus fibrocystic change. Differential characteristics. *Acta Cytol* 37:807, 1993. Abstract.

29. Davies CJ, Elston CW, Colton RG, et al: Preoperative diagnosis in carcinoma of the breast. *Br J Surg* 64:326–328, 1977.

30. Devitt JE, Curry RH: Role of aspiration breast biopsy. *Can J Surg* 20:450–451, 1977.

31. Dua NK, Montana J, Sirkin B, et al: Aspiration cytology of the breast: an analysis of 865 cases. *NY State J Med* 83:867–869, 1983.

32. Kline TS, Joshi LP, Neal HS: Fine needle aspiration of the breast. Diagnosis and pitfalls: a review of 3,545 cases. *Cancer* 44:1458–1464, 1979.

33. Layfield L, Glasgow BJ, Cramer H: Fine needle aspiration in management of breast mass. *Pathol Annu* 24:23–62, 1989.

34. Chen KTK: Aspiration cytology of breast fibroadenoma with atypia. *Diagn Cytopathol* 82:283–288, 1992.

35. Stanley MW, Tani EM, Skoog L: Fine needle aspiration of fibroadenomas of the breast with atypia: a spectrum including cases that cytologically mimic carcinoma. *Diagn Cytopathol* 6:375–382, 1990.

36. Kline TS: *Handbook of Fine Needle Aspiration Biopsy Cytology.* St Louis, Mo, CV Mosby Co, 1988.

37. Rogers LA, Lee KR: Breast carcinoma simulating fibroadenoma or fibrocystic change by fine needle aspiration. A study of 16 cases. *Am J Clin Pathol* 98:155–160, 1992.

38. Fischler D, Sneige N, Ordonez N, et al: Tubular cancer of the breast (TBC): cytological features in fine needle aspiration and application of monoclonal anti–smooth muscle actin in diagnosis. *Diagn Cytopathol* 10:120–125, 1994.

39. Deitos AP, Grustina DD, Martin DV, et al: Aspiration biopsy cytology of tubular carcinoma of the breast. *Diagn Cytopathol* 11:146–150, 1994.

40. Gupta RK, Simpson J: Carcinoma of the breast in a fibroadenoma: diagnosis by fine needle aspiration cytology. *Diagn Cytopathol* 7:60–62, 1991.

41. Simpson RHW, James KA, Kelly RM, et al: Carcinoma in a breast fibroadenoma. *Acta Cytol* 31:313–316, 1987.

42. Jensen ML, Johansen P, Noer H, et al: Ductal adenoma of the breast: the cytological features of six cases. *Diagn Cytopathol* 10:143–145, 1994.

43. Stanley MW, Tani EM, Rutquist LE, et al: Cystosarcoma phyllodes of the breast: a cytologic and clinicopathologic study of 23 cases. *Diagn Cytopathol* 5:29–34, 1989.

44. Dusenberry D, Frable WJ: Fine needle aspiration cytology of phyllodes tumor: potential diagnostic pitfalls. *Acta Cytol* 36:215–221, 1992.

45. Linsk JA, Franzen S: *Clinical Aspiration Cytology,* 6th ed. Philadelphia, Pa, JB Lippincott Co, 1980, pp. 132–133.

46. Rao CR, Narasimhamurthy NK, Jaganathan G, et al: Cystosarcoma phyllodes. Diagnosis by fine needle aspiration cytology. *Acta Cytol* 36:203–207, 1992.

47. Carter D: Intraductal papillary tumors of the breast. A study of 78 cases. *Cancer* 39:1689–1692, 1977.

48. Murad TM, Contesso G, Mouriesse H: Papillary tumors of large lactiferous ducts. *Cancer* 48:122–133, 1981.

49. Sara SS, Gottfried MR: Benign papilloma of the male breast following chronic phenothiazine therapy. *Am J Clin Pathol* 87:649–650, 1979.

50. Kraus FT, Neubecker RD: The differential diagnosis of papillary tumors of the breast. *Cancer* 15:444–455, 1962.

51. Rosen PP: AP Stout and papilloma of the breast. Comments on the occasion of his 100th birthday. *Am J Surg Pathol* 10(suppl 1):100–107, 1986.

52. Saphir O, Parker ML: Intracystic papilloma of the breast. *Am J Pathol* 16:189–210, 1940.

53. Nielsen BB: Oncocytic breast papilloma. *Virchows Arch A Pathol Anat Histopathol* 393:345–351, 1981.

54. Flint A, Oberman HAL: Infarction and squamous metaplasia of intraductal papilloma. a benign breast lesion that may simulate carcinoma. *Hum Pathol* 15:764–767, 1984.

55. Koss LG, Woyke S, Olszewski W: *Aspiration Biopsy: Cytologic Interpretation and Histologic Bases.* New York, NY, Igaku-Shoin, 1984.

56. Al-Kaisi N: The spectrum of the "gray zone" in breast cytology. A review of 186 cases of atypical and suspicious cytology. *Acta Cytol* 38:898–908, 1994.

57. Jones DB: Florid papillomatosis of the nipple ducts. *Cancer* 8: 315–319, 1955.

58. Perzin KH, Lattes R: Papillary adenoma of the nipple (florid papillomatosis, adenoma, adenomatosis): a clinicopathologic study. *Cancer* 29:996–1009, 1972.

59. Rosen PP, Caireo TA: Florid papillomatosis of the nipple: a study of 51 patients including nine with mammary carcinoma. *Am J Surg Pathol* 10:87–101, 1986.

60. Baghavan BS, Patchefsy A, Koss LG: Florid subareolar duct papillomatosis (nipple adenoma) and mammary carcinoma: report of three cases. *Hum Pathol* 4:289–295, 1973.

61. Smith EJ, Kron SD, Gross PR: Erosive adenomatosis of the nipple. *Arch Dermatol* 102:330–332, 1970.

62. Stormby N, Bondeson L: Adenoma of the nipple. *Acta Cytol* 28:729–732, 1984.

63. Sood N, Jayaram G: Cytology of papillary adenoma of the nipple: a case diagnosed on fine needle aspiration. *Diagn Cytopathol* 6:345–348, 1990.

64. Mazzara PF, Flint A, Naylor B: Adenoma of the nipple: cytopathologic features. *Acta Cytol* 33:188–190, 1989.

65. Rosen PP, Cantrell B, Mullen DZ, et al: Juvenile papillomatosis (Swiss cheese disease) of the breast. *Am J Surg Pathol* 4:3–12, 1980.

66. Kline TS: Masquerades of malignancy: a review of 4241 aspirations from the breast. *Acta Cytol* 25:263–266, 1981.

67. Ostrzega N: Fine needle aspiration cytology of juvenile papillomatosis of breast: a case report. *Diagn Cytopathol* 9:457–460, 1993.

68. Rosen PP, Holmes G, Lesser ML, et al: Juvenile papillomatosis and breast carcinoma. *Cancer* 55:1345–1352, 1985.

69. Bazzocchi F, Santini D, Martinelli G, et al: Juvenile papillomatosis (epitheliosis) of the breast. A clinical and pathologic study of 13 cases. *Am J Clin Pathol* 86:745–748, 1986.

70. Ferguson BT, MacCarty KS Jr, Filston HC: Juvenile secretory carcinoma and juvenile papillomatosis: diagnosis and treatment. *J Pediatr Surg* 22:637–639, 1987.

71. McDivitt R, Stewart F, Berg J: Tumors of the breast. In: *Atlas of Tumor Pathology* (2nd series, fascicle 2). Washington, DC, Armed Forces Institute of Pathology, 1968.

72. Clement PB, Azzopard JG: Microglandular adenosis of the breast, a lesion simulating tubular carcinoma. *Histopathology* 7:169–180, 1983.

73. Rosen PP: Microglandular adenosis: a benign lesion simulating invasive mammary carcinoma. *Am J Surg Pathol* 7:137–144, 1983.

74. Gherardi G, Bernardi C, Marveggio C: Microglandular adenosis of the breast: fine needle aspiration biopsy of two cases. *Diagn Cytopathol* 9:72–76, 1993.

75. Koss LG, Woyke S, Olszewski W: The breast. In: *Aspiration Biopsy. Cytologic Interpretation and Histologic Bases.* New York, NY, Igaku-Shoin, 1984, pp. 60–66.

76. Bloxham CA, Shrimankar JJ, Wadehra V, et al: Fine needle aspiration of a lactational focus in a non-pregnant woman. *Cytopathology* 4:243–246, 1993.

77. Nguyen GK, Neifer R: Aspiration biopsy cytology of secretory carcinoma of the breast. *Diagn Cytopathol* 3:234–237, 1987.

78. Linsk JA, Franzen S: Breast carcinoma. In: Linsk JA, Franzen S, eds. *Clinical Aspiration Cytology,* 2nd ed. Philadelphia, Pa, JB Lippincott Co, 1989, pp. 111–143.

79. Silverman JF: Breast. In: Bibbo M, ed. *Comprehensive Cytopathology.* Philadelphia, Pa, WB Saunders Co, 1991, pp. 738–746.

80. Hertel BF, Zaloudek C, Kempson RL: Breast adenomas. *Cancer* 37: 2891–2905, 1976.

81. O'Hara MF, Page LD: Adenomas of the breast and ectopic breast under lactational influences. *Hum Pathol* 16:707–712, 1985.

82. Tavassoli FA, Yeh IT: Lactational and clear cell changes of the breast in nonlactating, nonpregnant women. *Am J Clin Pathol* 87:23–29, 1987.

83. McDivitt EW: Breast carcinoma arising in solitary fibroadenoma. *Surg Gynecol Obstet* 125:572, 1967. Abstract.

84. Haas JF: Pregnancy in association with a newly diagnosed cancer: population based epidemiologic assessment. *Int J Cancer* 34:229–235, 1984.

85. White TT: Prognosis of breast cancer for pregnant and non-pregnant women. *Surg Gynecol Obstet* 10:661–666, 1955.

86. Novotny DB, Maygarden SJ, Shermar RW, et al: Fine needle aspiration of benign and malignant breast masses associated with pregnancy. *Acta Cytol* 35:678–686, 1991.

87. Hagensen CD: Cancer of the breast in pregnancy and during lactation. *Am J Obstet Gynecol* 98:141, 1967.

88. White TT, White WC: Breast cancer in pregnancy: report of 49 cases followed 5 years. *Ann Surg* 144:384, 1956.

89. Bottles K, Taylor R: Diagnosis of breast masses in pregnant and lactating women by aspiration cytology. *Obstet Gynecol* 66:76–78, 1985.

90. Finley JL, Silverman JF, Lannin DR: Fine needle aspiration cytology of breast masses in pregnant and lactating women. *Diagn Cytopathol* 5:255–259, 1989.

91. Gupta RK, Wakefield SJ, Lallu S, et al: Aspiration cytodiagnosis of breast carcinoma in pregnancy and lactation with immunocytochemical and electron microscopic study of an unusual mammary malignancy with pleomorphic giant cells. *Diagn Cytopathol* 8:352–356, 1992.

92. Grenko RT, Lee KP, Lee KR: Fine needle aspiration cytology of lactating adenoma of the breast: a comparative light and morphometric study. *Acta Cytol* 34:21–26, 1990.

93. Gupta RK, McHutchinson AGR, Dowle CS, et al: Fine needle aspiration cytodiagnosis of breast masses in pregnant and lactating women and its impact on management. *Diagn Cytopathol* 9:156–159, 1993.

94. Bondeson L: Aspiration cytology of radiation-induced changes of normal breast epithelium. *Acta Cytol (Praha)* 31:309-310, 1987.

95. Peterse JL, Koolman-Schellekens MA, Van de Peppel-van de Ham T, et al: Atypia in fine needle aspiration cytology of the breast: a histologic follow-up study of 301 cases. *Semin Diagn Pathol* 6:126–134, 1989.

96. Peterse JL, Thunnissen FB, Van Heerde P: Fine needle aspiration cytology of radiation-induced changes in non-neoplastic breast lesions. Possible pitfalls in cytodiagnosis. *Acta Cytol (Praha)* 33:176–180, 1989.

97. Dornfeld JM, Thompson SK, Shurbaji MS: Radiation-induced changes in the breast: a potential diagnostic pitfall on fine-needle aspiration. *Diagn Cytopathol* 8:79–81, 1992.

98. Filomena CA, Jordan AG, Ehya H: Needle aspiration cytology of the irradiated breast. *Diagn Cytopathol* 8:327–332, 1992.

99. Schnitt SJ, Connolly JL, Harris JR, et al: Radiation-induced changes in the breast. *Hum Pathol* 15:545–550, 1984.

100. Costa MJ, Stewart G, Perez E, et al: Fine needle aspiration cytology in locally advanced breast adenocarcinoma: a case with complete response to preoperative chemotherapy in association with granulomatous inflammatory reaction. *Diagn Cytopathol* 10:357–361, 1994.

101. Soyage-Rabie L, Fanning CV, Staerkel GA, et al: Fine needle aspiration cytology of breast lesions following lumpectomy and irradiation: a review of 100 cases. *Acta Cytol* 37:766, 1993.

102. Malberger E, Edoute Y, Toledano O, et al: Fine needle aspiration and cytologic findings of surgical scar lesions in women with breast cancer. *Cancer* 69:148–152, 1992.

103. Maygarden SJ, Johnson DE, Powers CN, et al: Suture granulomas of the breast: a potential pitfall in the fine needle aspiration cytologic diagnosis of recurrent breast carcinoma. *Acta Cytol* 34:719, 1990. Abstract.

104. Orell SR, Sterrett GF, Walters MN-I, et al: *Manual and Atlas of Fine Needle Aspiration Biopsy.* New York, NY, Churchill Livingstone Inc, 1986, p. 207.

105. Briffod M, Gentile A, Hebert H: Cytopuncture in the followup of breast carcinoma. *Acta Cytol* 26:195–200, 1982.

106. Kline TS, Toshi LP, Neal HS: Fine needle aspiration of the breast: diagnosis and pitfalls. *Cancer* 44:1458–1464, 1979.

107. Golough R, Us-Krasovec M: Differential diagnosis of the pleomorphic aspiration biopsy sample of nonepithelial lesions. *Diagn Cytopathol* 1:308–316, 1985.

108. Maygarden SJ, Novotny DB, Johnson DE, et al: Fine needle aspiration cytology of suture granulomas of the breast: a potential pitfall in the cytologic diagnosis of recurrent breast cancer. *Diagn Cytopathol* 10:175–179, 1994.

109. Jans LD: Cytopathology of mesenchymal repair. *Diagn Cytopathol* 1:91–104, 1985.

110. Zajicek J: Aspiration biopsy cytology, part I: supradiaphragmatic organs. In: Wied GL, ed. *Monographs in Clinical Cytology,* Vol 4. Basel, Switzerland, S Karger, 1974, p. 177.

111. Zajedela A, Ghossein NA, Pilleron JP, et al: The value of aspiration cytology in the diagnosis of breast cancer: experience at the Fondation Curie. *Cancer* 35:499–506, 1975.

112. Silverman JF, Geisinger KR, Frable WJ: Fine needle aspiration cytology of mesenchymal tumors of the breast. *Diagn Cytopathol* 4:50–58, 1988.

113. Stanley MW, Tani EM, Skoog L: Metaplastic carcinoma of the breast: fine needle aspiration cytology of seven cases. *Diagn Cytopathol* 5:22–28, 1989.

114. Stanley MW, Tani EM, Horwitz CA, et al: Primary spindle cell carcinomas of the breast: diagnosis by fine needle aspiration. *Diagn Cytopathol* 4:244–249, 1988.

115. Frable WJ: Thin needle aspiration biopsy. In: Bennington JL, ed. *Major Problems in Pathology Series,* Vol. 14. Philadelphia, Pa, WB Saunders Co, pp. 53–60, 1983.

116. Rupp M, Hafiz AM, Khalluf E, et al: Fine needle aspiration in stromal sarcoma of the breast: light and electron microscopic findings with histologic correlation. *Acta Cytol* 32:72–74, 1988.

117. Willen R, Urelin B, Cameron R: Pleomorphic adenoma in the breast of a human female. *Acta Chir Scand* 152:709–713, 1986.

118. Nguyen GK, Shnitka TK, Jewell L: Aspiration biopsy cytology of mammary myepithelioma. *Diagn Cytopathol* 3:335–338, 1987.

119. Ordi J, Riverola A, Sole M, et al: Fine needle aspiration of myofibroblastoma of the breast in a man: a report of two cases. *Acta Cytol* 36:194–198, 1992.

120. Dahl I, Akerman M: Nodular fasciitis: a correlative cytologic and histologic study of 13 cases. *Acta Cytol* 25:215–223, 1981.

121. Fritschs HG, Mullen EA: Pseudosarcomatous fasciitis of the breast: cytologic and histologic features. *Acta Cytol* 29:562–565, 1985.

122. Sorensen K: Fine needle aspiration of fibromatosis of the breast. *Diagn Cytopathol* 3:320–322, 1987.

123. Akerman M, Idvall I, Rydholm A: Cytodiagnosis of soft tissue tumors and tumor-like conditions by means of fine needle aspiration biopsy. *Arch Orthop Trauma Surg* 76:61–67, 1980.

124. Christie AJ, Weinberger KA, Dietrich M: Silicone lymphadenopathy and synovitis. *JAMA* 237:1463–1464, 1977.

125. Symmers WS: Silicone mastitis in "topless" waitresses and some other varieties of foreign body mastitis. *Br Med J* 3:19–22, 1968.

126. Cruz G, Gillooley JF, Waxman M: Silicone granulomas of the breast. *NY State J Med* 85:599–601, 1985.

127. Ben-Hur N, Ballantyne DL Jr, Rees TD, et al: Local and systemic effects of dimethylpolysilcoxane fluid in mice. *Plast Reconstr Surg* 39:423–426, 1967.

128. Travis WD, Balegh K, Abraham JL: Silicone granulomas: report of three cases and review of the literature. *Hum Pathol* 16:19, 1985.

129. Hausner RJ, Schoen FT, Mendez-Fernandez MA, et al: Migration of silicone gel to axillary lymph nodes after prosthetic mammoplasty. *Arch Pathol Lab Med* 105:371–372, 1981.

130. Tabatowski K, Elson CE, Johnson WW: Silicone lymphadenopathy in a patient with a mammary prosthesis: fine needle aspiration cytology, histology and analytical electron microscopy. *Acta Cytol* 34:10–14, 1990.

131. Highland KE, Finley JL, Neill JSA, et al: Collagenous spherulosis: report of a case with diagnosis by fine needle aspiration biopsy with immunocytochemical and ultrastructural observations. *Acta Cytol* 37:3–9, 1993.

132. Grignon DJ, Ro JY, Mackey BN, et al: Collagenous spherulosis of the breast: immunohistochemical and ultrastructural studies. *Am J Clin Pathol* 91:388–392, 1989.

133. Johnson TL, Kini SR: Cytologic features of collagenous spherulosis of the breast. *Diagn Cytopathol* 7:417–419, 1991.

134. Perez JS, Perez-Guillermo M, Bernal AB, et al: Diagnosis of collagenous spherulosis of the breast by fine needle aspiration cytology: a report of two cases. *Acta Cytol* 37:725–728, 1993.

135. Stanley MW, Tani EM, Rutquist LE, et al: Adenoid cystic carcinoma of the breast: diagnosis by fine-needle aspiration. *Diagn Cytopathol* 9:184–187, 1993.

136. Tyler X, Coghill SB: Fine needle aspiration cytology of collagenous spherulosis of the breast. *Cytopathology* 2:159–162, 1991.

137. Silverman JF, Dabbs DJ, Norris HT, et al: Localized primary amyloid tumor of the breast: cytologic, histologic, immunocytochemical and ultrastructural observations. *Am J Surg Pathol* 10:539–545, 1986.

138. Lew W, Seymour A: Primary amyloid tumor of the breast, case report and literature review. *Acta Cytol* 29:7–11, 1985.

139. Lipper S, Kahn LB: Amyloid tumor: a clinicopathologic study of four cases. *Am J Surg Pathol* 2:141–145, 1978.

140. O'Connor CR, Rubinow A, Cohen AS: Primary (AL) amyloidosis as a cause of breast masses. *Am J Med* 77:981–986, 1984.

141. Heller EL, Fleming JC: Fibrosing adenomatosis of the breast. *Am J Clin Pathol* 20:141–146, 1950.

142. Urban JA, Adair FE: Sclerosing adenosis. *Cancer* 2:625–634, 1949.

143. Haagensen CD: *Diseases of the Breast,* 3rd ed. Philadelphia, Pa, WB Saunders Co, 1989, pp.106–117.

144. Nielssen BB: Adenosis tumor of the breast: a clinicopathologic investigation of 72 cases. *Histopathology* 11:1259–1275, 1987.

145. Silverman JF, Dabbs DJ, Gilbert CF: Adenosis tumor of the breast: cytologic, histologic, immunocytochemical and ultrastructural observations. *Acta Cytol* 33:181–187, 1989.

146. MacEvlean DP, Nathan BE: Calcification in sclerosing adenosis simulating malignant breast calcification. *Br J Radiol* 45:944–945, 1972.

147. Wellings SR, Roberts P: Electron microscopy of sclerosing adenosis and infiltrating duct carcinoma of the human mammary gland. *J Natl Cancer Inst* 30:269–287, 1963.

148. Koss LG, Wayke J, Olszewski W: *Aspiration Biopsy: Cytologic Interpretation and Histologic Bases.* Tokyo, Japan, Igaku-Shoin, 1984.

149. Anderson JA, Carter D, Linell F: A symposium on sclerosing duct lesions of the breast. *Pathol Annu* 21:145–179, 1986.

150. Nielsen M, Jensen J, Andersen JA: An autopsy study of radial scar in the female breast. *Histopathology* 9:287–295, 1985.

151. Tavassoli FA: *Pathology of the Breast.* Norwalk, Conn, Appleton and Lange, 1992, pp. 107–114.

152. Anderson TJ, Battersby S: Radial scar of benign and malignant breast: comparative features and significance. *J Pathol* 147:23–32, 1985.

153. Fenoglio C, Lattes R: Sclerosing papillary proliferations in the female breast. A benign lesion often mistaken for carcinoma. *Cancer* 33:691–700, 1974.

154. Vazquez MF, Mitnick J, Waisman J, et al: Stereotaxic aspiration of radial scars. *Acta Cytol* 35:584, 1991. Abstract.

155. Frierson HJ, Iezzoni JC, Covell JL: Stereotaxic fine needle aspiration cytology of radial scars. *Acta Cytol* 37:814, 1993. Abstract.

CHAPTER SIX

Benign Mesenchymal Tumors

The breast consists of epithelial and myoepithelial cells as well as stroma. Within the stroma, there are fibroblasts, fat cells, nerve cells, nerve fibers, endothelial cells, and smooth muscle cells surrounding the vessels. Any of these elements can give rise to a variety of benign and malignant lesions. In addition, soft tissue sarcomas can metastasize to the breast, presenting a diagnostic challenge. Morphologic distinction between primary and secondary sarcoma of the breast is somewhat difficult.

Benign mesenchymal tumors include fibromatosis, myofibroblastoma, adenomyoepithelioma, granular cell tumor, neurofibroma, spindle cell lipoma, and lipoma. Several physiologic, inflammatory, and reactive conditions give rise to conspicuous spindle cell proliferation, which may mimic a neoplastic process cytologically. These include exuberant granulation tissue formation, subareolar abscess, juvenile hypertrophy of the breast, post–fine needle aspiration biopsy (FNAB) reactive stromal proliferation, nodular fasciitis, and stromal induction in proliferative breast disease. The cytologic features of these conditions may not be specific, and correlation with the patient's clinical presentation, age, and history may be required. For example, spindle cell proliferation and reactive changes may be caused by an inflammatory condition or a procedure such as a biopsy. Exuberant granulation tissue yields a cellular aspirate, with sheet-like arrangements of densely packed capillaries surrounded by endothelial cells. There may be atypical spindle cells in an inflammatory background.[1]

Juvenile hypertrophy is characterized by cohesive sheets of hyperplastic, ductal epithelium and a conspicuous number of well-preserved cells, singly and in clusters. These cells are often admixed with fibrillary stroma, reflecting the presence of abundant fibrous tissue of variable cellularity. Scattered, naked nuclei are also present.[2] In the absence of a clinical or his-

147

torical explanation for the presence of spindle cell proliferation, surgical excision of the lesion is most helpful in substantiating the aspirate diagnosis.

Fibromatosis

Fibromatosis is characterized by the formation of locally aggressive lesions consisting of a neoplastic proliferation of fibroblastic cells. It is most commonly encountered in the abdominal wall and only rarely seen in the breast. Nichols[3] reported the first case of breast fibromatosis in 1923. Since then many cases have been reported.[4–6] Fibromatosis occurs in an age range of 14 to 80; occasionally, patients with fibromatosis may present with a bilateral lesion. Fibromatosis may mimic carcinoma clinically and mammographically, and patients may present with skin dimpling, nipple retraction, and a stellate lesion.[7,8] Fibromatosis has been reported in association with Gardner's syndrome and at the site of a breast implant in a few patients.[8–10]

Despite its clinical presentation, fibromatosis may be almost indistinguishable from normal breast tissue and lacks the appearance of a cancer. Microscopically, lesions associated with fibromatosis are characterized by an infiltrating proliferation of uniform, plump, spindle cell fibroblasts around ducts and lobules. No calcification or necrosis is seen. Mitoses are rare. Local excision is the treatment of choice, unless the lesion is so large that it requires mastectomy. Tamoxifen therapy has been found to induce regression in cases of recurrent fibromatosis.[5,7,11] The risk of recurrence is higher in incompletely resected lesions; most recurrences develop within 3 years of diagnosis. The incidence of recurrence ranges from 21% to 27%.[7,8,12]

Preoperative diagnosis of fibromatosis by FNAB can be fraught with difficulty. A wide spectrum of both benign and malignant breast lesions should be considered before the diagnosis of fibromatosis is made. Only a few cases of fibromatosis of the breast have been studied by FNAB.[5,13–19] Although the cellularity of the aspirates may vary, in most cases the smears are cellular and contain isolated spindle cells; small groups of cohesive, benign epithelial cells; and scattered lymphocytes in a background of amorphous material. The spindle cells are uniform in appearance and devoid of atypical features (Images 6.1 through 6.5). The presence of lymphoid aggregates, primarily at the periphery of the lesion, has been described as a histologic feature of fibromatosis of the breast.[5–8,14] If the lesion is sampled adequately, lymphocytes may constitute a conspicuous component of the aspirate.

Spindle cell lesions of the breast that can mimic fibromatosis of the breast cytologically include fibrosarcoma, malignant fibrous histiocytoma, malignant phyllodes tumor, and metaplastic carcinoma. These lesions display pleomorphic, markedly atypical spindle cells with a conspicuous number of mitotic figures.[19–23] In addition to isolated, large spindle cells, many atypical epithelial cells, isolated and in clusters, are observed in metaplastic carcinoma. Demonstration of epithelial markers expressed in the cytoplasm of tumor cells by applying immunocytochemical stains to aspirated material often substantiates the diagnosis of metaplastic carcinoma.[23,24]

Cellular fibroadenoma and phyllodes tumor also have some cytologic features in common with fibromatosis. Clinical impression of a circumscribed mass, often of large size, and the presence of highly cellular, stromal fragments; isolated, bipolar, naked nuclei; and abundant epithelial cells are features that militate against a diagnosis of fibromatosis of the breast.[14,22,24] The cytologic appearance of mammary fibromatosis may also resemble that of nodular fasciitis. However, smears of nodular fasciitis are often more cellular and contain variably sized spindle cells; plump, ganglion-like cells; mitoses; and a polymorphous inflammatory infiltrate in a myxoid background.[25,26]

The cytologic distinction between fibromatosis and spindle cell adenomyoepithelioma can be difficult. Expression of vimentin, actin, and cytokeratin separates adenomyoepithelioma from fibromatosis, which does not show positive immunostaining for cytokeratin.[17,27] The nonmyoepithelial origin of fibromatosis can be further confirmed by electron microscopic study.[17]

In a clinically suspicious lesion, recognition of the cytologic features of fibromatosis, ie, bland spindle cells and small groups of benign epithelial cells and lymphocytes, may allow resection with a sufficiently wide local excision. This may prevent recurrence and avoid unnecessary surgery. Immunocytochemistry and electron microscopic study can also be used to arrive at a correct diagnosis. Extreme caution should be exercised in interpreting aspirates of fibromatosis of the breast, since a few groups of hyperchromatic epithelial cells were reportedly overdiagnosed as carcinoma in one case.[5]

Cytomorphology of Fibromatosis
Variable cellularity
Pronounced spindle cell proliferation
A few small groups of epithelial cells
Scattered lymphocytes
Amorphous material in the background

Myofibroblastoma

Myofibroblastoma is a well-circumscribed, solitary, palpable, firm mass occurring predominantly in men between the ages of 41 and 85 years. The mass generally measures from 1 to 5 cm and presents as a nodular, round, slightly lobulated lesion. Microscopically, myofibroblasts are arranged in a fascicular fashion and are associated with hyalinized collagen. The cells of this tumor consist of uniform, bipolar, ovoid to spindle cells arranged diffusely or in clusters. They are separated by broad bands of collagen. Mitotic figures are rare. Immunoreactivity for vimentin, actin, and desmin is reported. The cells are negative for S-100 and cytokeratin. Ultrastructurally, the tumor cells show features of fibroblasts or myofibroblasts.[28,29] Local excision is the treatment of choice.

Myofibroblastoma may be diagnosed by FNAB. Cytologically, the smears show the presence of spindle cells with naked, ovoid nuclei arranged in regular or vaguely fascicular clusters and the absence of epithelial cells.[30] Some of the cell clusters show a vacuolated, myxoid-appearing matrix. Nuclear grooves are occasionally seen in the tumor cells; nucleoli are inconspicuous (Images 6.6 through 6.10).

A greater degree of cellular pleomorphism and the presence of atypical spindle cells and epithelial cells distinguish myofibroblastoma from stromal

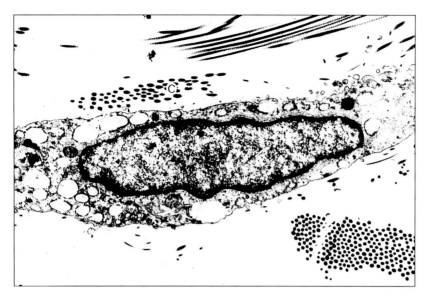

Figure 6.1
FNAB of myofibroblastoma. Ultrastructural features include a spindle cell surrounded by collagen fibers (C) (12,300X).

sarcoma and metaplastic carcinoma. Immunocytochemical and electron microscopic studies are important diagnostic adjuncts (Figure 6.1).

Cytomorphology of Myofibroblastoma
Variable cellularity
Proliferation of spindle cells with naked, oval nuclei
Absence of epithelial cells
Myxoid-appearing matrix
Inconspicuous nucleoli

Adenomyoepithelioma

Adenomyoepithelioma, a rare, solitary tumor of the breast, is characterized by proliferation of myoepithelial and admixed epithelial cells. This tumor is locally aggressive, with a potential for local recurrence. Occasionally, metastasis may also occur. Malignancy can be predicted by mitotic activity (1–4/10 hpf) and cytologic atypia.[7,31,32] The distinction between adenomyoepithelioma and fibromatosis is possible only by immunocytochemistry. Adenomyoepithelioma shows positive immunostaining for vimentin, actin, and cytokeratin. In contrast, no expression of cytokeratin is seen in fibromatosis.[27,33] Grossly, the lesion may appear as a well-circumscribed nodule with no evidence of cyst formation or hemorrhage. Microscopically, the tumor is composed of a predominant, solid mass of spindle cells admixed with a few epithelial-lined spaces. Mitoses are rare.

The importance of recognizing this lesion cannot be overemphasized, since a number of benign adenomyoepitheliomas have been misdiagnosed as infiltrating carcinomas, resulting in unnecessary mastectomies and axillary dissections.[34] Because adequate treatment is local excision with a wide margin, it is important to be familiar with the cytomorphology of adenomyoepithelioma. Reports on the cytomorphology of adenomyoepithelioma are sparse, and our own experience is limited to one case.[33,35] However, aspirates of adenomyoepithelioma are generally rich in cellularity, with a heterogeneous population of small, cohesive clusters of cells. In air-dried smears stained with May-Grünwald–Giemsa (MGG), Vielh et al[33] described the cells as large, with a gray-blue cytoplasm embedded in an abundant, fibrillary, myxoid substance or lying free in the background. Nuclei were eccentrically located and were either round, eccentric, or spindle shaped. The chromatin had a fine, reticular pattern and showed no evidence of mitosis. Hoch and Chan[35] reported cohesive groups of epithelial cells with a prominent rim of naked, bipolar nuclei; a small amount of fibrous stroma; and occasional apocrine cells.

In the one case of adenomyoepithelioma that we evaluated, the aspirate was cellular, consisting of sheets of crowded, cohesive clusters of smooth, uniform cells. In Papanicolaou-stained smears, the cells were round to oval, with a fine chromatin pattern and surrounded by many cells with naked nuclei. Scant stromal material could occasionally be seen (Images 6.11 through 6.13). In none of the cases described above was the diagnosis of adenomyoepithelioma made initially. Instead, interpretation of the aspirates ranged from proliferative breast disease to tumors of sweat gland origin, and surgical excision was recommended.

Myoepithelial lesions of the breast have recently been classified into myoepitheliosis, malignant myoepithelioma, and adenomyoepithelioma, including a spindle cell type, a tubular or lobulated type with clear or eosinophilic cells, and the rare carcinoma arising in adenomyoepithelioma.[34] The spectrum of biologic behavior of these lesions has also been studied.[36] Adjunct studies such as immunocytochemistry and electron microscopy complement morphologic findings in breast fine needle aspirates. Adenomyoepitheliomas demonstrate immunoreactivity for keratin, actin, and S-100 protein (Image 6.14).[35,37] Ultrastructurally, the spindle cells are joined by mature desmosomes with pinocytotic vesicles, keratin intermediate filaments, and actin filaments, as well as glandular formation.[35,37]

The cytologic differential diagnosis of adenomyoepithelioma includes tubular carcinoma, lobular carcinoma, and papillary neoplasms. The absence of complex branching and angulated epithelial cells and the presence of myoepithelial cell differentiation excludes the possibility of tubular carcinoma.[38,39] The absence of bipolar, naked nuclei and the presence of intracytoplasmic vacuoles are other features that militate against a diagnosis of lobular carcinoma.[38,39] Differentiating between adenomyoepithelioma and papillary lesions may be difficult. However, the absence of true papillary aggregates, foam cells, or apocrine cells and predominance of naked nuclei favor a diagnosis of adenomyoepithelioma. Malignant adenomyoepithelioma has been described histologically[34,36] and is characterized by cellular pleomorphism and, most important, mitotic activity. The cytologic features of malignant adenomyoepithelioma have yet to be defined.

Cytomorphology of Adenomyoepithelioma
Rich cellularity
Clusters of small cells with uniform nuclei and a fine chromatin pattern
Inconspicuous nucleoli
Bipolar, naked nuclei in the background and in the periphery of epithelial aggregates
Scanty stromal matrix

Granular Cell Tumor

Granular cell tumor, a well-recognized neoplasm of neural origin, occurs rarely in the breast. It occurs in a wide age range (21–75 years), with the average in the thirties.[40–42] Occasionally, granular cell tumor develops in a male breast. However, it occurs most often in women, suggesting a hormonal relationship. So far, no expression of estrogen or progesterone receptors has been reported in granular cell tumors.[43] While some granular cell tumors manifest as a well-defined mass clinically and mammographically, others may show skin retraction and satellite lesions mammographically, resembling carcinoma. This tumor can involve breast parenchyma as well as the nipple, enlarging it conspicuously.

Grossly, granular cell tumor is well circumscribed. However, occasionally areas of induration and irregularity can be seen in the outlines of the lesion.[44] Microscopically, granular cell tumor presents either as a well-defined lobulated mass or as a stellate lesion with an infiltrating pattern. The tumor is composed of infiltrating cords and clusters of uniform, round, polygonal cells with granular cytoplasm and centrally located nuclei. Immunostaining for S-100 confirms the diagnosis. Malignant granular cell tumors are generally large, with local invasion, extensive pleomorphism, and a high degree of mitotic activity. Granular cell tumor rarely metastasizes to axillary lymph nodes.[45]

Fine needle aspiration biopsies of granular cell tumors yield cellular smears containing large, cohesive sheets of cells with abundant, granular cytoplasm and indistinct cell borders. Nuclei are uniform in size, have an evenly dispersed chromatin pattern, and may contain nucleoli. Immunostaining for S-100 and carcinoembryonic antigen, as well as electron microscopic study, may help to substantiate the diagnosis of granular cell tumor (Figure 6.2 and Images 6.15 through 6.18). Ultrastructurally, there are granules resembling autophagosomes, which are osmophilic structures. Malignant granular cell tumors demonstrate all the nuclear features of malignancy.[46,47]

Cytomorphology of Granular Cell Tumor
Cellular smear
Cohesive clusters of epithelial cells
Abundant, granular cytoplasm
Evenly distributed chromatin pattern
Conspicuous nucleoli

Neurofibroma

Neurofibroma, or neurilemoma, is a rare benign lesion of the breast occurring in both women and men.[48,49] Neurofibroma may be associated with Recklinghausen's neurofibromatosis.[49] Cytologically, the tumor shows clusters of spindle-shaped cells with ill-defined cytoplasmic margins and nuclear palisades. Immunocytochemistry and electron microscopy substantiate the diagnosis (Images 6.19 through 6.22).[50–52]

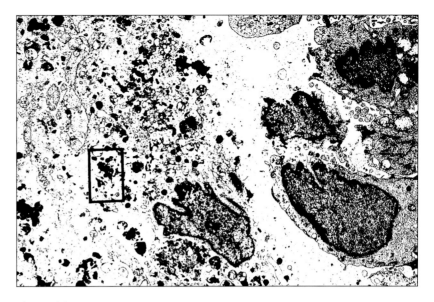

Figure 6.2
Ultrastructural findings in aspirate of granular cell tumor: abundant phagolysosomes (enclosed area) filled with heterogeneous osmiophilic material (6500X).

Cytomorphology of Neurofibroma
Moderate cellularity
Spindle-shaped cells
Ill-defined cytoplasmic margin
Nuclear palisades

Spindle Cell Lipoma

Spindle cell lipoma, a tumor indistinguishable from benign spindle cell tumor of the breast, was originally described in 1981 by Toker et al[53] and later reported by other investigators.[54,55] This lesion affects both men and women and follows a benign course. Local excision is curative.

Clinically, patients present with a single, palpable breast lesion. Multiple lesions are rare. Grossly, the lesion is well defined and white, grayish white, yellow-brown, brown, or reddish gray in color. The size may range from 2 to 9 cm in diameter.

Microscopically, spindle cell lipoma is composed of spindle-shaped fusiform and stellate cells with scant, ill-defined cytoplasm. The cells are characteristically arranged in a fasciculated or whorled pattern. Cytoplasmic vacuoles may also be present. Small groups of mature adipocytes, mast cells, and lymphocytes are seen in a collagenous or myxoid stroma.

In a 1992 report of a single case, Lew[56] described the cytomorphology of spindle cell lipoma. The smears in the case were hypocellular and showed atypical cells dispersed or in small aggregates in a myxoid background. The cells were pleomorphic and varied from round to oval to spindle shaped. Some of the nuclei had irregular nuclear membranes and prominent nucleoli. The amount of cytoplasm was variable. A few multinucleated giant cells were also present. The cytoplasm of some of the cells formed fine, elongated or fibrillary processes, and the multinucleated cells had a wreath-like pattern identical to that of the floret cells seen in pleomorphic liposarcoma.[57,58] The cytologic findings were reported as suspicious for malignancy and excisional biopsy was performed. This report highlights yet another diagnostic pitfall in FNAB of the breast. Awareness of spindle cell lipoma, with its atypical cytologic features, is important in preventing misdiagnosis of malignancy by FNAB.

Cytomorphology of Spindle Cell Lipoma
Hypocellular aspirate
Cells dispersed or in small aggregates
Pleomorphic cell population
Nuclear atypia
Multinucleated giant cells
Floret-like cells
Absence of lipoblasts

Lipoma

Lipoma occurs in the breast as a solitary, often unilateral mass in middle-aged women.[59,60] Patients with lipoma present with a circumscribed, well-formed, soft, movable lesion in the breast. Although the average size of the tumor is about 2.5 cm, it can be larger than 10 cm.[61] Grossly, the tumor is a well-demarcated, lobulated, yellow mass. Microscopically, the tumor is composed of typical round, mature lipocytes and surrounded by a delicate capsule.

Cytologically, breast elements are not seen unless, via aspiration, the surrounding breast tissue is sampled. The aspirate is composed of fragments of adipose tissue with small blood vessels, stromal cells, and a few inflammatory cells (Images 6.23 and 6.24). The cytologic impression of lipoma in a breast FNAB should be correlated with the clinical presentation of the lesion.

Image 6.1
Fibromatosis, spindle cells, and scattered lymphocytes in background of amorphous material (H&E, 100X).

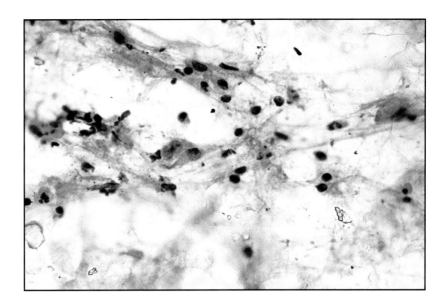

Image 6.2
Higher magnification of the same case shows uniform spindle cell proliferation (H&E, 200X).

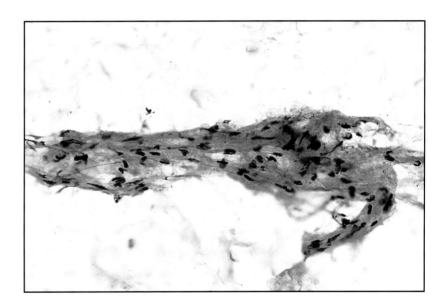

Image 6.3
Papanicolaou-stained smear of the same case shows similar features (400X).

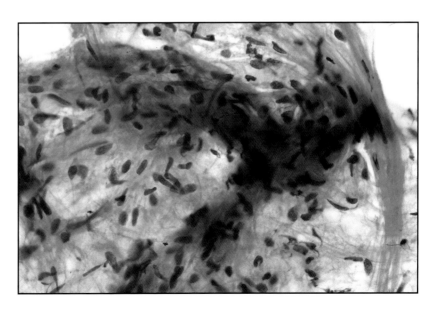

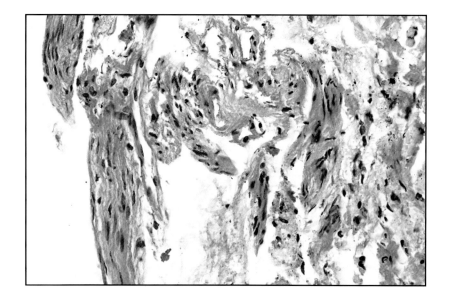

Image 6.4
Cell block preparation of the same case of fibromatosis demonstrates fragments of fibrous tissue with prominent spindle cell proliferation (H&E, 200X).

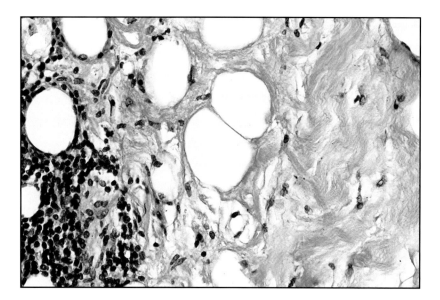

Image 6.5
Corresponding surgically excised lesion demonstrates scattered spindle cell fibroblasts embedded in amorphous, dense connective tissue with a collection of lymphocytes like those characteristically seen in fibromatosis (H&E, 200X).

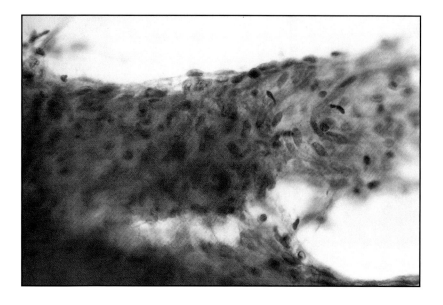

Image 6.6
Myofibroblastoma. Spindle cell proliferation in a hyalinized matrix arranged in a vaguely fascicular pattern (Papanicolaou, 200X).

Image 6.7
Another view of the same case of myofibroblastoma demonstrates naked, ovoid nuclei in a myxoid-appearing matrix (Papanicolaou, 200X).

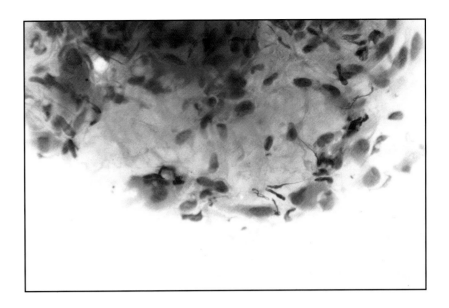

Image 6.8
Higher magnification of the same case. In contrast to fibromatosis, lymphocytes are absent (Papanicolaou, 400X).

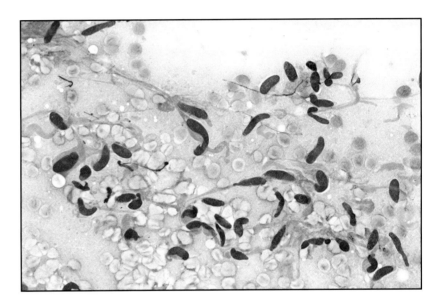

Image 6.9
Cell block preparation of the same case shows fragments of dense connective tissue containing spindle cells (H&E, 200X).

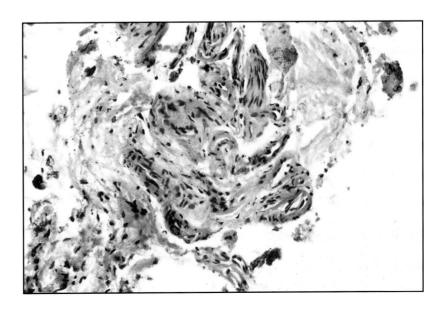

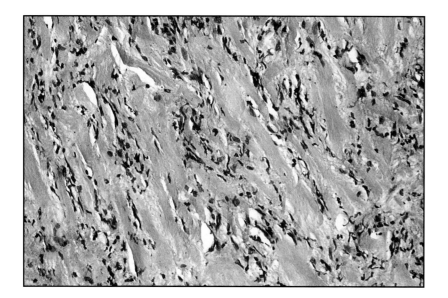

Image 6.10
Corresponding surgically excised lesion of myofibroblastoma demonstrates a diffuse proliferation of spindle cell fibroblasts separated by broad ribbons and bands of collagen (H&E, 200X).

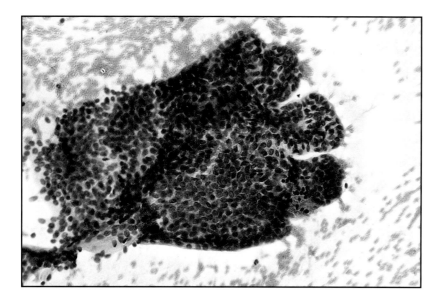

Image 6.11
Cellular aspirate of adenomyoepithelioma shows crowded clusters of rather uniform cells (Papanicolaou, 200X).

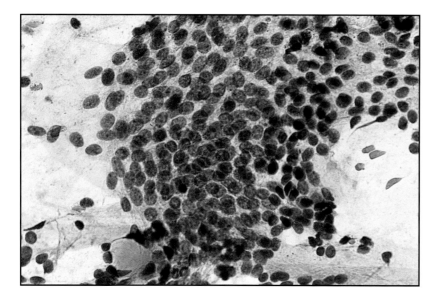

Image 6.12
Higher-power magnification of the same case demonstrates round- to oval-shaped cells with a fine chromatin pattern, inconspicuous nucleoli, and a scanty stromal matrix. The cellular aggregate is surrounded by isolated naked nuclei (Papanicolaou, 400X).

Image 6.13
Corresponding surgically excised lesion diagnosed as adenomyoepithelioma (H&E, 200X).

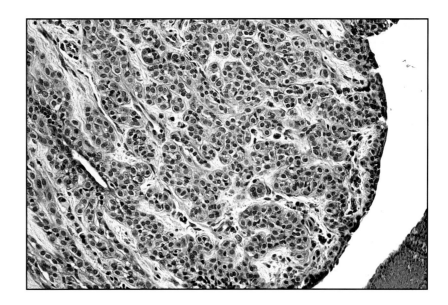

Image 6.14
Positive immunostaining for muscle specific actin in resected specimen confirms the myoepithelial origin of the tumor (Immunoperoxidase, 400X).

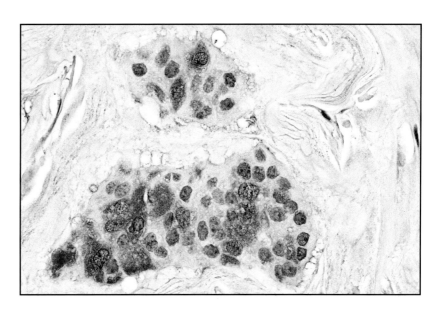

Image 6.15
Granular cell tumor. Clusters of epithelial cells with granular cytoplasm and indistinct cell borders (Diff-Quik®, 200X).

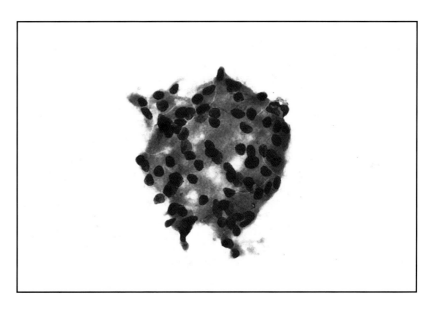

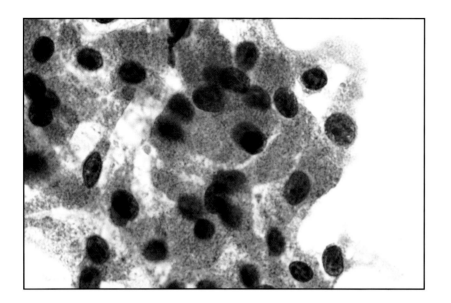

Image 6.16
Higher magnification of the same case of granular cell tumor demonstrates epithelial cells with abundant, granular cytoplasm; uniform-sized nuclei with an evenly dispersed chromatin pattern; and conspicuous nucleoli (Papanicolaou, 400X).

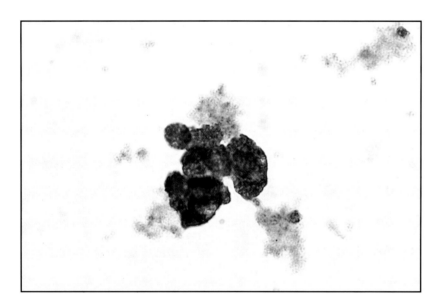

Image 6.17
Cell block preparation of the same case shows positive immunostaining for S-100 (Immunoperoxidase, 400X).

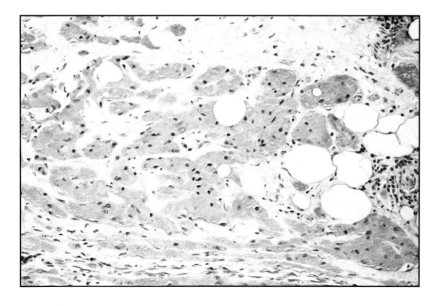

Image 6.18
Corresponding surgically excised lesion diagnosed as granular cell tumor (H&E, 200X).

Image 6.19
Neurofibroma of the breast. Cellular smear from FNAB of a patient with Recklinghausen's neurofibromatosis contains palisades of spindle-shaped cells with indistinct cell borders (H&E, 200X).

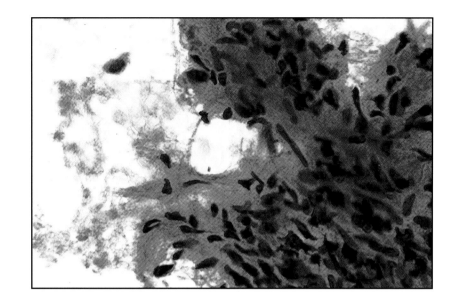

Image 6.20
Papanicolaou-stained smear of the same case showing the same features (400X).

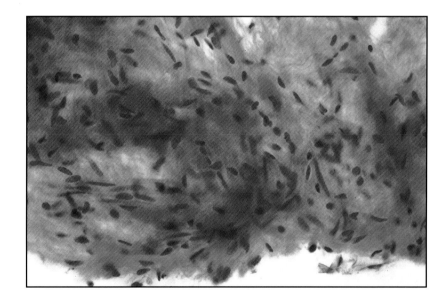

Image 6.21
Cell block preparation of the same case showing positive expression for neuron specific enolase (Immunoperoxidase, 400X).

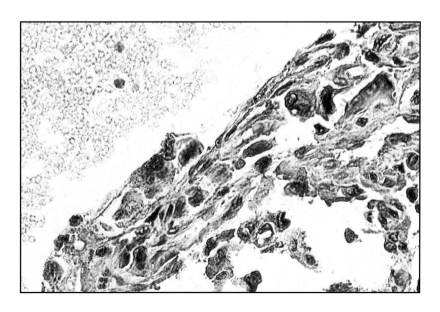

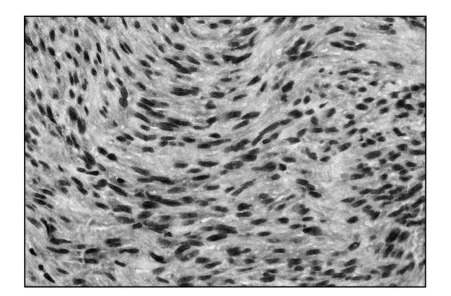

Image 6.22
Tissue section obtained from surgically excised lesion from the same case diagnosed as neurofibroma (H&E, 200X).

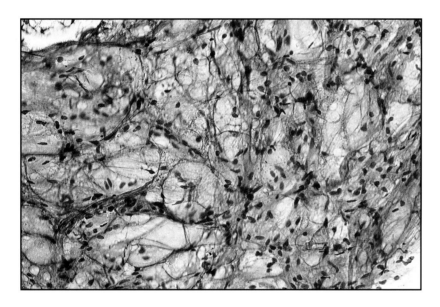

Image 6.23
Lipoma: fragments of adipose tissue with stromal cells and small blood vessels (Papanicolaou, 200X).

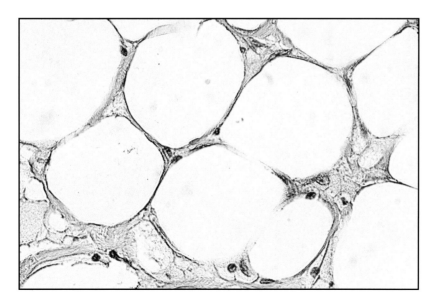

Image 6.24
Tissue sections obtained from corresponding surgically excised lesion diagnosed as lipoma (H&E, 400X).

References

1. Bardales R, Stanley M: Benign spindle and inflammatory lesions of the breast: diagnosis by fine needle aspiration. *Diagn Cytopathol* 12:126–130, 1995.

2. Silverman JF, Lannin DR, Unverferth M, et al: Fine needle aspiration cytology of subareolar abscess of the breast. Spectrum of cytomorphologic findings and potential diagnostic pitfalls. *Acta Cytol* 30:413–419, 1986.

3. Nichols RW: Desmoid tumors: a report of 31 cases. *Arch Surg* 7:227–236, 1923.

4. Gump F, Sternschein M, Wolf M: Fibromatosis of the shoulder girdle (extraabdominal desmoid). *Cancer* 20:1131–1140, 1967.

5. Bogomoletz W, Boulenger E, Simatos A: Infiltrating fibromatosis of the breast. *J Clin Pathol* 34:30–34, 1980.

6. Hanna W, Jambrosic J, Fish G: Aggressive fibromatosis of the breast. *Arch Pathol Lab Med* 109:260–262, 1985.

7. Gump FE, Sternschein MJ, Wolff M: Fibromatosis of the breast. *Surg Gynecol Obstet* 15:57–60, 1981.

8. Rosen PP, Ernsberger D: Mammary fibromatosis: a benign spindle-cell tumor with significant risk for local recurrence. *Cancer* 63:1363–1369, 1989.

9. Haggih RC, Booth JL: Bilateral fibromatosis of the breast in Gardner's syndrome. *Cancer* 25:161–166, 1970.

10. Jewett ST Jr, Mead JH: Extra-abdominal desmoid arising from a capsule around a silicone breast implant. *Plast Reconstr Surg* 63:577–579, 1979.

11. Kinzbrunner B, Ritter S, Domingo J, et al: Remission of rapidly growing desmoid tumors after tamoxifen therapy. *Cancer* 7:227–236, 1983.

12. Wargotz ES, Norris HJ, Austin RM, et al: Fibromatosis of the breast: a clinical and pathological study of 28 cases. *Am J Surg Pathol* 11:38–45, 1987.

13. Cederlund CG, Gustavsson S, Linell F, Moquist-Olsson I, Anderson I: Fibromatosis of the breast mimicking carcinoma at mammography. *Br J Radiol* 57:98–101, 1984.

14. El-Naggar A, Abdul-Karim FW, Marshalleck JI, et al: Fine needle aspiration of fibromatosis of the breast. *Diagn Cytopathol* 3:320–322, 1987.

15. Tani EM, Stanley MW, Skoog L: Fine needle aspiration cytology presentation of bilateral mammary fibromatosis. Report of a case. *Acta Cytol* 32:555–558, 1988.

16. Thomas T, Lorino C, Ferrara JJ: Fibromatosis of the breast: a case report and literature review. *J Surg Oncol* 35:70–74, 1987.

17. Pettinato G, Manivel JC, Petrella G, et al: Fine needle aspiration cytology, immunocytochemistry and electron microscopy of fibromatosis of the breast. Report of two cases. *Acta Cytol* 35:403–408, 1991.

18. Zaharopoulos P, Wong JY: Fine needle aspiration cytology in fibromatosis. *Diagn Cytopathol* 8:73–78, 1992.

19. Luzzatto R, Grossman S, Scholl JF, et al: Post-radiation pleomorphic malignant fibrous histiocytoma of the breast. *Acta Cytol* 30:48–50, 1986.

20. Remor S, Tartter PI, Schwartz IS: Malignant fibrous histiocytoma of the breast: a case report and review of the literature. *Breast Dis* 1:37–45, 1987.

21. Silverman JF, Geisinger KR, Frable WJ: Fine needle aspiration cytology of mesenchymal tumors of the breast. *Diagn Cytopathol* 4:50–58, 1988.

22. Stanley MW, Tani EM, Skoog L: Metaplastic carcinoma of the breast: fine needle aspiration cytology of seven cases. *Diagn Cytopathol* 5:22-28, 1989.

23. Gal R, Gukovsky-Oren S, Lehman JM, Schwartz P, et al: Cytodiagnosis of a spindle cell tumor of the breast using antisera to epithelial membrane antigen. *Acta Cytol* 31:317–321, 1987.

24. Stanley MW, Tani EM, Rutqvist LE, et al: Cytosarcoma phyllodes of the breast: a cytopathologic study of 23 cases. *Diagn Cytopathol* 5:29–34, 1989.

25. Dahl J, Akerman M: Nodular fasciitis: a correlative cytologic and histologic study of 13 cases. *Acta Cytol* 25:215–223, 1981.

26. Fritsches HG, Muller EA: Pseudosarcomatous fasciitis of the breast. Cytologic and histologic features. *Acta Cytol* 27:73–75, 1983.

27. Weidner N, Levine JD: Spindle-cell adenomyoepithelioma of the breast. A microscopic, ultrastructural and immunocytochemical study. *Cancer* 62:1561–1567, 1988.

28. Wargotz ES, Weiss S, Norris HJ: Myofibroblastoma of the breast. Sixteen cases of a distinctive benign mesenchymal tumor. *Am J Surg Pathol* 11:493–502, 1987.

29. Boger A: Benign spindle cell tumor of the male breast. *Pathol Res Pract* 178:395–398, 1984.

30. Ordi J, Riverol A, Sole M, et al: Fine needle aspiration of myofibroblastoma of the breast in a man. A report of two cases. *Acta Cytol* 36:194–198, 1992.

31. Hamperl H: The myoepithelioma (myoepithelial cells), normal state, regressive changes, hyperplasia, tumors. *Curr Top Pathol* 53:161–220, 1970.

32. Azzopardi JG: *Problems in Breast Pathology.* London, England, WB Saunders Co, 1979.

33. Vielh P, Thiery JP, Validire P, et al: Adenomyoepithelioma of the breast: fine needle sampling with histologic, immunohistologic and electron microscopic analysis. *Diagn Cytopathol* 9:188-193, 1993.

34. Tavassoli FA: Myoepithelial lesions of the breast: myoepitheliosis, adenomyoepithelioma and myoepithelial carcinoma. *Am J Surg Pathol* 15:554–568, 1991.

35. Hoch YL, Chan SY: Adenomyoepithelioma of the breast: a case report correlating cytologic and histologic features. *Acta Cytol* 38:953–956, 1994.

36. Loose JH, Patchefsky AS, Hollander IJ, et al: Adenomyoepithelioma of the breast. A spectrum of biologic behavior. *Am J Surg Pathol* 16:868–876, 1992.

37. Schurch W, Potvin C, Seemayer T: Malignant myoepithelioma (myoepithelial carcinoma) of the breast. An ultrastructural and immunocytochemical study. *Ultrastruct Pathol* 8:1–11, 1985.

38. Koss LG, Zajicek T: The breast. In: Koss LG, ed. *Diagnostic Cytopathology and Its Histologic Bases,* 4th ed. Philadelphia, Pa, JB Lippincott Co, 1992, pp.1293–1315.

39. Orell SR, Sterrett GF, Walters N, et al: *Manual and Atlas of Fine Needle Aspiration Cytology,* 2nd ed. Edinburgh, Scotland, Churchill Livingstone Inc, 1992, pp. 129–169.

40. Raju GC, O'Reilly AP: Immunohistochemical study of granular cell tumor. *Pathology* 19:402–406, 1987.

41. Armin A, Connelly EM, Rowden G: An immunoperoxidase investigation of S-100 protein in granular cell myoblastoma. Evidence of Schwann cell derivation. *Am J Clin Pathol* 79:37–44, 1983.

42. Bassett LW, Cove HC: Myoblastoma of the breast. *Am J Roentgenol* 132:122–123, 1979.

43. Ingram DL, Mossler JA, Snowhite I, et al: Granular cell tumors of the breast. Steroid receptor analysis and localization of carcinoembryonic antigen, myoglobin, and S-100 protein. *Arch Pathol Lab Med* 108:897–901, 1984.

44. Zemoura L, Contesso G, Caillou B, et al: Myoblastomas granleux du sein. A propos de sept observations. *Ann Pathol* 4:151–156, 1984.

45. DeMay RM, Kay S: Granular cell tumor of the breast. *Pathol Annu* 19:121–148, 1984.

46. Strobel SL, Shah NT, Lucas JG, et al: Granular cell tumor of the breast: a cytologic immunohistochemical and ultrastructural study of two cases. *Acta Cytol* 29:598–601, 1985.

47. Geisinger KR, Kawamoto EH, Marshall EB, et al: Aspiration and exfoliative cytology, including ultrastructure of a malignant granular cell tumor. *Acta Cytol* 29:593–597, 1985.

48. Collins R, Gan G: Neurilemoma presenting as a lump in the breast. *Br J Surg* 60:242–243, 1973.

49. Soloman L, Kim YH, Reiner L: Neurofibromatous pseudogynecomastia associated with prepubertal idiopathic gynecomastia. *NY State J Med* 76:932–934, 1976.

50. Ramzy I: Benign schwannoma: demonstration of Verocay bodies using fine needle aspiration. *Acta Cytol* 21:316–219, 1977.

51. Fisher PE, Estabrook A, Gatien MB: Fine needle aspiration biopsy of intramammary neurilemoma. *Acta Cytol* 34:35–37, 1990.

52. Onsunbe PM, Vaamonde EF, Gonzalez-Estechu A, et al: Neurilemoma of the breast in a man. A case report. *Acta Cytol* 36:4, 1992.

53. Toker C, Tang CK, Whitely JF, et al: Benign spindle cell breast tumor. *Cancer* 48:1615-1622, 1981.

54. Enzinger FM, Harvey A: Spindle cell lipoma. *Cancer* 36:1852-1859, 1975.

55. Chan KW, Chadially FN, Alagaratnam TT: Benign spindle cell tumour of breast. *Pathology* 16:331–337, 1984.

56. Lew WYC: Spindle cell lipoma of the breast: a case report and literature review. *Diagn Cytopathol* 9:434–437, 1993.

57. Allen PW: Tumours and proliferations of adipose tissue. In: Sternberg SS ed. *Masson Monographs in Diagnostic Pathology.* Chicago, Ill, Masson Publishing USA Inc, 1981, pp. 20–33.

58. Enzinger FM, Weiss SW: *Soft Tissue Tumours.* St Louis, Mo, CV Mosby Co, 1983, p. 215.

59. Brebner DM, Cosman B, Shapiro J: Lipoma of the breast diagnosed by film and xeromammography. *S Afr Med J* 50:685–688, 1976.

60. Haagensen CD: *Diseases of the Breast,* 3rd ed. Philadelphia, Pa, WB Saunders Co, 1986, pp. 333–335.

61. Tedesch CB: Mammary lipoma. *Arch Pathol Lab Med* 46:386–397, 1948.

◎ CHAPTER SEVEN

Fibrocystic Change, High Risk, and Premalignant Breast Disease

Fibrocystic change, the most commonly diagnosed benign breast disease, reflects a spectrum of changes ranging from normal physiologic alterations in the breast to proliferative changes approximating carcinoma in situ. These include cyst formation, apocrine metaplasia, stromal fibrosis, and various degrees of ductal hyperplasia (Image 7.1). It has been known for many years that women who undergo breast biopsy for so-called fibrocystic disease have an increased risk of breast cancer.[1,2] For this reason, attempts have been made to classify the spectrum of fibrocystic disease into reproducible and prognostically relevant categories.

Studies have evaluated the relative risk of subsequent development of breast disease in patients with fibrocystic disease based on the histologic features of their biopsy specimens. The results of these studies have been twofold. First, a new terminology of nonproliferative breast disease, proliferative breast disease without atypia, and proliferative breast disease with atypia (atypical hyperplasia) has been introduced. The term fibrocystic disease has also been abandoned and replaced by fibrocystic change. Second, the specific histologic changes associated with each category have been defined.[3–6] It is generally agreed that nonproliferative breast disease carries no increased risk. Patients with proliferative breast disease without atypia have a slightly increased risk (1.5–2× greater), and patients with proliferative breast disease with atypia have a moderately increased risk (4–5× greater) of subsequently developing breast cancer. Patients with carcinoma in situ have an 8 to 10 times greater risk of developing breast cancer.[7,8]

The risk profiles described above have given recognition of the spectrum of morphologic changes seen in breast disease a new significance. It is now possible to separate breast lesions into benign, premalignant, and malignant categories. The precise histologic features of each category of breast lesion have been well described.[9–11] However, despite the reliability of breast FNAB in separating benign from malignant lesions, the cytologic features of premalignant lesions have not yet been well defined.

In a prospective study of mammographically guided fine needle aspirations of 100 nonpalpable breast lesions, my colleagues and I assessed the reliability of a cytologic grading system in defining the cytologic features of proliferative and nonproliferative breast disease and differentiating between benign, premalignant, and malignant breast lesions. We developed a cytologic grading system to evaluate aspirates for cellular arrangement, the degree of cellular pleomorphism and anisonucleosis, the presence of myoepithelial cells and nucleoli, and the chromatin pattern. Values ranging from 1 to 4 were assigned to each criterion, and a score based on the sum of the individual values was calculated for each case. With scores ranging from a minimum of 6 to a maximum of 24, the cases were divided into four categories: nonproliferative breast disease without atypia (score 6–10), proliferative breast disease without atypia (score 11–14), proliferative breast disease with atypia (score 15–18), and cancer (score 19–24). When we compared the cytologic diagnosis with the histologic diagnosis obtained from needle localization biopsies, we found a high degree of concordance between the results (Tables 7.1 through 7.3). Based on this study, we believe that by using

Table 7.1
Cytologic Criteria/Grading System for Interpretation of Mammographically Guided Fine Needle Aspiration Biopsies[*]

Cellular Arrangement	Cellular Pleomorphism	Myoepithelial Cells	Anisonucleosis	Nucleoli	Chromatin Clumping	Score[†]
Monolayer	Absent	Many	Absent	Absent	Absent	1
Nuclear Overlapping	Mild	Moderate	Mild	Micronucleoli	Rare	2
Clustering	Moderate	Few	Moderate	Micro and/or rare macronucleoli	Occasional	3
Loss of cohesion	Conspicuous	Absent	Conspicuous	Predominantly micronucleoli	Frequent	4

[*]Reproduced with permission from: Masood S, Frykberg ER, McLellan GL, et al: Prospective evaluation of radiologically detected fine needle aspiration biopsy of nonpalpable breast lesions. *Cancer* 66:1480–1487, 1990.
[†]Total score: nonproliferative breast disease, 6–10; proliferative breast disease without atypia, 11–14; proliferative breast disease with atypia, 15–18; and carcinoma in situ and invasive cancer, 19–24.

Table 7.2
Cytologic Findings Compared with Histologic Diagnosis in 100 Mammographically Suspicious Cases[*]

Cytology	No. of Cases	Histologic Diagnosis				
		Nonproliferative Breast Disease	Proliferative Without Atypia	Proliferative With Atypia	Carcinoma in Situ (LCIS, DCIS)	Invasive Cancer
Insufficient cellular material	9	7	2	–	–, –	–
Nonproliferative breast disease	34	29	4	–	1[†], –	–
Proliferative without atypia	17	–	15	2	–, –	–
Proliferative with atypia	23	–	–	21	1[†], 1[†]	–
Carcinoma	17	–	–	–	–, 5	–
Total	100	36	21	23	2, 6	12

[*]Reproduced with permission from: Masood S, Frykberg ER, McLellan GL, et al: Prospective evaluation of radiologically detected fine needle aspiration biopsy of nonpalpable breast lesions. *Cancer* 66:1480–1487, 1990.
[†]False-negative cytologic interpretations.
LCIS, lobular carcinoma in situ; DCIS, ductal carcinoma in situ.

Table 7.3

Concordance Between Cytologic Evaluation and Histologic Diagnosis in
100 Mammographically Guided Fine Needle Aspirates*

Diagnosis	No. of Cases	Concordance (%)
Nonproliferative breast disease	29/34	85
Proliferative breast disease without atypia	15/17	88
Proliferative breast disease with atypia	21/23	91
Cancer	17/20	85

*Modified from: Masood S, Frykberg ER, McLellan GL, et al: Cytologic differentiation
between proliferative and nonproliferative breast disease in mammographically guided
fine-needle aspirates. *Diagn Cytopathol* 7:581–590, 1991.

strict cytologic criteria, it is possible to define the continuous spectrum of
changes in breast lesions and separate hyperplasia from neoplasia.[12,13]

Nonproliferative Breast Disease

In our study, the cell yield in aspirates from patients with nonproliferative breast disease was variable and depended on the nature of the lesion. In noncystic lesions, the cellularity of the aspirate was scant or moderate. Frequently, the aspirate consisted of clusters of small, uniform epithelial cells arranged in monolayered sheets with a honeycomb pattern. Foam cells, apocrine cells, naked single cells, and fragments of stromal cells were frequently observed. The cells had regular nuclei with a fine chromatin pattern. Nucleoli were not commonly seen. Myoepithelial cells were easily identified (Images 7.2 through 7.6).

Cytomorphology of Nonproliferative Breast Disease
Low cellularity
Fragments of stroma and/or adipose tissue
Monolayered clusters of uniform cell population with honeycomb pattern
Foam cells, apocrine cells
Myoepithelial cells

Proliferative Breast Disease Without Atypia

Proliferative breast disease differed from nonproliferative breast disease in its higher cell yield and unique cellular arrangement. Cellularity was moderate to high depending on the degree of proliferative epithelial changes. There was an increased number of tightly cohesive groups of ductal epithelial and myoepithelial cells with some overriding of the nuclei, occasional loss of polarity, and some variability in nuclear size. Micronucleoli were occasionally seen. Cytologic atypia was inconspicuous.

Apocrine cells, histiocytes, and occasional naked nuclei were the accompanying cells in these aspirates (Images 7.7 through 7.11).

Cytologic differentiation between proliferative breast disease, fibroadenoma, and papillary lesions was occasionally difficult. Utilizing the criteria of cellularity, fronds, naked nuclei, and stromal fragments, Linsk et al[14] and Bottles et al[15] found that these three conditions have overlapping cytologic features. We agree with Bottles et al that the presence of well-demarcated stroma containing spindle cells is the most important differentiating feature. The presence of an abundant number of naked nuclei favors a diagnosis of fibroadenoma. The absence of both hemosiderin-containing macrophages and a polymorphic population of tall columnar cells and ductal cells forming papillae may distinguish papillary breast lesions from proliferative breast disease.

Cytomorphology of Proliferative Breast Disease Without Atypia
Moderate to high cellularity
Conspicuous number of highly cohesive cell clusters
Overriding of nuclei, nuclear enlargement, and occasional micronucleoli
Apocrine cells, histiocytes, calcified particles
Focal loss of polarity
Myoepithelial cells

Proliferative Breast Disease With Atypia (Atypical Hyperplasia)

Aspirates of proliferative breast disease with atypia were frequently highly cellular and were composed of multiple clusters of epithelial cells. The crowded clusters of cells showed a conspicuous loss of polarity and overriding of the nuclei. Nuclei displayed a coarse, irregular chromatin pattern, and nucleoli were conspicuous. Variation in nuclear size and cellular pleomorphism were also present. Intermingled with crowded epithelial cells were spindle cells with morphologic evidence of myoepithelial cell differentiation (Images 7.12 through 7.20).

Cytomorphology of Atypical Hyperplasia
Cellular aspirate
Clustering and crowding of epithelial cells with overriding of the nuclei
Anisonucleosis and chromatin clumping
Occasional conspicuous nucleoli
Myoepithelial cells within the clusters of atypical epithelial cells
Rare apocrine cells and macrophages

Malignant Lesions

Malignant lesions were characterized cytologically by a loose cellular pattern and isolated single cells. Rich cellularity, pleomorphism, and a significant number of isolated single cells were frequent findings. Nuclear membrane abnormality, chromatin clumping, and macronucleoli were often present. Myoepithelial cells were absent. These cytologic features were common in both carcinoma in situ and invasive lesions, making cytologic differentiation between the two lesions impossible.

Cytomorphology of Malignant Breast Lesions
Cellular aspirate
Dispersed cell pattern
Pleomorphism and hyperchromasia
Anisonucleosis
Conspicuous nucleoli
Absent myoepithelial cells

Atypical Hyperplasia vs Neoplasia

As mentioned previously, the importance of recognizing atypical hyperplasia cannot be overemphasized because of the substantial risk it represents.[7,8] Atypical hyperplasia presents a diagnostic challenge for the pathologist, however. The term atypical hyperplasia has been used to describe noninfiltrating breast lesions with some but not all the features of cancer. Thus, atypical hyperplasia occupies an intermediate position between benign and malignant lesions. There may be a substantial degree of subjectivity and disagreement in making a diagnosis of atypical hyperplasia from histologic section. It is therefore reasonable to expect some difficulty in cytologically differentiating between atypical hyperplasia and carcinoma. Such differentiation is important, however, because of the very different clinical management each condition entails. The value of our grading system is that it provides an objective and reproducible method of diagnosis, augmenting the pathologist's judgment and enhancing overall diagnostic accuracy.

In our study, only 9 of 100 aspirates were insufficient for diagnosis. Nonproliferative breast disease scored between 6 and 10, and in the majority of cases did not present any diagnostic difficulty. Twenty-nine of 34 cytologic specimens (85%) with nonproliferative disease in the aspirate also had nonproliferative disease by biopsy. A monolayered cell arrangement and a lack of cytologic atypia were the predominant features of these lesions. Our missed diagnosis of lobular carcinoma in situ was most likely due to inaccurate localization and sampling, since lobular carcinoma in situ is often an incidental finding located outside the area of mammographic abnormality.[16] Furthermore, lobular carcinoma of the breast, particularly the noninvasive variety, is difficult to diagnose by cytologic examination because of its monomorphic, well-differentiated appearance.[17,18]

The aspirates from patients with proliferative breast disease in our study were cellular and scored between 11 and 14. Crowded clusters of epithelial cells with obvious overriding of the nuclei were the hallmarks of this condition. There was a discrepancy between histology and cytology in two cases where the degree of atypia in cytologic grading was underestimated. This probability should always be considered in cytologic diagnosis and may be the result of sampling error.

The aspirates from patients with proliferative breast disease with atypia (atypical hyperplasia) scored between 15 and 18. The aspirates showed crowded, three-dimensional cell clusters; moderate cellular pleomorphism and anisonucleosis; occasional chromatin clumping; frequent micronucleoli; and few myoepithelial cells. Of 23 cases, 2 cases of carcinoma in situ (9%) found on open biopsy were missed by FNAB. In both cases, a review of cytologic samples revealed myoepithelial cells, suggesting that the sample did not include the malignant lesion.

Increased cellularity, loss of cellular cohesion, significant pleomorphism, anisonucleosis, and a coarse chromatin pattern were the predominant features of malignant lesions in our study. Macronucleoli, when present, were associated with malignancy, but their absence did not indicate benignity. The presence of myoepithelial cells in the smears was quite significant, because these cells were absent in all cases of malignancy. However, they were found in nonproliferative breast disease, as well as in proliferative breast disease and atypical hyperplasia. Micronucleoli were common in both benign and malignant lesions and could not be used as a reliable indicator of malignancy. In our study, there were no false-positive results, which are generally considered the most important error to avoid, especially if definitive therapy is to be undertaken solely on the basis of cytology. Also, no invasive lesion was missed by cytologic diagnosis.

Our study supports the findings of other, similar studies. In 1979 Dziura and Bonfiglio[19] described cell changes in ductal neoplasia samples obtained by means of the Nordenstrom screw technique. Like us, they found anisonucleosis, the presence of macronucleoli, chromatin clumping, marked nuclear overlap, and cellular disarray to be cellular indicators of malignancy. However, only limited predictability of the degree of hyperplasia was possible with their morphologic criteria. Our study differed from theirs in two ways. First, in their experiment, samples were obtained from already excised lesions. Second, they utilized the screw technique of Nordenstrom. We used FNAB technique and obtained samples on site. Bibbo et al[20] also attempted to define the cytologic features of atypical hyperplasia in stereotaxic fine needle aspirates of clinically occult, malignant, and high-risk benign lesions. Like Dziura and Bonfiglio,[19] their ability to grade ductal hyperplasia was limited.

By far the most important aspect of our study is our cytologic grading system, which enabled us to define the continuous changes in breast lesions and separate hyperplasia from neoplasia. Ours is also the first study to advocate the use of the same terminology in cytologic diagnosis as in histologic diagnosis. This grading system should be tested by other investigators in order to assess its reproducibility in the interpretation of breast fine needle aspirates.

In a follow-up study, we used this cytologic grading system to evaluate 156 consecutive FNABs of palpable breast lesions.[21] Follow-up histology was available in 146 cases. The FNABs were interpreted by four pathologists in our institution who became familiar with the grading system through individual training. Despite the heterogeneity of a given palpable breast lesion, particularly of large tumors, we achieved a diagnostic accuracy of 95%. Distinguishing proliferative breast disease from fibroadenoma and papillary lesions remained difficult. Even though we considered the differentiating cytologic features, nine cases were still misdiagnosed. There were also five cases diagnosed as atypical hyperplasia by cytology that represented foci of atypical hyperplasia in fibroadenomas found in subsequent surgical excisions of the breast lesions. In addition, six cases of in situ and invasive carcinoma were misinterpreted as atypical hyperplasia. Review of these cases demonstrated absence of the cellular dyshesion seen in the usual mammary neoplasia. The tumors were also low grade.

Similar limitations were observed in a study conducted by Sneige and Staerkel.[22] They evaluated our grading system in a retroactive study of low-grade, in situ lesions of the breast. Sneige and Staerkel believe that our cytologic grading system should include architectural features such as cribriform and micropapillary patterns that facilitate differentiation between atypical hyperplasia and noncomedocarcinoma in situ. Silverman et al[23] and Abendroth et al[24] believe that separating the various stages of proliferative breast disease is still problematic, and they refrain from basing definitive diagnoses of atypical hyperplasia and carcinoma in situ on fine needle aspirates. However, they believe that in some cases, separation between ductal carcinoma in situ and atypical hyperplasia is possible. They diagnose atypical hyperplasia when cells are arranged in flat, cohesive sheets with distinct cell borders and myoepithelial cells. In contrast, ductal carcinoma in situ is characterized by single cells, which constitute more than 10% of atypical cells; cellular dyshesion; an inflammatory background; coarsely granular chromatin; and nuclear pleomorphism. Shiels et al[25] studied the cytomorphology of 15 cases of ductal carcinoma in situ. They consider the absence of myoepithelial cells in a cellular smear and the presence of conspicuous nuclear overriding and atypia the most important cytologic features distinguishing ductal carcinoma in situ from atypical hyperplasia.

Presently, most investigators advocate intraoperative consultation or excisional biopsy for any case diagnosed as atypical hyperplasia, suspicious or inconclusive for carcinoma.[13,23,26] Despite promising reports in the literature defining the cytomorphology of various lesions (ie, the spectrum of fibrocystic change and high-risk breast lesions), FNAB diagnosis of breast disease has limitations that do not necessarily result from inability to recognize different lesions. The heterogeneity of individual lesions is an important factor to be considered. For example, in 1994 Lennington et al[27] reviewed 100 sequentially collected cases of ductal carcinoma in situ from a consultation practice. Recognizing the bias of such a series toward the exclusion of easily recognizable comedocarcinomas, the authors studied the spectrum of mixed pattern lesions to identify variations and common features in the architectural arrangement of the various histologic patterns. Interestingly, atypical ductal hyperplasias were intermixed in 17 cases of ductal carcinoma in situ. Mixed patterns of comedo- and noncomedo-type ductal carcinoma in situ were seen in 33 cases. In every case of combined atypical ductal hyperplasia and ductal carcinoma in situ, the more advanced patterns of ductal carcinoma in situ were seen in the central portion of the lesion, while the components of atypical ductal hyperplasia were arranged peripherally. Thus, the presence of different patterns of ductal carcinoma in situ within individual lesions (46 of 100) and the coexistence of atypical ductal hyperplasia and ductal carcinoma in situ (17 of 100) strongly indicated the heterogeneity of a lesion.

In adequate samples, the spectrum of morphologic alterations in fibrocystic change, proliferative breast disease, and atypical hyperplasia are commonly seen in association with carcinoma in situ and/or invasive breast lesions. Multiple sampling of a breast lesion by FNAB may overcome the problem of heterogeneity of individual lesions to some extent. However, heterogeneity remains a limiting factor in FNAB interpretation and consequently in management of patients.

In addition to morphology, attempts have been made to utilize ancillary studies to distinguish between atypical hyperplasia and carcinoma in situ. We have already utilized flow cytometry and cell image analysis to assess the DNA ploidy pattern of breast fine needle aspirates as a means of differentiating between atypia and neoplasia. Although the frequency of aneuploidy in our study was higher in carcinoma than in atypical hyperplasia, the presence of aneuploidy in atypical hyperplasia limited the use of this technology (Table 7.4). Similar results were reported by Crissman et al,[28] who found that aneuploidy was more common in ductal carcinoma in situ, although 36% of cases of atypical ductal hyperplasia were aneuploid. Aneuploidy also correlated with poor nuclear grading. Teplitz et al[29] reported concordance in ploidy values for atypical ductal hyperplasia and concurrent carcinoma. Norris et al[30] used cell image analysis for DNA ploidy study as well as nuclear measurements in breast lesions. They concluded that neither DNA analysis nor nuclear measurements aided in making the difficult distinction between atypical hyperplasia and well-differentiated intraductal carcinoma.

Using 12 nuclear parameters, King et al[31] were able to correctly classify six of seven cases of moderate and atypical ductal hyperplasia as abnormal. Moderate hyperplasia, however, was within the spectrum of changes characteristic of usual intraductal hyperplasia without atypia. This image analysis study also had a low sensitivity for malignancy, which the authors ascribed to a large percentage of cases of in situ carcinoma. In a follow-up study, the same authors found that image cytometry could not be used to distinguish atypical hyperplasia from intraductal hyperplasia without atypia or ductal carcinoma in situ, although it could be used to separate atypical ductal hyperplasia from invasive carcinoma and nonproliferative lesions.[32] Thus, neither intra-active morphometry nor DNA ploidy study is likely to assist in differentiating between atypical ductal hyperplasia and ductal carcinoma in situ in cytologic specimens.

It is also intriguing to consider whether the study of oncogene expression can aid in differentiating between atypical hyperplasia and carcinoma in situ. We used standard immunocytochemistry to assess the pattern of expression of HER-2/*neu* oncogene in 65 cases of invasive carcinoma, 36

Table 7.4
DNA Ploidy Pattern of Atypical Hyperplasia, Carcinoma in Situ, and Invasive Breast Carcinoma

Histologic Type	No. of Cases	Flow Cyometry, No. of Aneuploid (%)	Image Analysis, No. of Aneuploid (%)
Atypical hyperplasia	28	8 (28.5)	10 (36)
Carcinoma in situ	8	4 (50)	4 (50)
Invasive carcinoma	32	19 (59)	21 (65)
Total	68	31 (45.5)	35 (51)

Concordance = 89%

Table 7.5

HER-2/*neu* Oncogene Expression in Premalignant and Malignant Breast Lesions*

Histologic Diagnosis	No. of Positive Cases (%)	No. of Negative Cases (%)	Total
Invasive carcinoma	28 (43)	37 (57)	65
Carcinoma in situ	14 (38)	22 (62)	36
Atypical ductal hyperplasia	4 (12)	28 (88)	32

*Modified from: Masood S: HER-2/*neu* oncogene expression in atypical ductal hyperplasia, carcinoma in situ and invasive breast cancer. *Mod Pathol* 4:12, 1991. Abstract.

cases of ductal carcinoma in situ, and 32 cases of atypical ductal hyperplasia. As shown in Table 7.5, positive immunostaining for HER-2/*neu* oncogene was observed in 43% (28/65) of cases of invasive carcinoma, 38% (14/36) of cases of carcinoma in situ, and 12% (4/32) of cases of atypical hyperplasia (Images 7.21 and 7.22). Naturally, these results discourage the use of oncogene study as an adjunct to distinguish hyperplasia from neoplasia. Among the different types of carcinoma in situ, comedocarcinoma had the highest frequency of HER-2/*neu* oncogene expression. This reinforces the concept that comedocarcinoma is biologically different from other in situ lesions. There was 92% concordance between the results of immunostaining for HER-2/*neu* oncogene of the in situ component and the invasive component of the same lesion. This may suggest that an expression of discordance between biopsies of carcinoma in situ and subsequent invasive carcinoma necessitates further study to evaluate the heterogeneity of HER-2/*neu* oncogene expression within the tumor.[33]

Attempts have also been made to define the immunoexpression of different breast lesions as a means of differentiating between benign and malignant lesions of the breast. The primary ones include epithelial membrane antigen, carcinoembryonic antigen, keratin, alphalactalbumin, S-100 protein, human chorionic gonadotropin, ABH, blood group isoantigens, neuron specific enolase, gross cystic disease fluid protein, actin, and tumor-associated monoclonal antibody (MAB) B72.3. Of all the antibodies, monoclonal antibody B72.3 is used most frequently as an adjunct in cytology. Monoclonal antibody B72.3 demonstrates selective reactivity for carcinoma cells rather than normal human adult tissue.[34] This is the basis of an immunocytochemical approach in which MAB B72.3 obtained by standard hybridoma technology is directed against a membrane protein of human breast cancer.[35,36] Using this immunoperoxidase technique on 50 breast fine needle aspirates, Lundy et al[37] reported a 10% increase in diagnostic accuracy. All cases considered cytologically malignant were confirmed by immunocytochemistry. Thus, they suggested, MAB B72.3 may be a valuable diagnostic adjunct in atypical and suspicious cases, particularly those in which hypocellular or cellular monomorphism precludes a diagnosis of malignancy by routine cytologic examination.

We used MAB 72.3 in 52 breast fine needle aspirates. Thirty-two were cytologically malignant and 20 were atypical. Every diagnosis was confirmed histologically. The results of this study demonstrated a diagnostic accuracy of 96%, sensitivity of 94%, and specificity of 100% (Images 7.23 and 7.24).[38]

Despite these promising reports, the use of MAB B72.3 as an aid in differentiating between atypical hyperplasia and carcinoma has remained limited. This is mainly due to scattered reports of false-positive immunostaining seen in fibrocystic change and apocrine cells.[39] We believe that the usual patterns of fibrocystic change and apocrine cells are recognizable morphologically. The use of MAB B72.3 should be limited to differentiation between atypical hyperplasia and carcinoma.

Muscle specific actin (MSA) immunostaining is another marker that may be useful in differentiating between atypical hyperplasia and carcinoma in situ. Actin is a contractile protein whose presence in muscular and normovascular cells is demonstrated using immunoperoxidase technique. Mukai et al[40] demonstrated actin in smooth and striated muscle, in pericytes, and in myoepithelial cells of the salivary glands, breast, and sweat glands. In another study, Papotti et al[41] used MSA immunostaining to differentiate between benign and malignant papillary lesions of the breast. In a similar study, Raju et al[42] demonstrated that lack of MSA immunostaining, which indicates that no myoepithelial layer is present, is strong evidence of papillary carcinoma.

We have also demonstrated the value of MSA in differentiating between atypical hyperplasia and carcinoma in situ in surgical cases (Images 7.25 and 7.26).[43] In these studies MSA was found to be a specific marker for detecting myoepithelial cells. In addition to the presence of cellular cohesion and the absence of a significant number of isolated single cells, we believe that the recognition of myoepithelial cells within clusters of atypical cells in a breast aspirate is a significant finding that can separate hyperplasia from neoplasia.[12,13,23]

Based on these observations, we assessed the feasibility of using MSA as a marker for myoepithelial cells in smears and cell block preparations of breast fine needle aspirates.[44,45] The staining of myoepithelial cells in benign and high-risk proliferative breast disease can be used as a strong differentiating feature in the interpretation of atypical breast fine needle aspirates. Muscle specific actin immunostaining can maximize the diagnostic accuracy of FNAB and reduce the number of inconclusive cytologic diagnoses (Images 7.27 and 7.28).

Our study confirms that morphologic distinction between myoepithelial cells and spindle cells of nonmyoepithelial origin is not always possible. Lack of immunostaining for MSA is strong evidence against the presence of myoepithelial cells (Images 7.29 and 7.30). Muscle specific actin–positive myoepithelial cells may also be seen in the background of malignant breast lesions due to passage of the needle through the benign component of a malignant breast lesion.

Ductal Carcinoma in Situ

Aspirates of ductal carcinoma in situ (DCIS) have variable cytologic features, reflecting the tumor's morphologic diversity. The two types of ductal carcinoma in situ, comedocarcinoma and noncomedocarcinoma, are very distinct cytologically.

Comedocarcinoma

It has been recognized for many years that in addition to its high-grade nuclear morphology, comedocarcinoma has a higher proliferative rate by cell kinetic study and is more frequently associated with microinvasion.[46-50] Comedocarcinoma is known to have a higher local recurrence rate than other types of DCIS, frequently expresses HER-2/*neu* oncogenes, and is often aneuploid.[51-53] In addition to nuclear grade, comedo-type necrosis contributes to the identification of comedocarcinoma that is more likely to produce local failure after excision. Of the two types of DCIS, it appears that comedocarcinoma is most closely related to invasive carcinoma.[23,53]

In our experience, fine needle aspirates of comedocarcinoma are usually cellular and display loosely cohesive clusters of malignant cells with individual cell necrosis and mitosis. Nuclear membrane abnormality, clumping of chromatin, and conspicuous nucleoli are often present. Nuclear pleomorphism and irregularly shaped nucleoli are characteristic features of comedocarcinoma. Microcalcifications may or may not be present (Images 7.31 through 7.33). Moriya et al[54] also found that aspirates of comedocarcinoma revealed necrosis, hypercellularity, marked nuclear atypia, and loss of cellular cohesion. In contrast, noncomedocarcinoma was characterized by minimal nuclear atypia, lack of single cells, a predominance of benign elements, and scant cellular yield. Malamud et al[55] showed that comedo-type DCIS is more likely to be diagnosed as positive on FNAB than is noncomedo-type DCIS. The authors of these two studies suggest that nuclear features are most helpful in differentiating between the two types of carcinoma in situ. Large, irregularly shaped nucleoli are the most characteristic feature of comedo-type lesions.

The presence of comedocarcinoma in fine needle aspirates often indicates a comedo-type DCIS, with or without invasion. Lilleng and Hagmar[56] compared invasive comedocarcinoma with minimally invasive and in situ lesions. They found that in situ and minimally invasive comedocarcinomas could be separated morphologically from invasive comedocarcinoma. Minimally invasive and in situ lesions demonstrated a background of necrotic cellular debris and tumor cells. In contrast, invasive comedocarcinoma revealed numerous single, scattered tumor cells intermingled with cell clusters and, in most cases, a background with inconspicuous or no necrotic material.

The interpretation of fine needle aspirates as a means of identifying high-risk and premalignant breast lesions presents a diagnostic dilemma for cytopathologists. It has been suggested that DCIS may be confused with atypical ductal hyperplasia,[57] and other evidence indicates that the distinction between DCIS and infiltrating carcinoma is virtually impossible.[58] This latter pitfall does not have significant clinical implications for patients with malignant, palpable breast masses, since most masses of this type are infiltrating carcinomas. Palpable DCIS often represents extensive disease, for which mastectomy is considered the appropriate therapy. However, a considerable percentage of nonpalpable breast lesions are small and in situ and may not require mastectomy.[59] In contrast, recognition of comedocarcinoma is important since it requires more aggressive therapy than noncomedocarcinoma.

Cytomorphology of Comedocarcinoma
Highly cellular aspirate

Pleomorphic population of neoplastic epithelial cells
Necrotic background
Individual cell necrosis
Mitosis
Absence of myoepithelial cells

Noncomedocarcinoma

Aspirates from noncomedo-type DCIS vary in cellularity and are characterized by a monomorphic cell population of small- to medium-sized epithelial cells arranged singly or in loosely cohesive clusters. The cell clusters may have a solid, cribriform, or papillary pattern with no accompanying myoepithelial cells. This is in contrast with atypical hyperplasia, in which the myoepithelial cells are intermingled with the groups of atypical cells and part of the cellular aggregate. Microcalcified particles, foamy histiocytes, and a few isolated myoepithelial cells may be seen in the background (Images 7.34 through 7.39).

Cytomorphology of Noncomedocarcinoma
Variable cellularity
Monomorphic population of small- to medium-sized epithelial cells
Cell clusters display solid, cribriform, or papillary pattern
Absence of myoepithelial cells

In Situ vs Invasive Carcinoma

The cytologic features of DCIS are not exclusive and are often seen in invasive carcinomas. We have not yet been able to define any cytomorphologic criteria to distinguish in situ from invasive carcinoma. However, invasive lesions are more cellular and more frequently display conspicuous loss of cell cohesion. It is not surprising that FNAB cannot provide a reliable basis for a diagnosis of carcinoma in situ, since this diagnosis requires careful study of the overall architecture and basement membrane integrity of the lesion, both of which can only be evaluated histologically. Nevertheless, it may be possible to maximize the utility of FNAB and arrive at a correct diagnosis by combining FNAB results with specific mammographic features and defined clinical presentations. This includes recognizing the cytologic features of special subtypes of ductal carcinoma, such as mucinous, medullary, sarcomatoid, and small cell carcinoma, which are most often present as invasive lesions, although in situ mucinous carcinoma and small cell carcinoma can occur, rarely. Neoplastic cells in a breast aspirate plus the presence of skin retraction, a fixed nipple, ulceration, inflammatory carcinoma, and/or evidence of metastasis are also indicative of advanced invasive breast carcinoma. Similarly, intracystic papillary carcinoma often appears as a cystic lesion in mammograms or sonograms. The aspirates are often bloody, rich in cellularity, and contain three-dimensional cell clusters with small or large papillae and scattered single epithelial cells.

Since the clinical management of DCIS may be similar to that of invasive ductal carcinoma at some institutions, differentiating between the two lesions may not be critical. However, the decision to perform a lumpectomy or a modified radical mastectomy often is based on the size of the lesion, the extent of in situ carcinoma, and/or the status of the lumpectomy margins. In addition, the distinction between DCIS and invasive ductal carcinoma is essential for patients selected for preoperative chemotherapy or radiotherapy. For such patients, we recommend assessment of tumor invasion by confirmatory surgical biopsy.

Lobular Carcinoma in Situ

Lobular carcinoma in situ (LCIS) is often an incidental finding in the pathologic study of tissue removed from palpable breast lesions or by needle localization of a mammographic abnormality.[60,61] In published series, LCIS has been found in 0.8% to 3.6% of breast biopsy specimens. A similar incidence has been reported for LCIS discovered by mammographic localization of nonpalpable breast lesions (1%–2%).[62,63] It is important to distinguish between LCIS and infiltrating lobular carcinoma (ILC), since the management of these two entities is quite different. LCIS is now considered only a marker for the subsequent development of breast cancer with close observation as appropriate management. However, in some cases, based on the patient's request, bilateral mastectomy may be a management option. In contrast, treatment for ILC is similar to that for other invasive cancers.

My colleagues and I agree with other investigators that the cytomorphologic distinction between atypical lobular hyperplasia (ALH), LCIS, and infiltrating lobular carcinoma may be difficult, and it may advisable to refer to them all as lobular neoplasia.[23,64,65] Aspirates of LCIS and ALH may show loosely cohesive groups of small, uniform cells with eccentric, regular nuclei and occasional intracytoplasmic lumina. The nuclei are hyperchromatic with fine chromatin clumping and occasional inconspicuous nucleoli. Occasionally, small groups of cells that form cell balls similar to the acini of lobular neoplasia may be seen (Images 7.40 through 7.47). Aspirates of ILC show features similar to those of ALH but are more cellular and contain more single, atypical cells. Characteristic cytomorphologic findings in ILC include low to moderate cell yield and a relatively uniform population of small- to medium-sized cells. The cells have scant, ill-defined cytoplasm with an increased N/C ratio. They tend to occur in small, Indian-file groups, in cords or singly. The cytoplasm may contain sharply punched-out vacuoles. Occasionally, signet ring forms may be seen (Image 7.48). We believe that cellular aspirates that contain a significant number of small, uniform cells characteristic of ILC should be diagnosed accordingly, and definitive therapy should be begun immediately. However, patients whose aspirates show scant cellularity should undergo an excisional biopsy to establish the diagnosis.

Summary

Based on our own studies,[12,13] we believe it is possible to distinguish between nonproliferative and proliferative breast disease cytologically. In the majority of cases, cytologic distinction between atypical hyperplasia and neoplasia is also possible. Immunostaining with MSA to detect myoepithelial cells is also a valid diagnostic adjunct.[44,45] However, cytologic differentiation between atypical hyperplasia and low-grade breast carcinomas remains difficult. Similarly, it is difficult to cytologically separate an in situ carcinoma from an invasive cancer. Thus, it is necessary to recommend a confirmatory biopsy as an intraoperative consultation in cases diagnosed cytologically as atypical hyperplasia or as suspicious for carcinoma.[66]

The potential value of cytologic recognition of atypical hyperplasia is in identifying high-risk breast cancer patients by fine needle aspiration biopsy. This recognition has significant clinical implications and is important in the design of chemoprevention trials.[66] Chemoprevention is an intriguing concept, full of possibility. The components necessary for the design and analysis of chemoprevention trials include accurate prediction of breast cancer risk, flexibility of tissue sampling and monitoring, selection of appropriate biologic markers as surrogate endpoints, and reproducibility of results. Initial phase II trials will involve women at high risk for breast cancer with morphologic evidence of atypical hyperplasia and carcinoma in situ.[67]

The breast is uniquely suited to sampling via fine needle aspiration biopsy. If adequately cellular, aspirates can easily be used to assess potential high-risk molecular markers, DNA ploidy and proliferation rate, hormone receptors, oncogenes, and tumor suppressor genes.[67-69] It has already been shown that morphologic and molecular abnormalities occur in random needle aspirates or nipple aspirates of women at increased risk for breast cancer.[69,70] Cytologic and biomarker abnormalities detected by random fine needle aspiration of high-risk women have intriguing potential for risk assessment and may also serve as surrogate indicators of response to chemopreventive agents.

Recently, it has become possible to test for genetic susceptibility for breast cancer. Epidemiologic studies have consistently shown that a history of breast cancer in a first-degree relative increases a woman's risk of developing breast cancer. Although the exact nature of the underlying risk factors cannot always be ascertained, complex segregation analysis of breast cancer aggregation in high-risk families suggests that breast cancer susceptibility is due to autosomal dominant inheritance of one or more rare genes.[71]

A breast cancer susceptibility gene named BRCA1 has recently been discovered. It is localized to the chromosomal region 17q12-q21 on the long arm of chromosome 17.[72] Shortly after this discovery, researchers announced the discovery of a second familial breast cancer gene, BRCA2, on the short arm of chromosme 13.[73,74] In contrast to BRCA1, which is also responsible for a large proportion (more than 75%) of inherited predisposition to ovarian cancer,[75] mutations in BRCA2 are found in at least one third of cases of familial breast (but not ovarian) cancer. This suggests that BRCA2 may also be an important breast cancer gene.

The identification of susceptibility genes in high-risk families can assist in risk estimation for genetic counseling and serve as a guide in choosing candidates for clinical trials of breast cancer screening and chemoprevention. Breast tissue samples obtained via FNAB provide an excellent resource for studying genetic mutations in high-risk women.

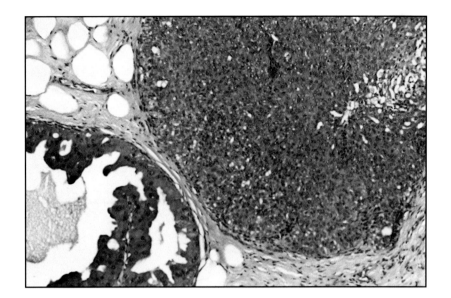

Image 7.1
Spectrum of morphologic features seen in fibrocystic change, ranging from apocrine metaplasia and cyst formation to atypical hyperplasia (H&E, 200X).

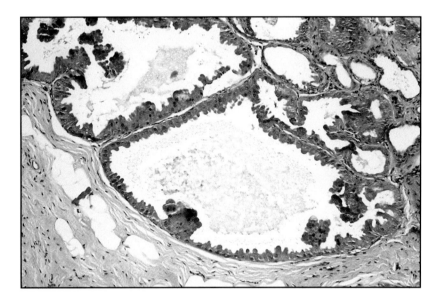

Image 7.2
Histopathologic features of nonproliferative breast disease (H&E, 100X).

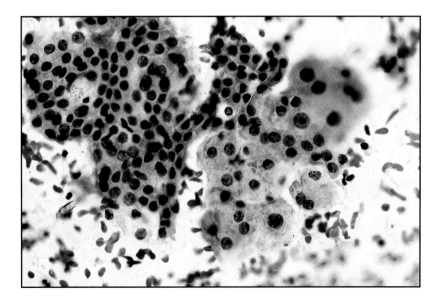

Image 7.3
Cytomorphology of nonproliferative breast disease: a monolayer cell arrangement with a few clusters of apocrine cells (Papanicolaou, 400X).

Image 7.4
Cytomorphology of nonproliferative breast disease: myoepithelial and ductal epithelial cells with no cytologic atypia (Papanicolaou, 200X).

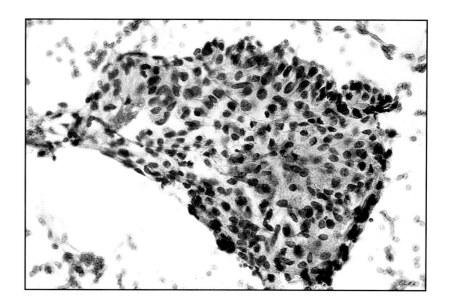

Image 7.5
Cytomorphology of nonproliferative breast disease: a microcalcified particle (H&E, 400X).

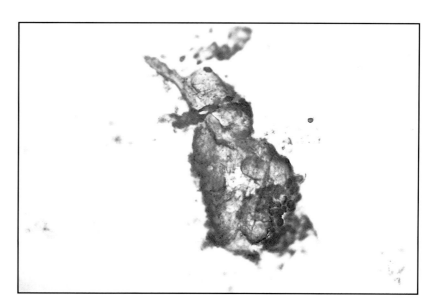

Image 7.6
Cytology of nonproliferative breast disease: cluster of ductal epithelial cells with apocrine cells and minute fragments of stroma (Papanicolaou, 200X). Reproduced with permission from: Masood S, Frykberg ER, McLellan GL, et al: Cytologic differentiation between proliferative and nonproliferative breast disease in mammographically guided fine-needle aspirates. *Diagn Cytopathol* 7:581–590, 1991.

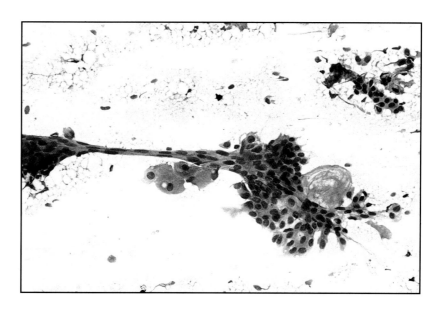

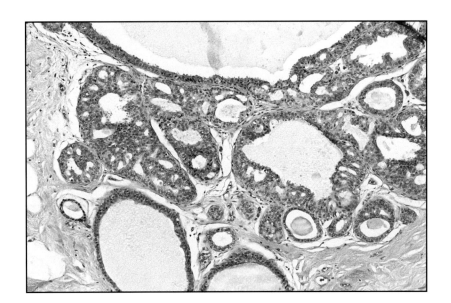

Image 7.7
Histopathologic features of proliferative breast disease without atypia (H&E, 100X).

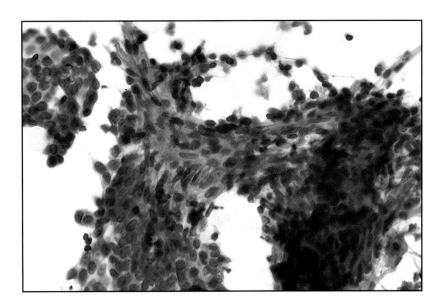

Image 7.8
Cytomorphology of proliferative breast disease without atypia: tightly clustered ductal epithelial cells with overriding of the nuclei (Papanicolaou, 400X). Reproduced with permission from: Masood S, Frykberg ER, McLellan GL, et al: Cytologic differentiation between proliferative and nonproliferative breast disease in mammographically guided fine-needle aspirates. *Diagn Cytopathol* 7:581–590, 1991.

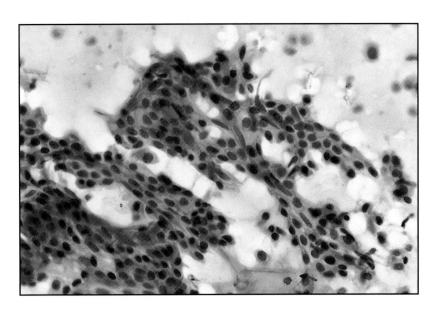

Image 7.9
Cytomorphology of proliferative breast disease without atypia: abundant spindle cells resembling myoepithelial cells (Papanicolaou, 400X). Reproduced with permission from: Masood S, Frykberg ER, McLellan GL, et al: Cytologic differentiation between proliferative and nonproliferative breast disease in mammographically guided fine-needle aspirates. *Diagn Cytopathol* 7:581–590, 1991.

Image 7.10
Cytomorphology of proliferative breast disease without atypia: a sheet-like arrangement of cells with microcalcifications (Papanicolaou, 200X). Reproduced with permission from: Masood S, Frykberg ER, McLellan GL, et al: Cytologic differentiation between proliferative and nonproliferative breast disease in mammographically guided fine-needle aspirates. *Diagn Cytopathol* 7:581–590, 1991.

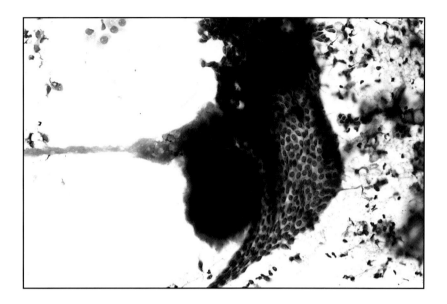

Image 7.11
Cytomorphology of proliferative breast disease without atypia: variability in nuclear size, fine chromatin pattern, and occasional micronucleoli (Papanicolaou, 400X). Reproduced with permission from: Masood S, Frykberg ER, McLellan GL, et al: Cytologic differentiation between proliferative and nonproliferative breast disease in mammographically guided fine-needle aspirates. *Diagn Cytopathol* 7:581–590, 1991.

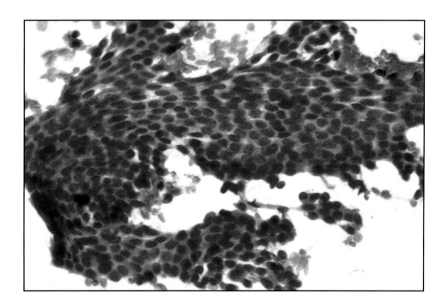

Image 7.12
Histopathology of proliferative breast disease with atypia (H&E, 400X). Reproduced with permission from: Masood S, Frykberg ER, McLellan GL, et al: Cytologic differentiation between proliferative and nonproliferative breast disease in mammographically guided fine-needle aspirates. *Diagn Cytopathol* 7:581–590, 1991.

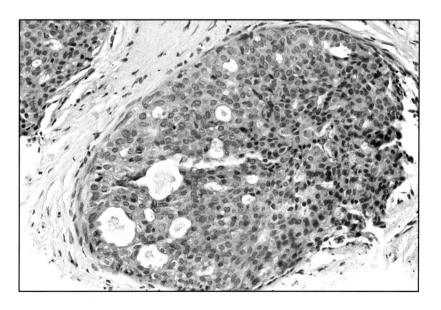

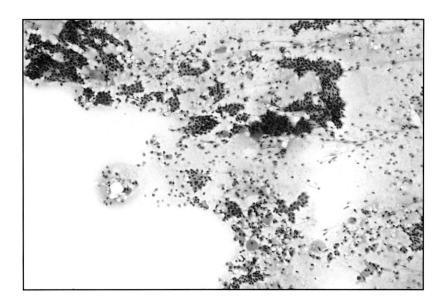

Image 7.13
Cytomorphology of proliferative breast disease with atypia: a highly cellular aspirate. The differential diagnosis includes noncomedo-type ductal carcinoma in situ (Papanicolaou, 100X). Reproduced with permission from: Masood S, Frykberg ER, McLellan GL, et al: Cytologic differentiation between proliferative and nonproliferative breast disease in mammographically guided fine-needle aspirates. *Diagn Cytopathol* 7:581–590, 1991.

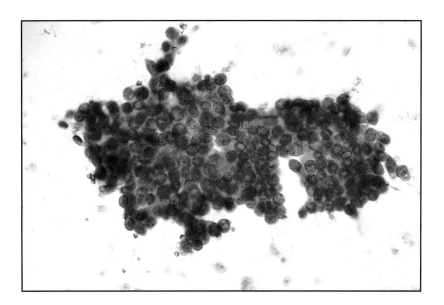

Image 7.14
Cytomorphology of proliferative breast disease with atypia: marked crowding of the nuclei and cytologic atypia (Papanicolaou, 400X). Reproduced with permission from: Masood S, Frykberg ER, McLellan GL, et al: Cytologic differentiation between proliferative and nonproliferative breast disease in mammographically guided fine-needle aspirates. *Diagn Cytopathol* 7:581–590, 1991.

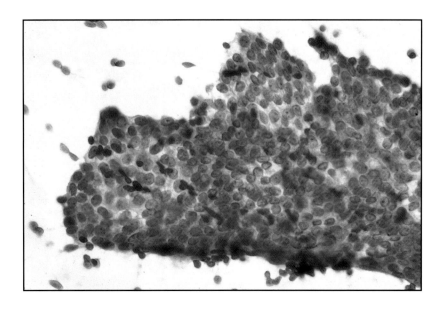

Image 7.15
Cytomorphology of proliferative breast disease with atypia: clusters of ductal epithelial cells mixed with cells resembling myoepithelial cells (Papanicolaou, 400X). Reproduced with permission from: Masood S, Frykberg ER, McLellan GL, et al: Cytologic differentiation between proliferative and nonproliferative breast disease in mammographically guided fine-needle aspirates. *Diagn Cytopathol* 7:581–590, 1991.

Image 7.16
Cytomorphology of proliferative breast disease with atypia: clusters of atypical cells with micronucleoli (Papanicolaou, 400X). Reproduced with permission from: Masood S, Frykberg ER, McLellan GL, et al: Cytologic differentiation between proliferative and non-proliferative breast disease in mammographically guided fine-needle aspirates. *Diagn Cytopathol* 7:581–590, 1991.

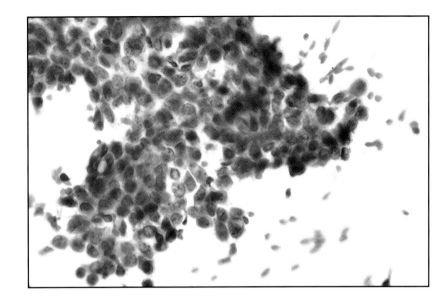

Image 7.17
Cytomorphology of proliferative breast disease with atypia: three-dimensional structures simulating papillary lesions (Diff-Quik®, 400X).

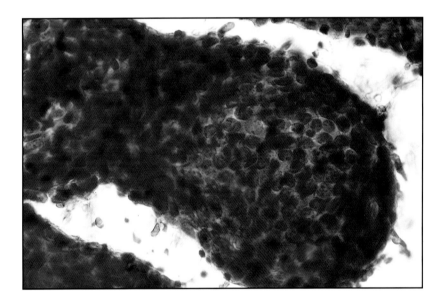

Image 7.18
Corresponding histopathology of the same case: proliferation of atypical epithelial cells forming papillae within the ductal structure (H&E, 400X).

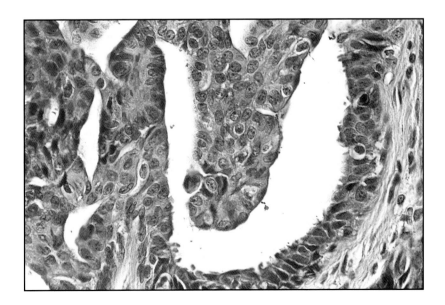

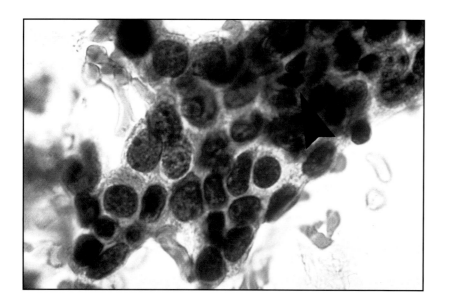

Image 7.19
Cluster of highly atypical cells with features simulating those of carcinoma. However, the presence of myoepithelial cells (arrow) excludes the possibility of a neoplasm (Papanicolaou, 1000X). Reproduced with permission from: Masood S: Cytomorphology of fibrocystic change, high risk and premalignant breast lesions. *Breast J* 1:210–221, 1995.

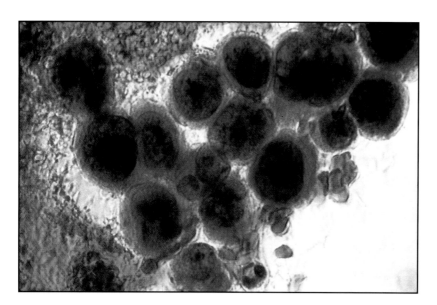

Image 7.20
In contrast, no myoepithelial cells are seen within the cluster of neoplastic cells in a primary breast carcinoma (Papanicolaou, 1000X). Reproduced with permission from: Masood S: Cytomorphology of fibrocystic change, high risk and premalignant breast lesions. *Breast J* 1:210–221, 1995.

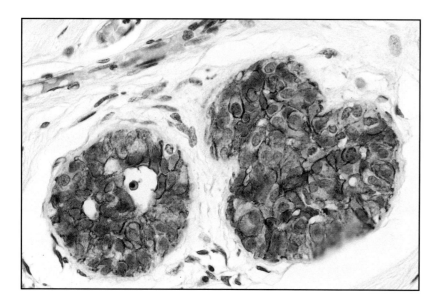

Image 7.21
Expression of HER-2/*neu* oncogene in atypical hyperplasia (Immunoperoxidase, 400X).

Image 7.22
HER-2/*neu* oncogene expression is also seen in comedocarcinoma (Immuno-peroxidase, 400X).

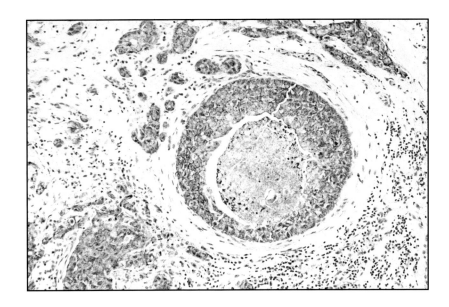

Image 7.23
Cell block preparation of a breast fine needle aspirate with a few malignant cells (H&E, 400X). Reproduced with permission from: Masood S: Cyto-morphology of fibrocystic change, high risk, and premalignant breast lesions. *Breast J* 1:210–221, 1995.

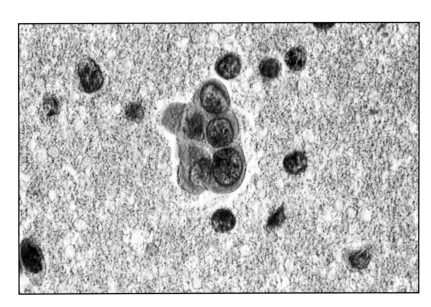

Image 7.24
Positive immunostaining reaction with MAB B72.3 in neoplastic epithelial cells (400X). Reproduced with per-mission from: Masood S: Cyto-morphology of fibrocystic change, high risk, and premalignant breast lesions. *Breast J* 1:210–221, 1995.

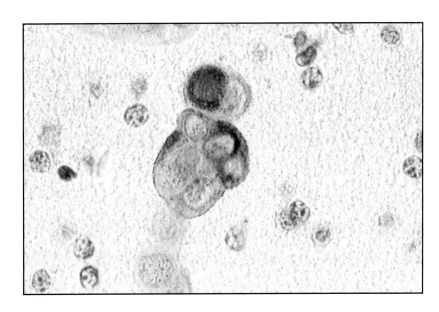

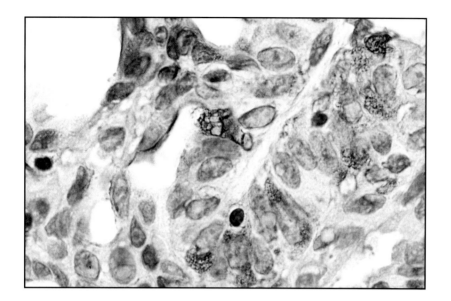

Image 7.25
Expression of muscle specific actin in atypical hyperplasia, indicating the presence of myoepithelial cells (Immunoperoxidase, 400X).

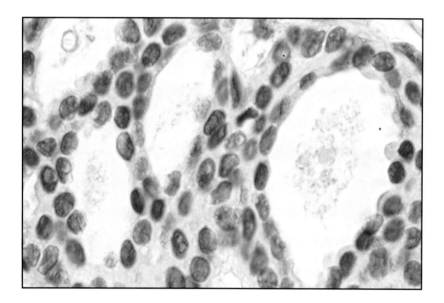

Image 7.26
Absence of expression of muscle specific actin in carcinoma in situ (Immunoperoxidase, 400X).

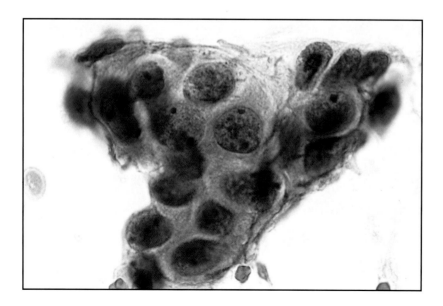

Image 7.27
Breast aspirate: a cluster of atypical epithelial cells with features similar to those of carcinoma (Papanicolaou, 400X). Reproduced with permission from: Masood S, Lu L, Assaf-Munasifi N: Application of immunostaining for muscle specific actin in detection of myoepithelial cells in breast fine needle aspirates. *Diagn Cytopathol* 13:71–74, 1995.

Image 7.28

Expression of muscle specific actin in cell blocks of the same case, indicating the presence of myoepithelial cells (Immunoperoxidase, 400X). Reproduced with permission from: Masood S, Lu L, Assaf-Munasifi N: Application of immunostaining for muscle specific actin in detection of myoepithelial cells in breast fine needle aspirates. *Diagn Cytopathol* 13:71–74, 1995.

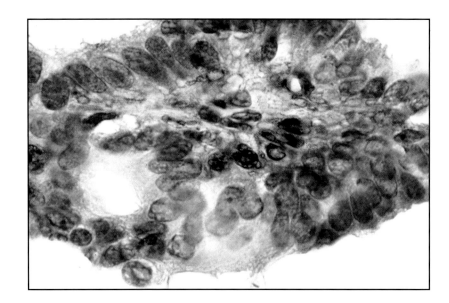

Image 7.29

Breast aspirate: a cluster of atypical myoepithelial cells suggestive of malignancy (Papanicolaou, 400X). Reproduced with permission from: Masood S, Lu L, Assaf-Munasifi N: Application of immunostaining for muscle specific actin in detection of myoepithelial cells in breast fine needle aspirates. *Diagn Cytopathol* 13:71–74, 1995.

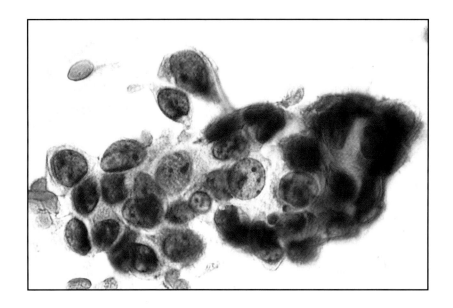

Image 7.30

Absence of muscle specific actin expression confirms the neoplastic nature of the lesion (Immuno-peroxidase, 400X). Reproduced with permission from: Masood S, Lu L, Assaf-Munasifi N: Application of immunostaining for muscle specific actin in detection of myoepithelial cells in breast fine needle aspirates. *Diagn Cytopathol* 13:71–74, 1995.

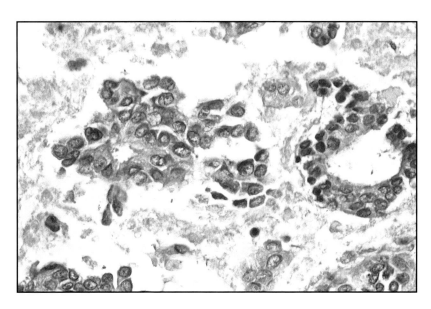

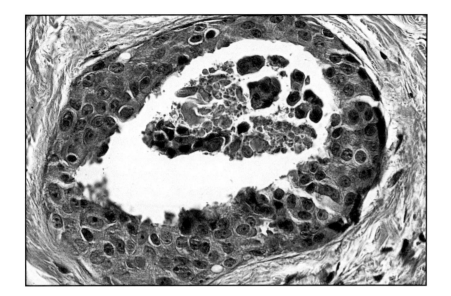

Image 7.31
Histopathology of comedocarcinoma (H&E, 400X).

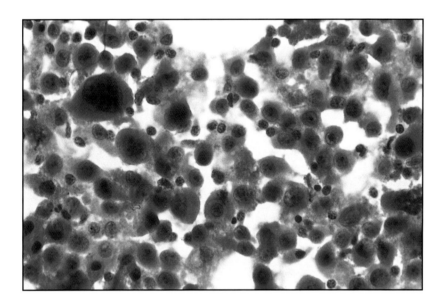

Image 7.32
Aspirate of comedocarcinoma shows clusters of highly atypical epithelial cells with a few neutrophils (Papanicolaou, 400X). Reproduced with permission from: Masood S: Cytomorphology of fibrocystic change, high risk and premalignant breast lesions. *Breast J* 1: 210–221, 1995.

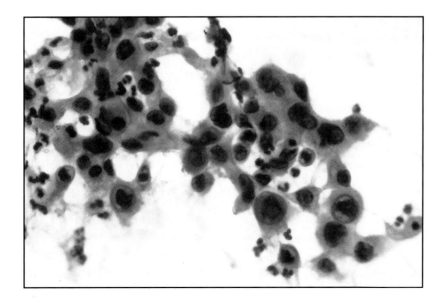

Image 7.33
Aspirate of comedocarcinoma shows pleomorphic population of neoplastic cells with evidence of individual cell necrosis (H&E, 400X). Reproduced with permission from: Masood S: Cytomorphology of fibrocystic change, high risk and premalignant breast lesions. *Breast J* 1:210–221, 1995.

Image 7.34
Histopathology of noncomedocarcinoma in situ (H&E, 400X). Reproduced with permission from: Masood S, Frykberg ER, McLellan GL, et al: Cytologic differentiation between proliferative and nonproliferative breast disease in mammographically guided fine-needle aspirates. *Diagn Cytopathol* 7:581–590, 1991.

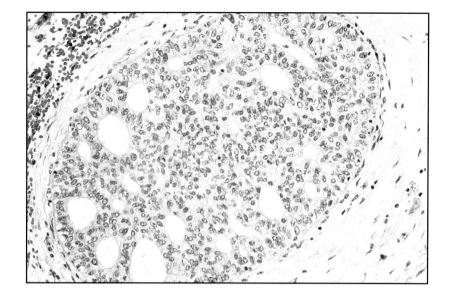

Image 7.35
Noncomedocarcinoma: breast aspirate shows cohesive clusters of bland epithelial cells (Papanicolaou, 200X). Reproduced with permission from: Masood S: Cytomorphology of fibrocystic change, high risk and premalignant breast lesions. *Breast J* 1:210–221, 1995.

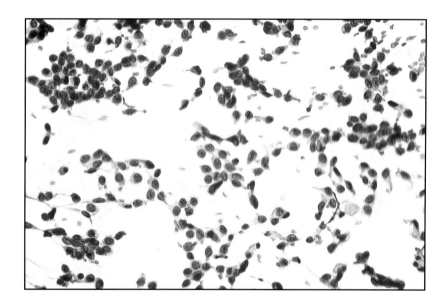

Image 7.36
Higher magnification of the same case demonstrates groups of epithelial cells forming a cribriform pattern. No myoepithelial cells are present (Papanicolaou, 400X). Reproduced with permission from: Masood S: Cytomorphology of fibrocystic change, high risk and premalignant breast lesions. *Breast J* 1:210–221, 1995.

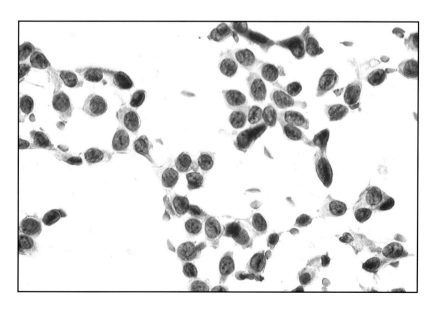

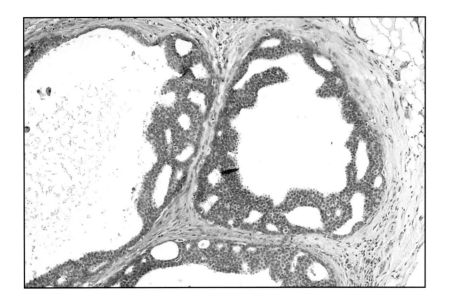

Image 7.37
Histopathology of noncomedocarcinoma in situ, micropapillary type (H&E, 100X).

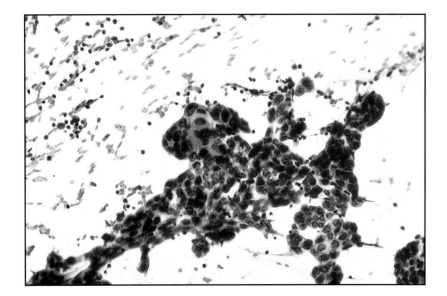

Image 7.38
Cytomorphology of micropapillary carcinoma in situ: loosely arranged clusters of epithelial cells forming three-dimensional structures (Papanicolaou, 100X).

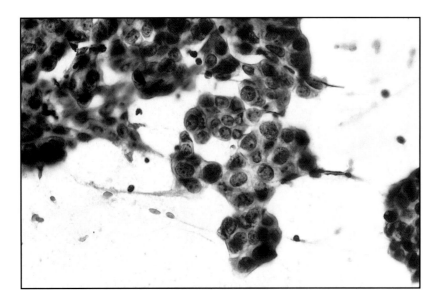

Image 7.39
Different view of the same case shows nuclear atypia, cribriform formation, and the presence of small papillae (Papanicolaou, 200X).

Image 7.40
Histopathology of atypical lobular
hyperplasia (H&E, 200X).

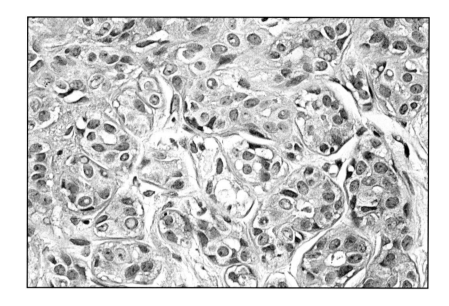

Image 7.41
Cytomorphology of atypical lobular
hyperplasia: acinar proliferation consisting of small cells with a uniform
appearance (Papanicolaou, 100X).

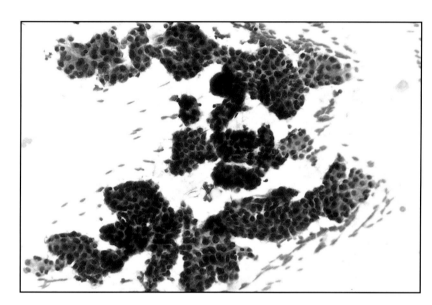

Image 7.42
Cell balls simulating acini in aspirate of
atypical lobular hyperplasia (Papanicolaou, 200X). Reproduced with permission from: Masood S: Cytomorphology
of fibrocystic change, high risk and
premalignant breast lesions. *Breast J*
1:210–221, 1995.

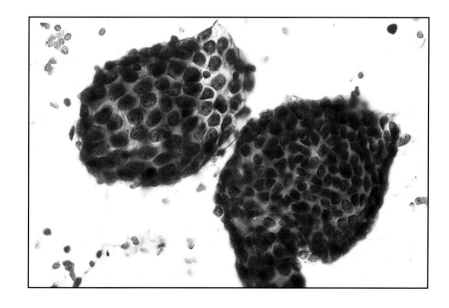

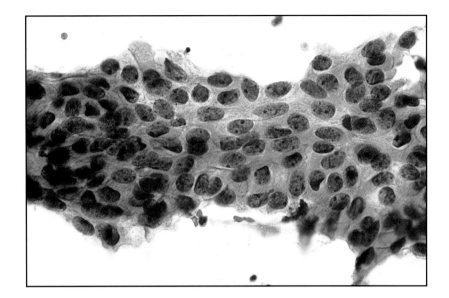

Image 7.43
Monotonous, bland, small epithelial cells, characteristic of lobular neoplasia (Papanicolaou, 200X).

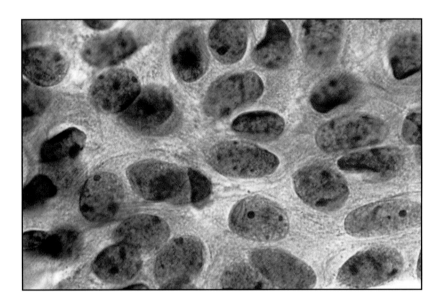

Image 7.44
Higher magnification shows fine chromatin pattern and inconspicuous nucleoli in aspirate of lobular neoplasia (Papanicolaou, 400X).

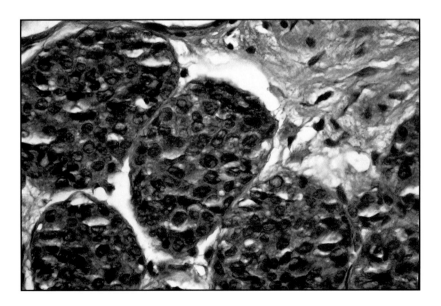

Image 7.45
Histopathology of lobular carcinoma in situ (H&E, 400X).

Image 7.46
Loosely arranged acini with a tightly cohesive population of small cells in aspirate of lobular carcinoma in situ (Papanicolaou, 200X).

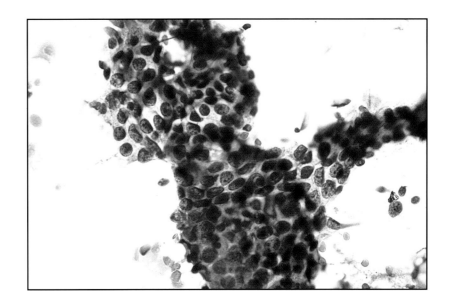

Image 7.47
Diff Quik–stained slide of an aspirate of lobular carcinoma in situ demonstrates loosely cohesive epithelial cells with insignificant atypia (200X).

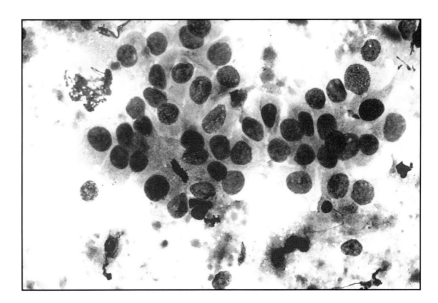

Image 7.48
Cytomorphology of infiltrating lobular carcinoma: chain of small, uniform cells and presence of intracytoplasmic lumens (Papanicolaou, 200X).

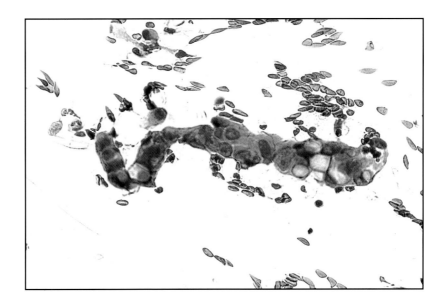

References

1. Emsler VL: The epidemiology of benign breast disease. *Epidemiol Rev* 3:184–202, 1981.

2. Lov SM, Gelman RS, Silen W: Fibrocystic "disease" of the breast—a nondisease? *N Engl J Med* 307:1010–1014, 1982.

3. Page DL, Vander Z, Weig R, et al: Relation between component parts of fibrocystic disease complex and breast cancer. *J Natl Cancer Inst* 61:1055–1063, 1978.

4. Kodlin D, Winger EE, Morgenstern NL, et al: Chronic mastopathy and breast cancer, a follow-up study. *Cancer* 39:2603–2607, 1977.

5. Hutchinson WB, Thomas DB, Hamlin WB, Roth GJ, Peterson AR, Williams B: Risk of breast cancer in women with benign breast disease. *J Natl Cancer Inst* 65:13–20, 1980.

6. Bach MM, Barclay THC, Cutler SJ, et al: Association of atypical characteristics of benign breast lesions with subsequent risk of breast cancer. *Cancer* 29:338–343, 1972.

7. Page DL: Cancer risk assessment in benign breast biopsies. *Hum Pathol* 17:871–878, 1986.

8. Dupont WD, Page DL: Risk factors for breast cancer in women with proliferative breast disease. *N Engl J Med* 312:146-151, 1985.

9. Azzopardi JG: Benign and malignant proliferative epithelial lesions of the breast: a review. *Eur J Cancer Clin Oncol* 19:1717–1720, 1983.

10. Wellings SR: Development of human breast cancer. *Adv Cancer Res* 31:287–314, 1980.

11. Ashikari R, Huros AG, Snyder RE, et al: A clinicopathologic study of atypical lesions of the breast. *Cancer* 33:310–317, 1974.

12. Masood S, Frykberg ER, McLellan GL, et al: Prospective evaluation of radiologically detected fine needle aspiration biopsy of nonpalpable breast lesions. *Cancer* 66:1480–1487, 1990.

13. Masood S, Frykberg ER, McLellan GL, et al: Cytologic differentiation between proliferative and nonproliferative breast disease in mammographically guided fine-needle aspirates. *Diagn Cytopathol* 7:581–590, 1991.

14. Linsk JA, Krunzer G, Zajicek J: Cytologic diagnosis of mammary tumors from aspiration biopsy smears, II. Studies on 210 fibroadenomas and 210 cases of benign dysplasia. *Acta Cytol* 16:130–138, 1972.

15. Bottles K, Chan JS, Holly EA, et al: Cytologic criteria for fibroadenoma. A stepwise logistic regression analysis. *Am J Clin Pathol* 89:707–713, 1988.

16. Schwartz GF, Feig SA, Patchefsky AS: Significance and staging of nonpalpable carcinomas of the breast. *Surg Gynecol Obstet* 166:6–10, 1988.

17. Wanebo HJ, Feldman PS, Wilhelm MC, et al: Fine needle aspiration cytology in lieu of open biopsy in management of primary breast cancer. *Ann Surg* 199:569–578, 1984.

18. Gent HJ, Sprenger E, Dowlatshahi K: Stereotaxic needle localization and cytological diagnosis of occult breast lesions. *Ann Surg* 204:580–584, 1986.

19. Dziura BR, Bonfiglio TA: Needle cytology of the breast. *Acta Cytol* 23:332–340, 1979.

20. Bibbo M, Scheiber M, Cajulis R, et al: Stereotaxic fine needle aspiration cytology of occult malignant and premalignant breast lesions. *Acta Cytol* 32:193–201, 1988.

21. Masood S, Hardy NM, Assaf-Munasifi N: Cytologic grading system in diagnosis of high-risk and malignant breast lesions. Merits and pitfalls. *Acta Cytol* 38:797–798, 1994. Abstract.

22. Sneige N, Staerkel GA: Fine needle aspiration cytology of ductal hyperplasia with and without atypia and ductal carcinoma in situ. *Hum Pathol* 25:485–492, 1994.

23. Silverman J, Masood S, Ducatman BS, et al: Can FNA biopsy separate atypical hyperplasia, carcinoma in situ, and invasive carcinoma of the breast? Cytomorphologic criteria and limitations in diagnosis. *Diagn Cytopathol* 9:713–728, 1993.

24. Abendroth CS, Wang HH, Ducatman BS: Comparative features of carcinoma in situ and atypical ductal hyperplasia of the breast on fine needle aspiration biopsy. *Am J Clin Pathol* 96:654–659, 1991.

25. Shiels LA, Mulford D, Dawson AG: Cytomorphology of proliferative breast disease. *Acta Cytol* 37:768, 1993. Abstract.

26. Stanley MW, Henry-Stanley MJ, Zera R: Prospective study of high risk proliferative lesions of breast duct epithelium by fine needle aspiration. *Acta Cytol* 35:611, 1991. Abstract.

27. Lennington WJ, Jensen RA, Dalton LW, et al: Ductal carcinoma in situ of the breast: heterogeneity of individual lesions. *Cancer* 73:118–124, 1994.

28. Crissman JD, Visscher DW, Kubus J: Image cytophotometric DNA analysis of atypical hyperplasia and intraductal carcinomas of the breast. *Arch Pathol Lab Med* 114:1249–1253, 1990.

29. Teplitz RL, Butler BB, Tesluk H, et al: Quantitative DNA patterns in human preneoplastic breast lesions. *Anal Quant Cytol Histol* 12:98–102, 1990.

30. Norris HJ, Bahr GF, Mikel UV: A comparative morphometric and cytophotometric study of intraductal hyperplasia and intraductal carcinoma of the breast. *Anal Quant Cytol Histol* 10:1–9, 1988.

31. King ER, Chen KL, Duarte L, et al: Image cytometric classification of premalignant breast disease in fine-needle aspirates. *Cancer* 62:114–124, 1988.

32. King ER, Chen KL, Hem JD, et al: Characterization of image cytometry of ductal epithelial proliferative disease of the breast. *Mod Pathol* 4:291–296, 1991.

33. Masood S: HER-2/*neu* oncogene expression in atypical ductal hyperplasia, carcinoma in situ and invasive breast cancer. *Mod Pathol* 4:12, 1991. Abstract.

34. Johnson WW, Szpak CA, Thor A, et al: Applications of immunocytochemistry to clinical cytology. *Cancer Invest* 5:593–611, 1987.

35. Nuti M, Teramoto YA, Mariani-Constantini R, et al: A monoclonal antibody (B72.3) defines patterns of distribution of a novel tumor-associated antigen in human mammary carcinoma cell populations. *Int J Cancer* 29:539–545, 1982.

36. Colchen D, Hovan Hand P, Nuti M, et al: A spectrum of monoclonal antibodies reactive with mammary tumor cells. *Proc Natl Acad Sci U S A* 78:3199–3203, 1981.

37. Lundy J, Lozowski M, Mishviki Y: Monoclonal antibody B72.3 as a diagnostic adjunct in fine needle aspirates of breast masses. *Ann Surg* 203:399–402, 1986.

38. Masood S: Use of monoclonal antibody B72.3 in breast fine needle aspirates. *J Breast Cancer Treat* 14:154, 1989.

39. Lundy J, Kline TS, Lozowski M, et al: Immunoperoxidase studies by monoclonal antibody B72.3 applied to breast aspirates: diagnostic considerations. *Diagn Cytopathol* 4:95–98, 1988.

40. Mukai K, Schollmeyer JV, Rosai J: Immunohistochemical localization of actin. *Am J Surg Pathol* 5:71–97, 1981.

41. Papotti M, Eusebi V, Gagliotta P, et al: Immunohistochemical analysis of benign and malignant papillary lesions of the breast. *Am J Surg Pathol* 7:451–461, 1983.

42. Raju VB, Lee MW, Zarbo RJ, et al: Papillary neoplasia of the breast: immunohistochemically defined myoepithelial cells in the diagnosis of benign and malignant papillary breast neoplasms. *Mod Pathol* 2:569–576, 1989.

43. Masood S, Sim SJ, Lu L: Immunohistochemical differentiation of atypical hyperplasia versus carcinoma in situ of the breast. *Cancer Detect Prev* 16:225–235, 1992.

44. Masood S, Lu L, Assaf-Munasifi N, et al: Application of immunostaining for muscle specific actin in detection of myoepithelial cells in breast fine needle aspirates. *Diagn Cytopathol* 13:71–74, 1995.

45. Masood S, Assaf-Munasifi N, Hardy NM: The value of muscle specific actin immunostaining in differentiation between atypical hyperplasia and carcinoma in breast fine needle aspirates. *Acta Cytol* 38:860–861, 1994. Abstract.

46. Rosai J: Breast. In: Rosai J, ed. *Ackerman's Surgical Pathology.* St Louis, Mo, CV Mosby Co, 1989, pp. 1219–1226.

47. Carter D, Smith RRL: Carcinoma in situ of the breast. *Cancer* 40: 1189–1193, 1977.

48. Meyer JS: Cell kinetics of histologic variants of in situ breast carcinoma. *Breast Cancer Res Treat* 7:171–180, 1986.

49. Patchefsky AS, Schwartz GF, Finkelstein SD, et al: Heterogeneity of intraductal carcinoma of the breast. *Cancer* 63:731–741, 1989.

50. Lagios MD, Westdahl PR, Margopin FR, et al: Duct carcinoma in situ. Relationship of extent of noninvasive disease to the frequency of occult invasion, multiplicity, lymph node metastasis and short-term treatment failures. *Cancer* 50:1309–1314, 1982.

51. Micale MA, Visscher DW, Gulino SE: Chromosomal aneuploidy in proliferative breast disease. *Hum Pathol* 25:29–35, 1994.

52. Bellamy COC, McDonald C, Salter PM, et al: Noninvasive ductal carcinoma of the breast. The relevance of histologic categorization. *Hum Pathol* 24:16–23, 1993.

53. Frykberg ER, Masood S, Copeland EM, et al: Ductal carcinoma in situ of the breast. *Surg Gynecol Obstet* 177:425–440, 1993.

54. Moriya T, Sidawy MK, Silverberg SG: Detection of ductal carcinoma in situ of the breast in cytologic samples. *Acta Cytol* 37:767, 1993. Abstract.

55. Malamud YR, Ducatman BS, Wang HH: Comparative features of comedo and noncomedo ductal carcinoma in situ of the breast on fine needle aspiration biopsy. *Diagn Cytopathol* 8:571–576, 1992.

56. Lilleng R, Hagmar B: The comedo subtype of intraductal carcinoma. Cytologic characteristics. *Acta Cytol* 36:345–352, 1992.

57. Masood S: Recent updates in breast fine needle aspiration biopsy. *Breast J* (In press).

58. Wang HH, Ducatman BS, Eich D: Comparative features of ductal carcinoma in situ and infiltrating ductal carcinoma of the breast on fine needle aspiration biopsy. *Am J Clin Pathol* 92:736–740, 1989.

59. Bradley SJ, Weaver DW, Bouwman DL: Alternatives in the surgical management of in situ breast cancer. A meta-analysis of outcome. *Ann Surg* 56:428–432, 1990.

60. Rosen PP, Lieberman PH, Braun DW, et al: Lobular carcinoma in situ of the breast. *Am J Surg Pathol* 2:225–250, 1978.

61. Anderson JA: Lobular carcinoma in situ: A long term follow up in 52 cases. *Acta Pathol Microbiol Scand (A)* 82:519, 1974.

62. Meyers J, Kopans PE, Stomper PC, et al: Occult breast abnormalities; percutaneous preoperative needle localization. *Radiology* 150: 333–337, 1984.

63. Rosenberg AL, Schwartz GF, Feig SA, et al: Clinically occult breast lesions: localization and significance. *Radiology* 162:167–170, 1987.

64. Kline TS, Kline IK: *Breast: Guides to Clinical Aspiration Biopsy.* New York, NY, Igaku-Shoin, 1989, pp. 235–248.

65. Salhany K, Page DL: Fine needle aspiration of mammary lobular carcinoma in situ and atypical lobular hyperplasia. *Am J Clin Pathol* 92:22–26, 1989.

66. Masood S: Cytomorphology of fibrocystic change, high risk, and premalignant breast lesions. *Breast J* 1:210–221, 1995.

67. Boone CW, Kelloff G: Biomarkers of premalignant breast disease and their use as surrogate endpoints in clinical trials of chemopreventive agents. *Breast J* 1:228–235, 1995.

68. Visscher D: Biomarkers of proliferative breast disease. *Breast J* 1:222–227, 1995.

69. Fabian CJ, Kamel S, Kimler BF, et al. Potential use of biomarkers in breast cancer risk assessment and chemoprevention trials. *Breast J* 1:236–242, 1995.

70. Wrensch M, Petrakis NL, King EB, et al. Breast cancer risk associated with abnormal cytology in nipple aspirates of breast fluids and prior history of breast biopsy. *Am J Epidemiol* 137:829–833, 1993.

71. Eby N, Chang-Claude J, Bishop DJ: The familial and genetic susceptibility for breast cancer. *Cancer Causes Control* 5:458–470, 1994.

72. Miki Y, Swensen J, Shattuck-Eidens D, et al: A strong candidate for the breast and ovarian cancer susceptibility gene BRCA1. *Science* 266:66–71.

73. Wooster R, Neuhausen SL, Mansion J, et al: Localization of a breast cancer susceptibility gene, BRCA2, to chromosome 13q12-13. *Science* 265:2088–2090, 1994.

74. Wooster R, Bignell G, Lancaster J, et al: Identification of the breast cancer susceptibility gene BRCA2. *Nature* 378:789–791, 1995.

75. Narod SA, Ford DA, Devilee P, et al: An evaluation of genetic heterogeneity in 145 breast-ovarian cancer families. Breast Cancer Linkage Consortium. *Am J Hum Genet* 56:254–264, 1995.

76. Lemoine NR: Molecular biology of breast cancer. *Ann Oncol* 4(suppl 5):31–37, 1994.

CHAPTER EIGHT

Primary Breast Carcinoma, Common Types

Infiltrating Duct Cell Carcinoma

Infiltrating duct cell carcinoma, also referred to as not otherwise specified (NOS) carcinoma, is the most common type of breast cancer, accounting for up to 75% of all invasive breast carcinomas. The frequency of this tumor varies in different countries. The largest percentage of patients are from the United States, while Japanese women are the least affected.[1–4]

Infiltrating duct cell carcinoma occurs most frequently in women in their mid to late fifties; however, it has been reported in women from their twenties to their nineties.[2] Infiltrating duct cell carcinoma is detected clinically or by the use of mammography. Patients may present with a mass, skin retraction, edema, peau d'orange, nipple retraction and/or discharge, or ulceration. Infiltrating duct cell carcinoma manifests either as a well-circumscribed mass or as a stellate lesion with infiltrating borders or a combination of invasive and pushing borders. The more common variety is the stellate lesion, which is characterized by extensive fibrosis and is also known as scirrhous carcinoma.[5] Stellate tumors consist of a central mass that radiates into the surrounding breast tissue. They are often larger than tumors with well-circumscribed borders and are more likely to metastasize to the axillary lymph nodes.[6]

Microscopically, infiltrating duct cell carcinoma is characterized by a spectrum of changes that vary according to the degree of differentiation, extent of stromal reaction, presence or absence of necrosis, and presence or absence of inflammatory cells. A lymphocytic infiltrate of T-cell type is seen in about 20% of infiltrating duct cell carcinomas and seems to be associated with a favorable prognosis.[2,7,8] Histologic differentiation of infiltrating duct cell carcinoma is based on the degree of tubule formation, nuclear appearance, and mitotic activity. The histologic and nuclear grades of infiltrating duct cell carcinoma are important prognostic indicators.[9] The majority of infiltrating duct cell carcinomas are estrogen receptor (ER) positive.[10] Positivity for progesterone receptor ranges from 33% to 70% of cases.[11] There is an inverse correlation between hormone-receptor expression and the degree of histologic differentiation of infiltrating duct cell carcinoma.[12,13]

Infiltrating duct cell carcinoma is the type of breast cancer most frequently diagnosed by fine needle aspiration biopsy (FNAB). The cellularity of the aspirate is variable and depends on the stromal content of the tumor. Aspirates of scirrhous-type infiltrating duct cell carcinoma may be hypocellular and may contain few neoplastic cells (Images 8.1 through 8.4).

FNAB smears of infiltrating duct cell carcinoma are cellular, with epithelial cells showing conspicuous loss of cohesion. Scattered individual tumor cells and aggregates of various-sized cells characterize the neoplasm. Three-dimensional clusters, syncytial groupings, or, occasionally, gland-like arrangements are also observed. The background is rarely clean. It may contain cellular debris, microcalcified particles, and numerous red blood cells. Cell size varies; however, in the majority of cases, the tumor cells are large and pleomorphic, with hyperchromatic nuclei and irregular nuclear membranes. The N/C ratio is high, and prominent nucleoli and occasional mitoses may also be seen (Images 8.5 through 8.10).

The small cell variant of duct cell carcinoma may be difficult to diagnose cytologically because of its small size. The presence of many intact single cells with hyperchromatic nuclei and the absence of myoepithelial cells may provide diagnostic clues. The small cell variant of infiltrating duct cell carcinoma is similar to infiltrating lobular carcinoma but is more cellular, with more hyperchromatic nuclei. FNAB smears obtained from older women may occasionally show modest numbers of neoplastic cells with poorly delineated nuclei and a plasmacytoid appearance that is best appreciated in Diff-Quik® (Images 8.11 through 8.13).

Infiltrating duct cell carcinoma can form multinucleated tumor giant cells. In FNAB smears of these cases, bizarre, multinucleated giant cells with marked nuclear pleomorphism are intermingled with mononuclear neoplastic epithelial cells. Positive immunostaining for epithelial markers substantiates the epithelial origin of the giant cells (Images 8.14 through 8.20).[14]

Giant cells may occur in several types of breast lesions.[1] For example, giant malignant epithelial cells are seen in infiltrating duct cell, medullary, and squamous cell carcinomas.[2] Stromal giant cells are seen in response to infiltrating duct cell carcinoma.[3] Giant cells are also seen in atypical fibrous histiocytoma,[4] extraosseous osteogenic sarcoma, and metaplastic breast cancer.[5] Osteoclastoma is a benign giant cell tumor of soft tissue when it occurs in the breast.[15-18] Clinical presentation, the cytomorphology of accompanying cells, immunostaining, and electron microscopic study often help to assess the nature of giant cells in an aspirate.

Generally, benign epithelial components and bipolar, naked nuclei are not seen in FNAB smears of infiltrating duct cell carcinoma unless the surrounding benign tissue is also aspirated or the cancer has arisen from a benign process. Overall, the incidence of false-negative diagnosis of infiltrating duct cell carcinoma is relatively low. False-negative diagnosis may be due either to faulty aspiration biopsy technique or the presence of prominent sclerosis in the tumor.

Cytomorphology of Infiltrating Duct Cell Carcinoma
Cellular smear
Variable cell pattern
Necrotic background
Conspicuous loss of cellular cohesion
Pleomorphic, isolated single cells
Occasional small cells with plasmacytoid appearance
Rare multinucleated tumor giant cells
Anisonucleosis

Infiltrating Lobular Carcinoma

Infiltrating lobular carcinoma (ILC) accounts for 0.7% to 14% of all invasive breast carcinomas.[19,20] This range may reflect differences in the criteria used for diagnosis of this tumor. Lobular carcinoma is the least well defined of the breast cancer subtypes,[21] and recognizing its cytologic features can be difficult.[22,23]

Invasive lobular carcinomas occur in patients between the ages of 26 to 86 years, with the median age ranging from 45 to 57 years.[23,24] The clinical presentation of this tumor is similar to that of other infiltrating lesions; however, Paget's disease is not seen in association with infiltrating lobular carcinoma. Because of their diffuse growth pattern, ILCs characteristically fail to produce a well-defined mass and therefore are hard to detect clinically and mammographically. Compared with other invasive breast carcinomas, infiltrating lobular carcinomas are associated with a higher incidence of bilaterality and multiplicity.[21,24] Lobular carcinomas have a different metastatic pattern than other breast tumors and have a tendency to involve skeletal, visceral, serosal, and meningeal areas. Ovary, uterus, and bone marrow are the other sites that infiltrating lobular carcinoma commonly involves.[25,26] Infiltrating lobular carcinomas are often hormone-receptor positive.[27]

Macroscopically, this tumor presents as an irregular, poorly defined area of increased density. Rarely, minute, firm, discrete nodules simulating grains of sand are seen in the breast tissue.[28] The classic microscopic features of infiltrating lobular carcinoma are diffuse infiltration of mammary stroma and normal ductal structures with neoplastic cells in a pagetoid growth pattern. In approximately 90% of cases, an associated lobular in situ carcinoma is present.[20] Tumor cells are small, with scant cytoplasm and occasional intracytoplasmic lumens. Other variants of infiltrating lobular carcinoma include solid pattern, alveolar pattern, and mixed solid/alveolar pattern.[29] In the solid pattern, the closely packed tumor cell nests and trabeculae are separated by delicate vascular channels. In the alveolar variant, the same type of cells form rounded nests and islands separated by minimal stroma. The mixed pattern combines the features of the solid and alveolar variants.

Breast fine needle aspirates of lobular carcinoma are associated with a high false-negative rate. The reports indicate that between 37% and 100% of lobular carcinomas are unrecognized by cytology.[30,31] However, by using strict criteria, Kline et al[32,33] showed that it is possible to correctly diagnose lobular carcinoma in up to 75% of cases. Characteristic cytomorphologic findings in ILC include low to moderate cell yield and a relatively uniform population of small- to medium-sized cells. The cells have scant, ill-defined cytoplasm with an increased N/C ratio. They tend to occur in small groups, Indian file, in cords, or singly. The cytoplasm may contain sharply punched-out vacuoles, and occasional signet ring forms may be seen. The nuclei have a fine chromatin pattern, small nucleoli, and often are eccentric. Anisonucleosis is minimal (Images 8.21 through 8.28).

Pleomorphic lobular carcinoma, a variant of infiltrating lobular carcinoma, is an aggressive neoplasm associated with short survival.[3,29] Histologically, the tumor is characterized by infiltration in the form of single files of tumor cells, prominent pagetoid patterns, occasional apocrine cytoplasmic features, and the presence of in situ lobular carcinomas.[34,35] In contrast to the darkly stained uniform small cells typical of classic infiltrating lobular carcinoma, pleomorphic lobular carcinoma shows conspicuous nuclear enlargement, hyperchromasia, marked variation in cell size, and occasional nucleoli.[36] These features simulate the cytomorphology of duct cell carcinoma and may create diagnostic difficulty. A careful search for single files of tumor cells or the typical small infiltrating lobular carcinoma may lead to correct diagnosis (Images 8.29 through 8.33).[37–39] We also agree with the suggestion that in contrast to classic lobular carcinomas, which are typically monotonous and are collectively regarded as low nuclear grade tumors, pleomorphic lobular carcinoma should be assigned a high nuclear grade.[36]

In a study of 31 cases of histologically proven ILC, Nguyen[40] suggests that eccentricity of nuclei and the presence of poorly cohesive small and large groups of cells with nuclear overlap are the features most useful in the evaluation of scant aspirates. As previously mentioned, ILCs, with their typically low cellularity and insignificant cellular atypia, are often misdiagnosed as fibrocystic change. Cytomorphologic distinction between atypical lobular hyperplasia, lobular carcinoma in situ, and infiltrating lobular carcinoma may also be difficult.[41–44] Aspirates of infiltrating lobular carcinoma and atypical lobular hyperplasia (better known as lobular neoplasia) may show loosely cohesive groups of small uniform cells with eccentric, regular nuclei and occasional intracytoplasmic lumens. Aspirates of infiltrating lobular carcinoma show overlapping features but are more cellular and contain more atypical single cells. We believe that cellular aspirates that contain a significant number of small uniform cells arranged in small groups, Indian files, cords, or singly are characteristic of infiltrating lobular carcinoma and warrant proceeding to definitive therapy. However, as previously mentioned, patients whose aspirates are scant in cellularity should undergo an excisional biopsy to establish the diagnosis.

The distinction between infiltrating lobular carcinoma and lobular carcinoma in situ is crucial in the management of patients with breast lesions. Lobular carcinoma in situ is now considered only a marker for the subsequent development of breast cancer, with bilateral mastectomy or close observation as management. In contrast, treatment for ILC is similar to that for other invasive breast cancers.[13]

Cytomorphology of Infiltrating Lobular Carcinoma
Low to moderate cell yield
Individual cells, small chains, strands, and small groups
Uniform population of small cells with mild atypia
Small nucleoli
Occasional signet ring cell

Tubular Carcinoma

Recognized more than 100 years ago,[45] tubular carcinoma is a distinct variant of breast carcinoma with a deceptively bland appearance. Tubular carcinoma previously represented only about 1% of all breast cancers in large series.[2,46] However, the increased use of mammography, which permits detection of smaller carcinomas, has resulted in a significant increase in the diagnosis of tubular carcinoma. In studies of nonpalpable malignant breast lesions, the percentage of tubular carcinomas is as high as 20%.[47,48] Some investigators suggest that tubular carcinoma represents a transitional phase of neoplasia that progresses to a less-differentiated growth phase and ultimately becomes obscured by ductal overgrowth.[49]

Tubular carcinoma typically occurs in a younger age group than regular infiltrating carcinoma[50] and is associated with a higher incidence of bilaterality and multiplicity.[51,52] There is also a family history of breast carcinoma in 40% of patients with tubular carcinoma.[51] Because of their small size and the rarity of axillary node metastasis, tubular carcinomas are associated with a good prognosis and are most suitable for conservative therapy.[53]

Tubular carcinomas range in size from 0.2 to 12 cm. However, in one study the majority of pure carcinomas were 1 cm or less in diameter.[52] Grossly, they present with different patterns ranging from stellate or scirrhous to areas of gray–white discoloration with induration and retraction.[54] Microscopically, tubular carcinoma is characterized by haphazard proliferation of angulated, oval, or elongated tubules surrounded by a dense, reactive, fibroblastic stroma. The lumens are lined by a single layer of epithelial cells. Atypia is minimal and mitotic activity is rare (Image 8.34).

Smears from FNABs of tubular carcinomas are moderately cellular with a background that has a littered appearance, perhaps due to the mixture of mesenchymal cells and stromal elements. Tumor cells are typically seen in cohesive clusters and only occasionally is pronounced dissociation observed. The cells form monolayer sheets with blunt and angular branching and three-dimensional tubular structures. Characteristically, tumor cells are uniform and have regularly shaped nuclei with finely dispersed chromatin and small nucleoli. There may be cellular atypia, such as angular nuclear membranes; irregular, grooved nuclei; uneven deposition of chromatin on the nuclear membrane; and, occasionally, a large, solitary, intracytoplasmic vacuole. Myoepithelial cells in the background are a common finding (Images 8.35 through 8.43).[55–61]

In contrast to what is commonly seen in other infiltrating duct cell carcinomas, well-differentiated tubular carcinomas do not show significant cytologic atypia. In addition, due to the complex nature of the lesion, it is not uncommon to find malignant components mixed with benign elements. These may contribute to the difficulty of diagnosing tubular carcinoma by FNAB. However, Bondeson and Lindholm,[55] in a review of the cytomorphology of 34 tubular carcinomas, suggest that the presence of grooved nuclei or cytoplasmic vacuoles of the same type seen in lobular carcinoma are warning signals. They found the most striking feature of aspirates of tubular carcinoma to be the structural pattern of highly cohesive, angular tubules, reflecting the histologic appearance of the tumor, which has open glands. However, this pattern can occasionally be seen in aspirates of benign lesions such as radial scars, which mammographically are very similar to small tubular carcinoma.[62]

Comparisons of the cytomorphology of tubular carcinoma and radial scar have shown that the two lesions have overlapping features, including cellularity, pleomorphism, nucleoli, dissociated cells, myoepithelial cells, tubular structures, acinar structures, and elastoid material. However, radial scars are characterized by lower cellularity, a higher prevalence of myoepithelial cells, and absence of nucleoli.[60,61] We have experienced diagnostic difficulty when radial scar is associated with areas of atypical hyperplasia (Images 8.44 and 8.45). When needle sampling is limited to hyperplastic areas only, the smears are cellular. Branching epithelial cells, loss of polarity, anisonucleosis, and nucleoli are features that militate against a diagnosis of typical radial scar and may raise the possibility of a neoplastic process. Positive immunostaining for muscle specific actin (MSA) and demonstration of myoepithelial cells within the atypical clusters substantiate the benign nature of the lesion (Images 8.46 through 8.51). Correlation of mammographic appearance with cytomorphologic features should aid in diagnosis of radial scar.

Minimal nuclear abnormality and relatively well-maintained cell cohesion in tubular carcinoma create a pattern reminiscent of fibroadenoma. However, the complex branching of ductal epithelial cells seen in fibroadenoma is not seen in tubular carcinoma. Instead, the ductal epithelial cells are arranged in angulated glandular or tubular structures with occasional intracytoplasmic lumens present. In tubular carcinoma, bipolar, naked nuclei are not seen within the clusters of epithelial cells, although they may be scattered in the background. Other features that may suggest a diagnosis of tubular carcinoma are nuclei with regular features and placement and distinctly enlarged but uniform nucleoli (Images 8.52 and 8.53).

The rate of unsatisfactory cytologic specimens of tubular carcinoma is as high as 20% in mammographically detected lesions.[55] However, the majority of tubular carcinomas can be clearly recognized as malignant in fine needle aspirates. Cytologic diagnosis of tubular carcinoma warrants proceeding to definitive therapy.

Cytomorphology of Tubular Carcinoma
Variable cellularity
Sheets of epithelial cells forming angulated glandular or tubular structures
Nuclear regularity and enlargement
Relatively uniform nuclei
Grooved nucleus
Cytoplasmic vacuoles

Papillary Carcinoma

Papillary carcinoma accounts for about 1% to 2% of breast cancers in postmenopausal women and is associated with good prognosis.[63-66] Papillary carcinoma may also develop in the male breast.[66] A variant of intraductal carcinoma, papillary carcinoma may cause bloody nipple discharge. A palpable tumor is present in up to 90% of patients. Skin dimpling, nipple retraction, or deviation may also occur. The tumor usually appears as a papillary nodule with a shaggy surface and is often associated with hemorrhage. Microscopically, myoepithelial cell layers are absent from the papillary processes proliferating into the distended duct lumen. The proliferating epithelial cells may assume a variety of patterns, such as cribriform or micropapillary, or they may display stratification. Tumor cells may be atypical, with a conspicuous number of mitoses present, but more often the cells exhibit a monotonous appearance (Images 8.54 and 8.55). The most important morphologic feature of papillary carcinoma is the absence of a myoepithelial cell layer, which may be assessed by immunostaining for muscle specific actin.[67] Papillary carcinomas rarely metastasize and are associated with a relatively high survival rate, making conservative therapy appropriate.

The cytomorphology of papillary carcinoma has been well described.[31,68-73] Characteristically, aspirates of papillary carcinoma are highly cellular and may have a bloody background with hemosiderin-containing macrophages. The presence of single papillae and three-dimensional papillary clusters similar to those described in papillary carcinoma of the thyroid gland are distinctive features. However, in contrast to thyroid carcinoma, nuclear pseudoinclusion is rarely seen. Additionally, mucin production can sometimes be seen in invasive papillary cancers and in micropapillary DCIS. Naked nuclei and tall columnar epithelial cells are frequent. The degree of anisonucleosis and nuclear membrane abnormality varies (Images 8.56 and 8.61).

To assess the distinctive features of papillary carcinoma, Dei Tos and Della-Giustina[72] reported their experience using a multiparametric morphologic analysis. The parameters studied included hypercellularity, cellular dissociation, necrosis, monomorphism, single papillae, three-dimensional aggregates with papillary configuration, low columnar cells, tall columnar cells, naked nuclei, microcalcifications, nuclear pseudoinclusions, hemorrhagic diathesis, cribriform structures, and signs of mucin production. Dei Tos and Della-Giustina found that the majority of aspirates were cellular, with tissue fragments, small clusters of cells, a significant number of single cells, and a hemorrhagic diathesis. Occasionally, necrotic debris was seen in the background. The tumor cell population invariably had a monotonous appearance. The cell population consisted of low to tall columnar cells, single papillae, and three-dimensional aggregates. The papillae were characterized by rich vascularization and the presence of a thin stromal network. Occasionally, the three-dimensional aggregates had a cribriform pattern. Bare nuclei were an infrequent finding. However, when present, they had the same morphology as the nuclei in neoplastic cells. Microcalcification was not an important diagnostic finding. Based on the results of their study, Dei Tos and Della-Giustina[72] suggest that the presence of a monotonous cell population indicates a malignant process. This seems reasonable, since the striking variation in cellular size and shape in benign papillary lesions is believed to be the result of divergent (epithelial and myoepithelial) differentiation.[74]

Some of the above features may also be seen in fibroadenoma or papilloma.[32,69] However, fibroadenomas are more common in younger women and cytologically are characterized by numerous naked nuclei. In addition, the naked nuclei in fibroadenoma are typically smaller than the naked nuclei in papillary carcinoma, which are irregularly rounded and are almost twice the size of those in fibroadenoma (Images 8.62 and 8.63). Furthermore, fibroadenomas do not have the bloody diathesis with hemosiderin-laden macrophages and the tall columnar cells seen in papillary carcinoma.

The distinction between papilloma and papillary carcinoma is difficult and warrants excisional biopsy unless a conclusive diagnosis of cancer can be made by demonstrating a conspicuous number of cytologically malignant single cells with a monotonous pattern (Images 8.64 and 8.65). Diagnostic adjuncts include immunocytochemistry for detection of carcinoembryonic antigen and muscle specific actin, as well as electron microscopy for visualization of intracytoplasmic, neurosecretory-type granules (Image 8.66).[32,64,67–70] Mucin production can sometimes be seen in invasive papillary carcinoma and in micropapillary ductal carcinoma in situ.[75,76] Cytologic distinction between pure papillary ductal carcinoma in situ and intracystic papillary carcinoma in situ is not possible, nor is cytologic distinction between in situ and invasive forms.[72,77]

It should also be remembered that infiltrating duct cell carcinoma may be confused with papillary carcinoma if the malignant component contains cells resembling low columnar cells or if focal papillary formation can be seen. In these circumstances, the near absence of naked nuclei and the presence of a bloody diathesis with hemosiderin-containing macrophages are useful differentiating features.

Cytomorphology of Papillary Carcinoma

Cell-rich aspirate
Bloody background with hemosiderin-containing macrophages and necrotic debris
Papillary clusters of atypical cells enriched by a fibrovascular core
Large, atypical, naked nuclei
Absence of myoepithelial cells
Tall columnar cells

Mucinous (Colloid) Carcinoma

Mucinous carcinoma, also known as colloid, mucoid, gelatinous, and mucin-producing carcinoma, has been recognized since the nineteenth century: by Robinson in 1852,[78] Lavrey in 1853,[79] and Lange in 1896.[80] Subsequently, other investigators demonstrated that mucinous carcinoma has a better prognosis than infiltrating duct cell carcinoma.[81,82] Characteristically, the neoplastic epithelial cells in mucinous carcinoma produce a large amount of extracellular mucus and have a gelatinous appearance.[83] Mucinous carcinomas account for 1% to 6% of all breast carcinomas.[84,85] The tumor affects an older population: the mean age of patients with mucinous carcinoma is over 60 years.[86]

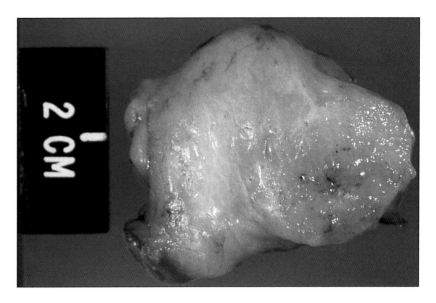

Figure 8.1
Gross appearance of mucinous carcinoma of the breast. Note the tumor's gelatinous quality and the focal hemorrhage.

Grossly, colloid carcinomas are known for their bulky, gelatinous appearance and their soft consistency. They are well circumscribed and vary from 0.5 to 20 cm in size (Figure 8.1). Microscopically, the tumor cells are round and uniform in appearance, with pale cytoplasm and vesicular nuclei. The cells appear in cohesive groups and often demonstrate cribriform patterns, tubules, cords, and papillae. The tumor cell clusters appear to be swimming in lakes of abundant mucin and are connected by delicate bands of fibrovascular connective tissue. Necrosis and calcification are rare, but atypia, mitosis, and signet ring forms may occur (Image 8.67).

Mucinous carcinomas are divided into pure and mixed. This categorization has significant clinical implications because of the favorable prognosis associated with the pure variant. At least 50% of a pure mucinous carcinoma should be extracellular mucin.[87] Infiltrating duct cell carcinoma is the tumor most commonly associated with mucinous carcinoma in mixed variants. Another mucin-producing adenocarcinoma in the breast is signet ring carcinoma. Signet ring carcinomas are associated with a poor prognosis and should be viewed as a separate entity. The majority of tumor cells in signet ring carcinoma show intracytoplasmic mucin production, resulting in the typical signet ring appearance.[88] Electron microscopic study of mucinous carcinoma reveals microvillous cytoplasmic processes, mucin vacuoles, round to pleomorphic dense core granules, and aggregates of intracytoplasmic filaments. Intracytoplasmic lumens are rare, and most of the mucin is extracellular.[89] Colloid carcinomas are often hormone-receptor positive and have a diploid DNA pattern. In contrast, the mixed variety of mucinous carcinoma usually has an aneuploid DNA pattern similar to that of infiltrating duct cell carcinoma.[90,91]

In the pure form of colloid carcinoma, the mucoid, glistening appearance of the aspirated material may be diagnostic.[92,93] The smears show abundant mucin and clusters of relatively small, uniform epithelial cells with bland cytologic features. The mucin appears brightly metachromatic in Diff-Quik® and pale green to yellow in Papanicolaou. Mucin shows positive reactions with periodic acid–Schiff, alcian blue, and mucicarmine (Image 8.68). Against a background of extracellular mucin, the tumor cells appear in three-dimensional clusters, monolayered sheets, or as dissociated groups of cells and isolated cells. The neoplastic cells are relatively uniform and have wispy cytoplasm with ill-defined margins. The nuclei may have a vesicular chromatin pattern with mild anisonucleosis or nuclear irregularity. Macronucleoli and naked nuclei are rare. A slight degree of cytologic atypia in tumor cells of mucinous carcinoma has been reported.[94,95] The cellularity of mucinous carcinoma is variable.[92,93] In hypocellular aspirates, the scanty nature of the cellular material and the bland appearance of the tumor cells may lead to a false-negative diagnosis of malignancy. If extracellular mucinous material is present in the background, the possibility of mucinous carcinoma should be considered (Images 8.69 through 8.72).

Mucinous carcinomas must be distinguished from mucocele-like tumors and myxoid fibroadenomas. Mucocele-like tumor, a rare benign condition of the breast, occurs in premenopausal women.[96] Mucinous carcinoma, in contrast, occurs in postmenopausal women.[86] Thus, extreme caution should be exercised when considering a diagnosis of mucinous carcinoma in a premenopausal woman. Mucocele-like tumors can also be distinguished from hypocellular variants of mucinous carcinoma by the types of cells embedded in the mucus. In mucocele-like tumors both epithelial and myoepithelial cells are present, whereas in mucinous carcinomas only epithelial cells are seen. Immunostaining for muscle specific actin easily demonstrates the presence of myoepithelial cells in mucocele-like tumors.

Cytologically, mucocele-like tumors display abundant mucin and a few clusters and sheets of regular epithelium that lack nuclear atypia. No intact single cells are present (Images 8.73 and 8.74).[97,98] Mucocele-like lesions can be associated with ductal hyperplasia or breast carcinoma. In a recent study reported by Hamele-Bern et al,[99] the neoplastic component in these lesions was micropapillary duct cell carcinoma in situ or mucinous carcinoma. There was no significant difference in patient age, tumor size, bilaterality, or patient outcome. Mucocele-like tumors with carcinomas differed from those with no malignancy only in their more prominent calcification, which led to earlier detection by mammography.

Another differential diagnosis is fibroadenoma with myxoid stroma, which may mimic the appearance of mucus. Clues to the correct diagnosis are young age of the patient and the presence of two cell populations, bare nuclei, and antler horns in fibroadenoma. Nuclei are reportedly significantly larger in mucinous carcinoma than in benign lesions of the breast.[100]

Colloid carcinomas are well-circumscribed lesions and should be distinguished from poorly defined, high-grade, mucin-producing infiltrating duct cell carcinomas. In mixed mucinous carcinomas, cytologic features of both mucinous and infiltrating duct cell carcinomas are present. In both the pure and the mixed form of mucinous carcinoma, mucin is the essential ingredient for diagnosis. Based on a comparative cytologic study of mucinous breast carcinoma and mixed mucinous infiltrating duct cell carcinoma, Stanley et al[101] suggested that necrosis, a scant amount of mucin, and one or more smears totally without mucin are features indicative of a mixed form of mucinous carcinoma. Features indicative of pure mucinous carcinoma included abundant mucin in all smears and absence of pleomorphism or necrosis. Stanley et al also suggested that cases that are not typical of either pure mucinous carcinoma or a mixed form of mucinous carcinoma should be designated carcinoma with a mucinous component.[100,101]

Cytomorphology of Mucinous Carcinoma
Variable cellularity
Abundant mucin
Tumor cells isolated and in clusters, often with insignificant atypia
Occasional signet ring cells
Fragments of stroma with small blood vessels

Signet Ring Carcinoma

Signet ring carcinomas account for 2% to 4% of all breast carcinomas and occur in patients in their mid to late fifties.[102,103] Signet ring carcinoma was classified by Saphir[104] as an unusual variant of mucinous carcinoma. However, these two lesions are not only morphologically different but show a significant difference in clinical behavior. Signet ring carcinomas have also been described as a variant of infiltrating lobular carcinoma.[105] Since the in situ phase associated with signet ring carcinoma may be lobular or ductal, the exact origin of the tumor remains controversial. However, because the presence of signet ring cells in a carcinoma appears to make the lesion behave more aggressively, signet ring carcinoma should be regarded as a high-risk carcinoma.[54]

The criteria for diagnosis of pure signet ring carcinoma vary. The reported series include tumors in which more than 90% of cells were signet rings and a variety of carcinomas, ranging from tumors in which 20 signet ring cells per high-power field were seen in multiple foci to tumors in which signet ring cells composed 20% or more of the carcinoma (Image 8.75).[3,54] In our experience, fine needle aspirates of signet ring carcinoma are characterized by a moderate to rich cellular yield. The cells are arranged singly or in small, loose groups. The cells are predominantly small, with crescent-shaped nuclei compressed to the cell periphery by mucin (Images 8.76 and 8.77).

The differential diagnosis includes metastatic carcinoma, most likely from the gastrointestinal tract; infiltrating lobular carcinoma; secretory carcinoma; and lipid-secreting carcinoma. Metastatic carcinoma should be excluded by obtaining detailed clinical information and employing ancillary studies such as immunocytochemistry and electron microscopy. For example, immunostaining for gross cystic disease fluid protein–15 (GCDFP-15) has been found to be a sensitive marker for primary signet ring carcinoma of the breast (Image 8.78).[106]

Infiltrating lobular carcinomas contain cells other than the signet rings that may display the characteristic Indian file pattern. The cytologic features of secretory carcinoma include numerous large, branching sheets of neoplastic cells with cytoplasmic vacuoles and extracellular lumens. The background shows erythrocytes, cellular debris, and a large number of round, naked nuclei. Tumor cells vary in size, with moderate to abundant granular or lacy cytoplasm. Numerous signet ring cells may also be seen intermingled with the tumor cells. However, a background with tumor diathesis and multivacuolated lacy elements is not a feature of signet ring carcinoma (Images 8.79 and 8.80).[107-109] Secretory carcinoma is associated with good prognosis in children and adolescents. For young patients, local excision is considered adequate to control the disease. In contrast, secretory carcinoma in adults should be treated like any other primary carcinoma because of the high incidence of nodal metastasis associated with the tumor.[110,111] Signet ring carcinoma should be distinguished from lipid-secreting or lipid-rich carcinoma, which contains abundant intracytoplasmic lipid material but does not contain PAS-positive secretions. The presence of lipid material can be easily demonstrated on air-dried smears and by the use of oil red O staining.[112]

Cytomorphology of Signet Ring Carcinoma
Moderate to rich cellular yield
Small- to medium-sized cells, isolated or in clusters
Crescent-shaped nuclei with mucin-filled cytoplasmic vacuoles

Medullary Carcinoma

In 1945, Geschikter[113] defined medullary carcinoma as a specific entity. He concluded that despite its size and microscopic appearance, medullary carcinoma is associated with an excellent prognosis. This observation was supported by Moore and Foote[114] in 1949. Medullary carcinomas account for 5% to 7% of all breast carcinomas and occur in patients between 21 and 95 years old, with a mean of 50 years.[115-117] Medullary carcinoma presents as a well-defined, soft lesion and may resemble a fibroadenoma clinically and mammographically. Grossly, medullary carcinoma is fleshy and bulges out on cut section, in contrast to scirrhous carcinoma, which has a shrunken appearance on cut section.

Microscopically, medullary carcinoma is characterized by a syncytial growth pattern in which anastomosing cords and sheets are separated by small amounts of loose connective tissue and surrounded by a lymphoplasmacytic infiltrate (Image 8.81). This syncytial pattern characterizes 75% of the tumor.[118] The tumor cells are large and pleomorphic, with abundant cytoplasm, vesicular nuclei, and one or multiple prominent nucleoli. Abnormal mitoses are frequent, and in 10% of cases multinucleated giant cells are seen. Necrosis may be present and form a cyst in the center of the tumor.[119,120] Rarely, a granulomatous reaction may occur in the stroma.[121] Up to two thirds of medullary carcinomas are hormone-receptor negative. Despite their favorable prognosis, medullary carcinomas usually have an aneuploid DNA pattern.[122,123]

Ultrastructural studies do not show any pathognomonic features in medullary carcinoma.[124] Tumor cells have the same morphologic characteristics seen in tissue sections. The tumor cells have generous amounts of homogeneous cytoplasm and nuclei that vary in size, with nuclear membrane abnormalities and conspicuous macronucleoli. Bizarre naked nuclei are frequent, and numerous lymphocytes and plasma cells are present.

Aspirates of medullary carcinoma are generally cellular, with a necrotic background, many highly neoplastic epithelial cells, and numerous lymphocytes and plasma cells. In some cases, the smears may show predominantly lymphoid elements; in others, clumps of malignant epithelial cells are surrounded by a few lymphoid and plasma cells (Images 8.82 through 8.86). The differential diagnosis includes poorly differentiated duct cell carcinoma with lymphocytic infiltrate and malignant lymphoma.[125]

Aspirates of duct cell carcinoma commonly show a single cell pattern and/or several multilayered, dyshesive aggregates rather than the mono-layered syncytia seen in medullary carcinoma. In duct cell carcinoma the cells are smaller, with less cytoplasm and no bizarre naked nuclei. To avoid a false-negative diagnosis of a cystic lesion, look closely for the occasional tumor cells, which tend to be obscured by the inflammatory cells in the background. Cytocentrifugation and cell block preparation of the cyst fluid may help to concentrate the diluted tumor cells.[120] Malignant lymphomas are characterized by a monomorphic pattern with no accompanying malignant epithelial cells. Immunophenotypic analysis of aspirated material by either flow cytometry or immunocytochemistry may substantiate the correct diagnosis.

Cytomorphology of Medullary Carcinoma
Cellular smear
Necrotic background
Pleomorphic cells isolated and in syncytial aggregates
Abundant cytoplasm with marked nuclear abnormalities
Bizarre naked nuclei
Occasional multinucleation
Lymphocytes and plasma cells

Mammary Carcinoma With Carcinoid Features

First described by Feyrter and Hartman in 1963,[126] mammary carcinoma with carcinoid features, also known as mammary carcinoid or argyrophilic carcinoma, constitutes approximately 5% of all breast carcinomas.[127] Considered a variant of conventional breast carcinoma, mammary carcinoma with carcinoid features has a distinct morphology, histochemistry, and prognosis.[128–130]

Clinically, as with other cancers, patients present with a breast mass with no manifestations of carcinoid syndrome. Mammary carcinoma with carcinoid features is associated with a higher incidence of bilaterality and rarely occurs in men.[127,129,131] The overall prognosis for mammary carcinoma with carcinoid features appears to be comparable to that for other primary breast carcinomas. Some authors further classify neuroendocrine tumors of the breast into several subtypes with different prognoses.[132] In individual cases, however, the biologic behavior of this tumor may be unpredictable. Features such as tumor size, mitotic activity, cell morphology, and presence or absence of necrosis have been found to influence the behavior of this tumor.[133]

The histologic features are typical of a carcinoid tumor supported by a delicate fibrovascular stroma, with tumor cells arranged in a variety of patterns, including solid nests, ribbon-like tubular and glandular configurations, and cribriform-like arrangements. The tumor cells contain uniform, round to oval nuclei with a fine chromatin pattern and occasional nucleoli. They may show positive immunostaining reactions to antibodies against serotonin, neuron-specific enolase, chromogranin, and norepinephrine. They are also hormone-receptor positive. Ultrastructurally, the tumor cells contain membrane-bound, dense core neurosecretory granules in the cytoplasm.[90,129,134,135]

The cytologic features of mammary carcinoma with carcinoid features are well documented.[135,136–139] The smears are characteristically cell rich, with cells predominantly in a dispersed pattern. The neoplastic cells are small and uniform and have regular, round to oval nuclei with moderately abundant cytoplasm. The nuclei are frequently eccentric, and the cytoplasm may contain granules. No necrotic background has been reported (Images 8.87 through 8.90).

The differential diagnosis of mammary carcinoma with carcinoid features includes carcinoid tumor metastatic to the breast, infiltrating lobular carcinoma, and non-Hodgkin's lymphoma of the breast. Although extremely rare, carcinoid tumor metastatic to the breast has been reported.[140,141] Morphologic distinction between a primary carcinoid tumor and a metastatic lesion is not possible (Figure 8.2 and Images 8.91 through 8.93). However, since primary mammary carcinoma with carcinoid features is argentaffin negative, whenever neoplastic cells from a breast tumor with carcinoid features are shown to contain argentaffin granules, the diagnosis of carcinoid tumor metastatic to the breast should be considered.[141] In addition, careful attention should be given to the patient's medical history and the laboratory findings. The small size and plasmacytoid appearance of the neoplastic cells seen in mammary carcinoma with carcinoid features may closely resemble the appearance of neoplastic cells in lobular carcinoma of the breast. However, lobular carcinomas typically have a lower cell yield, with tumor cells that are more pleomorphic. The nuclei in lobular carcinoma are more hyperchromatic and do not have a stippled chromatin pattern. Cytoplasmic granules are absent in lobular carcinoma. In addition, lobular carcinoma may contain mucin-positive intracytoplasmic vacuoles and may have an Indian file pattern.

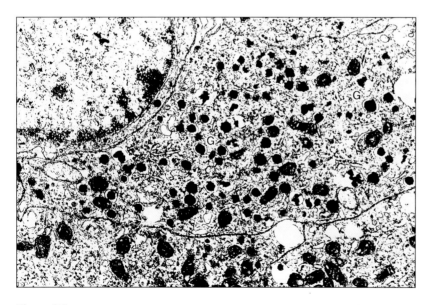

Figure 8.2
Electron microscopic picture of a carcinoid tumor shows numerous membrane-bound granules (G) with acinar central cores and electron-lucent halos (18,200X).

Mammary carcinoma with carcinoid features may also resemble non-Hodgkin's malignant lymphoma of the breast. Primary lymphoma of the breast, a form of extranodal non-Hodgkin's lymphoma, is well-recognized.[142-144] Cytologically, primary lymphoma is characterized by a monotonous population of atypical lymphoid cells with scant cytoplasm. In contrast to carcinoid tumors, the nuclei in malignant lymphomas are hyperchromatic, often irregular, and display a coarse, granular chromatin pattern. Immunophenotypic analysis of aspirates via flow cytometry or immunocytochemistry facilitates differentiation between malignant lymphoma and mammary carcinoma with carcinoid features.

Cytomorphology of Mammary Carcinoma With Carcinoid Features
Rich cellularity
Dispersed cell pattern with occasional acinus-like clusters
Uniform cells with eccentric nuclei and granular cytoplasm
Fine, stippled chromatin pattern

Intracystic Carcinoma

Intracystic carcinoma is a rare breast tumor accompanying 0.7% of all breast carcinomas. It most frequently occurs in elderly, obese black women, with bloody nipple discharge as the only presenting symptom. This tumor should be suspected clinically if a cystic lesion is seen in a postmenopausal woman not taking estrogen. Radiologically, it appears as a sharply circumscribed cystic mass that persists following fine needle aspiration biopsy (Figure 8.3). The smears are cellular, with a hemorrhagic background.

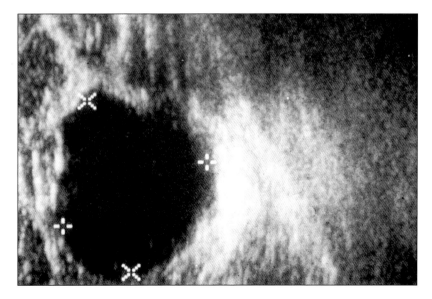

Figure 8.3
Ultrasound demonstration of a cystic lesion characteristically seen in intracystic carcinoma. Reproduced with permission from: Silverman J, Masood S, Ducatman B, et al: Can FNA biopsy separate atypical hyperplasia, carcinoma in situ and invasive carcinoma of the breast? Cytomorphologic criteria and limitations in diagnosis. *Diagn Cytopathol* 9:713–728, 1993.

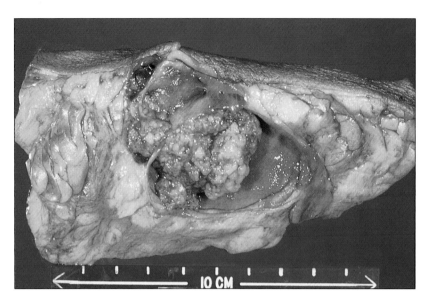

Figure 8.4
Photograph of a surgically resected breast lesion with macroscopic features of intracystic carcinoma.

Loosely arranged atypical cells in a monomorphic pattern are intermingled with papillary clusters and/or cribriform configurations and numerous single epithelial cells (Figure 8.4 and Images 8.94 through 8.96). The tumor cells are cuboidal or columnar and are often aneuploid. Thus, DNA ploidy study of cells obtained from the bloody cyst fluid of a postmenopausal woman can assist in confirming a diagnosis of malignancy.[145,146]

Cytomorphology of Intracystic Carcinoma
Cellular aspirates
Hemorrhagic background with hemosiderin-containing macrophages or foamy cells
Monomorphic cell population in clusters and dispersed
Mild to moderate pleomorphism
Absence of naked nuclei
Papillary and/or cribriform pattern

Image 8.1
Fine needle aspiration biopsy of infiltrating duct cell carcinoma, scirrhous type. Low magnification reveals only a few clusters of epithelial cells (Diff-Quik, 200X).

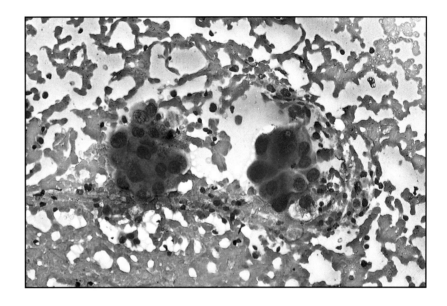

Image 8.2
Higher magnification of the same case reveals a cluster of atypical epithelial cells (Diff-Quik, 400X).

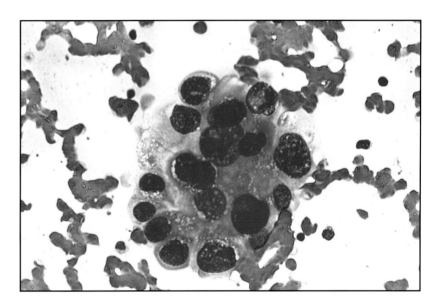

Image 8.3
Papanicolaou-stained smear of the same case demonstrates significant hyperchromasia, anisonucleosis, and a lack of myoepithelial cells (400X).

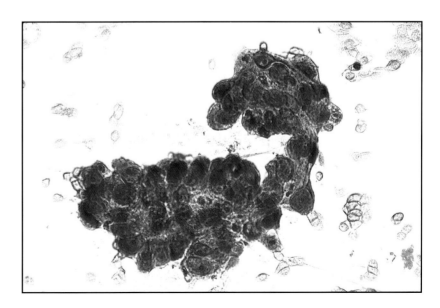

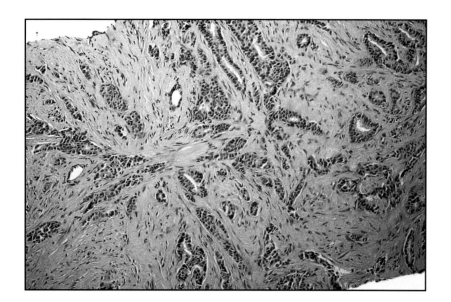

Image 8.4
Corresponding tissue section diagnosed as infiltrating duct cell carcinoma, scirrhous type (H&E, 200X).

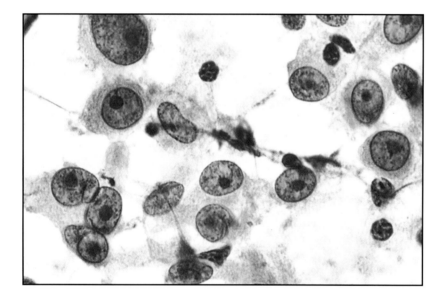

Image 8.5
Infiltrating duct cell carcinoma not otherwise specified (NOS). Direct smear shows conspicuous loss of cellular cohesion, anisonucleosis, and macronucleoli (H&E, 400X).

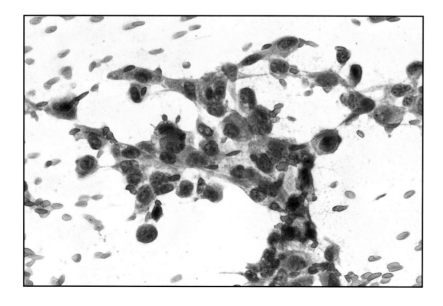

Image 8.6
Papanicolaou stain of another case of duct cell carcinoma NOS demonstrates a loosely arranged cell pattern and conspicuous pleomorphism (200X).

Image 8.7
Higher magnification of the same case shows loss of polarity, with scattered, isolated cells; anisonucleosis; and hyperchromasia (Papanicolaou, 400X).

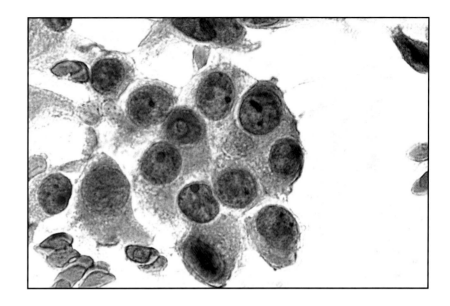

Image 8.8
Corresponding surgically excised lesion of the same case (H&E, 400X).

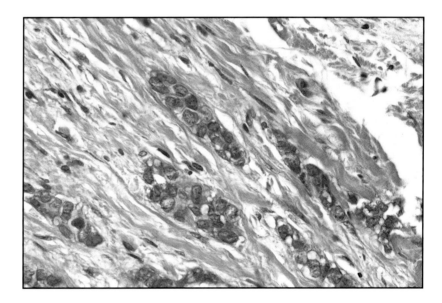

Image 8.9
Neoplastic cells in an aspirate diagnosed as poorly differentiated infiltrating duct cell carcinoma with necrotic background (Papanicolaou, 400X).

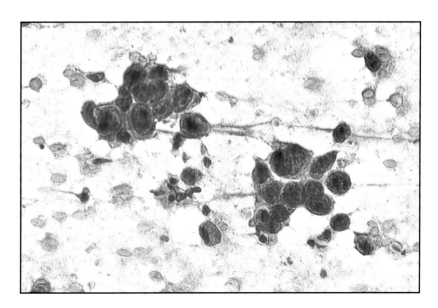

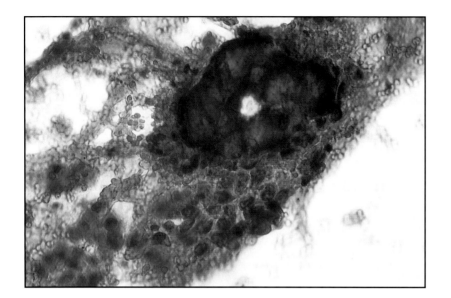

Image 8.10
Red blood cells and microcalcified particles in an aspirate of duct cell carcinoma (Papanicolaou, 400X).

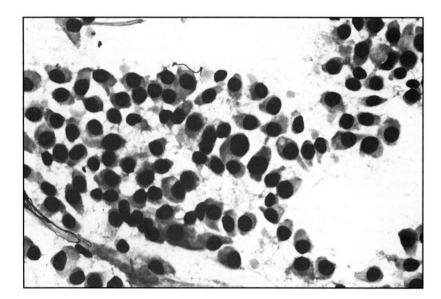

Image 8.11
Small cell variant of duct cell carcinoma yields a cellular aspirate with a dispersed cell pattern and eccentric nuclei (Diff-Quik, 200X).

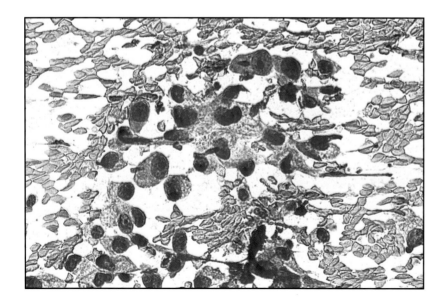

Image 8.12
Papanicolaou-stained slide of the same case demonstrates similar features (200X).

Image 8.13
Corresponding tissue section with the characteristic features of the small cell variant of duct cell carcinoma (H&E, 400X).

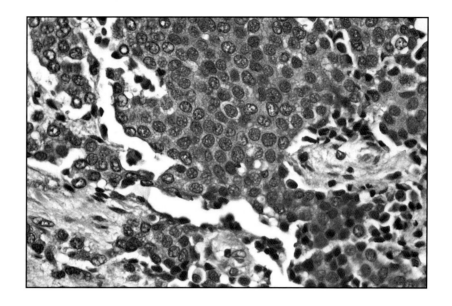

Image 8.14
Diff-Quik stain of an infiltrating duct cell carcinoma shows pleomorphism and multinucleated tumor cells (1000X).

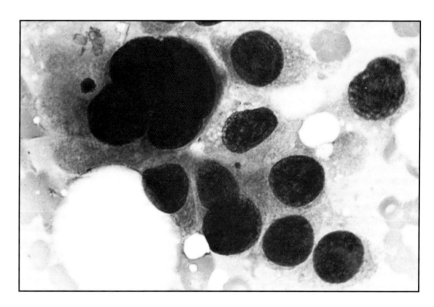

Image 8.15
Papanicolaou-stained smear of the same case demonstrates neoplastic mononuclear cells and tumor giant cells (200X).

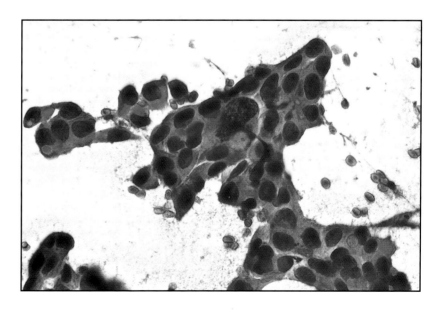

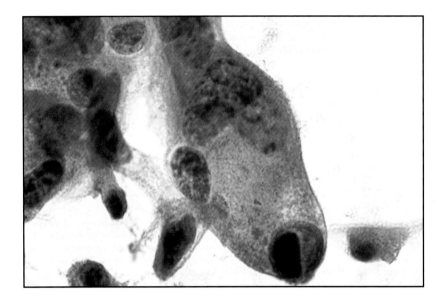

Image 8.16
Higher magnification of the same features shown in Image 8.15 (Papanicolaou, 1000X).

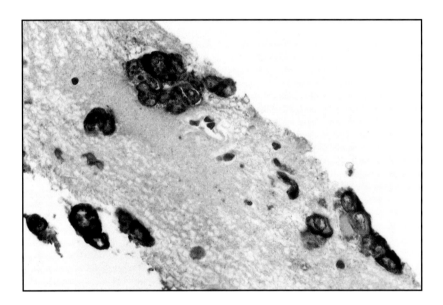

Image 8.17
Cell block preparation of the infiltrating duct cell carcinoma shown in Images 8.14–8.16. Positive expression for epithelial membrane antigen confirms the epithelial nature of the lesion (200X).

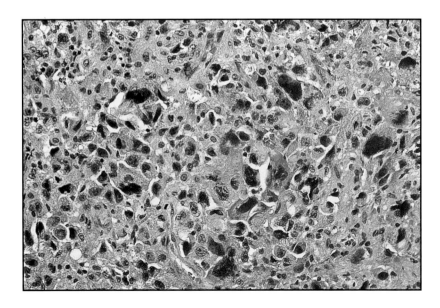

Image 8.18
Corresponding surgically excised lesion in the same case shows poorly differentiated carcinoma with marked pleomorphism (H&E, 400X).

Image 8.19
Another view demonstrates the presence of giant cells similar to those seen in the original aspirate (Images 8.14–8.17) (H&E, 400X).

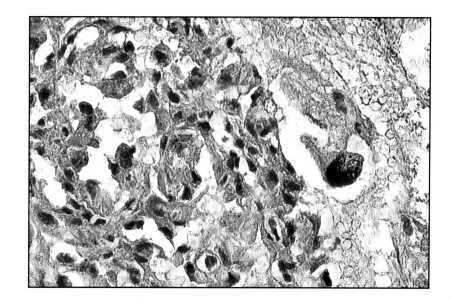

Image 8.20
Positive immunostaining for epithelial membrane antigen in tissue section of the same case (400X).

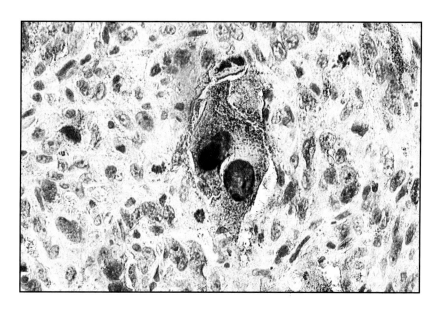

Image 8.21
Low cell yield in an aspirate of infiltrating lobular carcinoma (Diff-Quik, 200X).

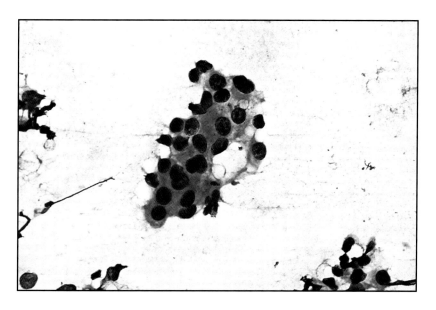

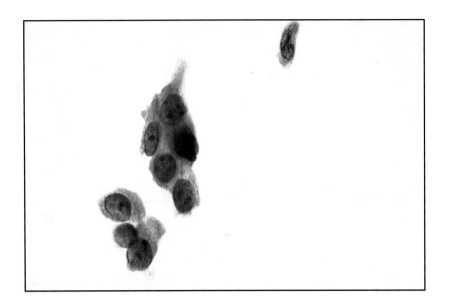

Image 8.22
Different view of the same case shows sparse cell clusters composed of uniform small cells with regular nuclei (Papanicolaou, 400X).

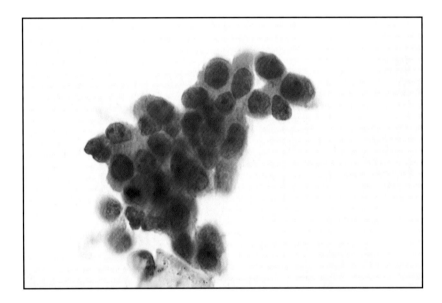

Image 8.23
Another cluster of small cells in the same case reveals regular, round nuclei with a fine chromatin pattern. Note the absence of myoepithelial cells (Papanicolaou, 400X).

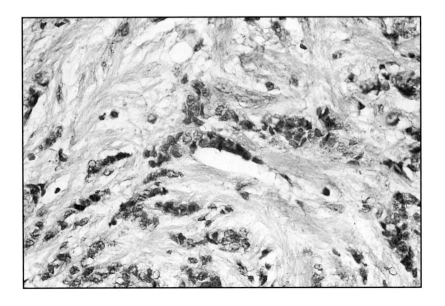

Image 8.24
Corresponding surgically resected specimen, diagnosed as infiltrating lobular carinoma (H&E, 400X).

Image 8.25
Moderately cellular aspirate of infiltrating lobular carcinoma shows small cells with hyperchromatic, eccentric nuclei (Papanicolaou, 200X).

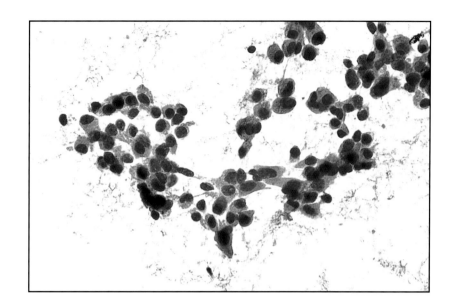

Image 8.26
Different view of the same case reveals a necrotic background, nuclear molding, and small cells forming strands (Papanicolaou, 200X).

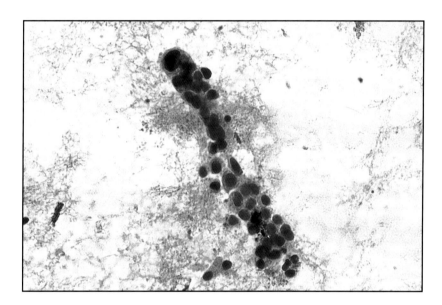

Image 8.27
Tumor cells from the same case in chains and strands with conspicuous nuclear molding (Papanicolaou, 200X).

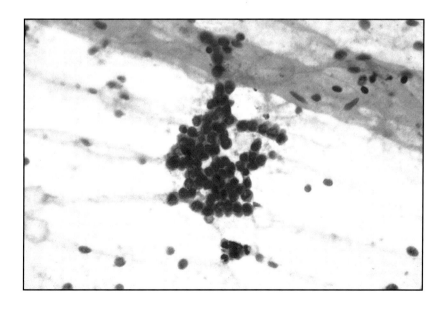

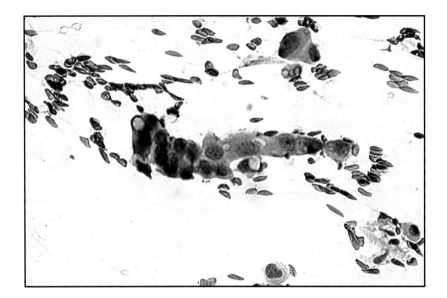

Image 8.28
Indian file pattern and intracytoplasmic lumens characteristic of lobular carcinoma (Papanicolaou, 400X).

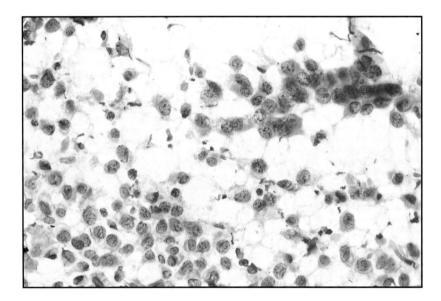

Image 8.29
Cellular smear of a breast lesion diagnosed histologically as pleomorphic lobular carcinoma (Papanicolaou, 200X).

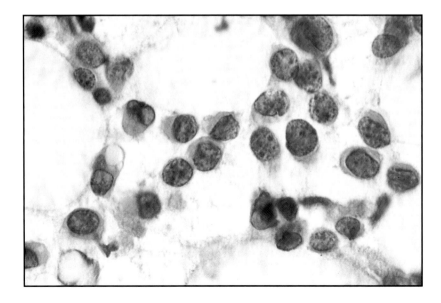

Image 8.30
Higher magnification of the same case shows cells isolated and in small groups. The cells are typically larger than those in classic infiltrating lobular carcinoma and have cytoplasmic vacuoles (Papanicolaou, 200X). Reproduced with permission from: Masood S: Cytomorphology of fibrocystic change, high risk and premalignant breast lesions. *Breast J* 1:210–221, 1995.

Image 8.31
In contrast to classic infiltrating lobular carcinoma, variation in nuclear size and nuclear membrane irregularity in pleomorphic lobular carcinoma can simulate duct cell carcinoma (Papanicolaou, 400X).

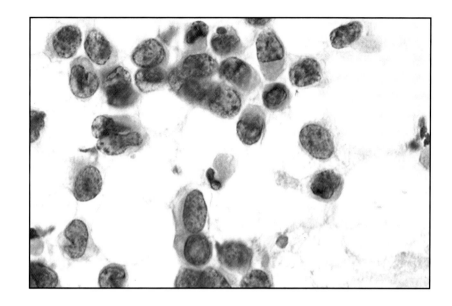

Image 8.32
Single files of cells suggest a diagnosis of lobular carcinoma (Papanicolaou, 400X). Reproduced with permission from: Masood S: Cytomophology of fibrocystic change, high risk and pre-malignant breast lesions. *Breast J* 1:210–221, 1995.

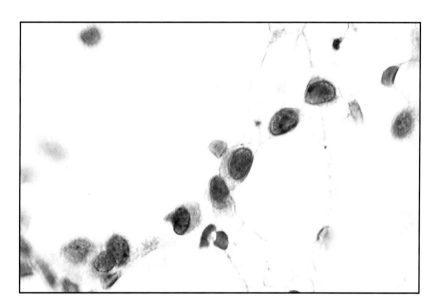

Image 8.33
Corresponding tissue section demonstrates variation in nuclear size (H&E, 400X).

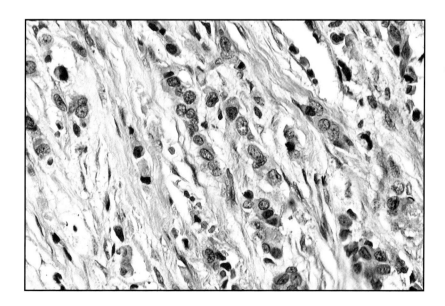

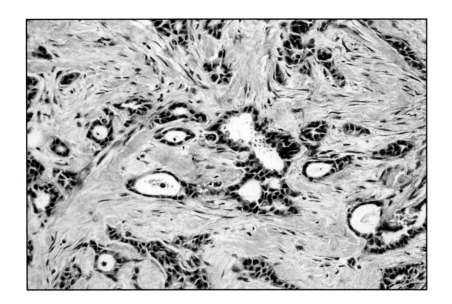

Image 8.34
Microscopic section of tubular carcinoma shows glandular structures with open lumens. Some glands are pointed and appear to split the dense, fibroelastic stroma. The lumens are lined by a single layer of epithelial cells (H&E, 200X).

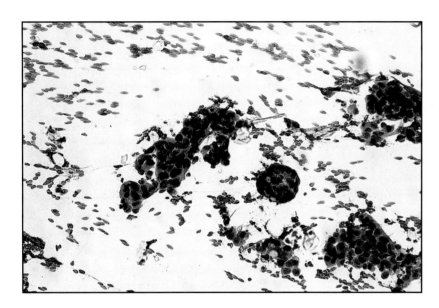

Image 8.35
Low-power magnification of an aspirate of tubular carcinoma of the breast shows cohesive clusters of epithelial cells (Papanicolaou, 100X).

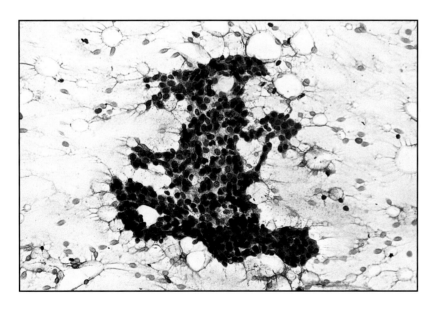

Image 8.36
A complex tubular structure with an open lumen and a blunted, angular structure in the same case shown in Images 8.34 and 8.35 (Papanicolaou, 200X).

Image 8.37
Slender, tubular epithelial clusters against a littered background (Papanicolaou, 200X).

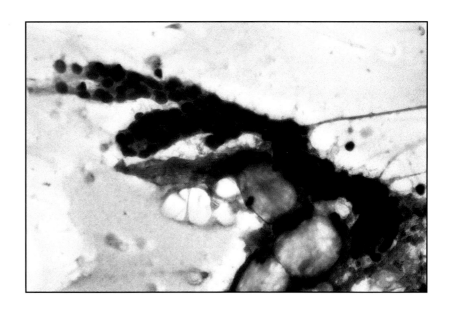

Image 8.38
Tubular structure with adjacent dense connective tissue and rare naked nuclei in the background (Papanicolaou, 400X).

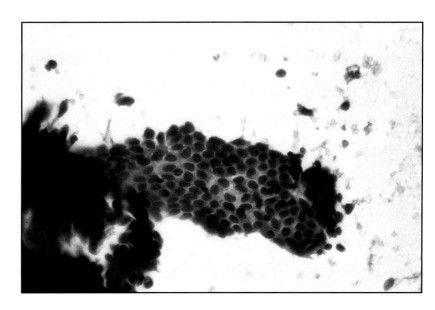

Image 8.39
An isolated tubular structure shows polarity of epithelial cells with minimal nuclear atypia (Papanicolaou, 400X).

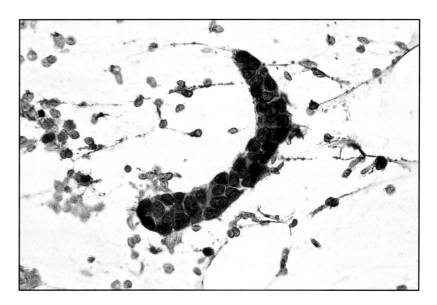

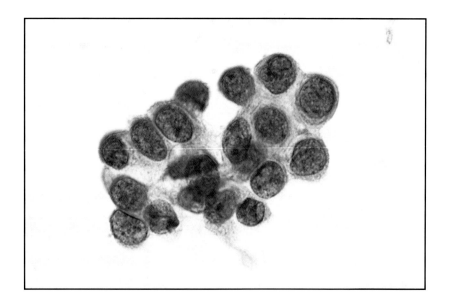

Image 8.40
A cluster of epithelial cells with uniform nuclei and small nucleoli (Papanicolaou, 400X).

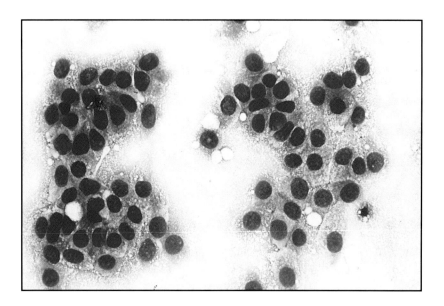

Image 8.41
Diff Quik–stained aspirate of tubular carcinoma shows loosely cohesive cells (200X).

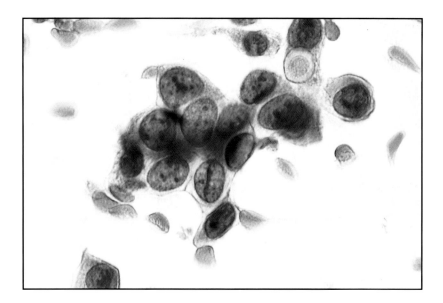

Image 8.42
Higher magnification demonstrates nuclear grooves and solitary intracytoplasmic vacuoles (Papanicolaou, 400X).

Image 8.43
Fibrillary material corresponding to the elastic material often seen in tubular carcinoma (Papanicolaou, 200X).

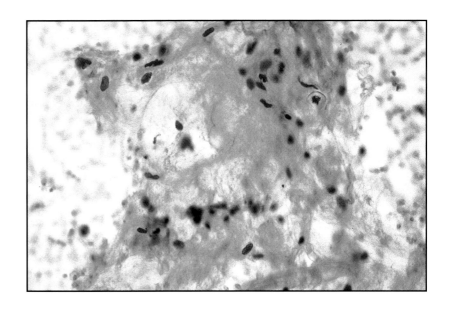

Image 8.44
Tissue section of a radial scar with areas of atypical ductal hyperplasia (H&E, 100X).

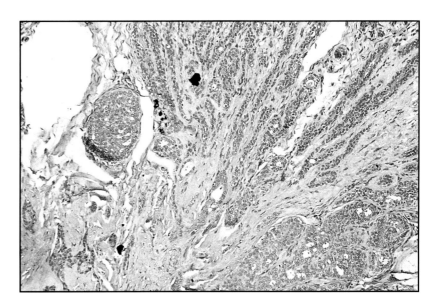

Image 8.45
Higher magnification demonstrates hyperplastic areas (H&E, 400X).

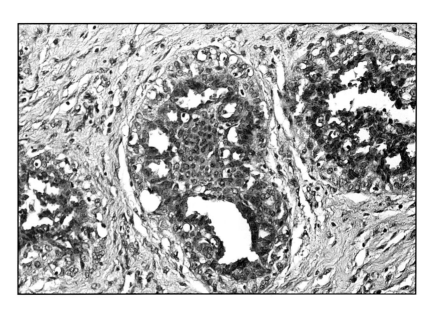

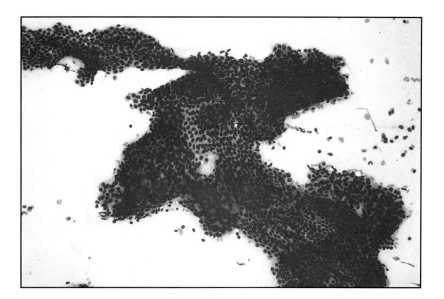

Image 8.46
Cellular aspirate of the same case shows exuberant clusters not typically seen in radial scar (Diff-Quik, 100X).

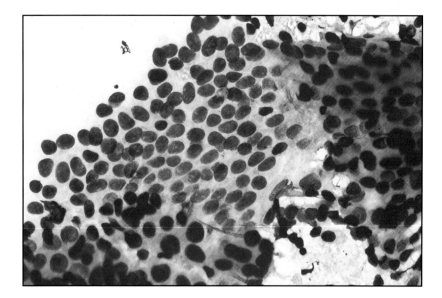

Image 8.47
Higher magnification of the same case demonstrates focal loss of polarity with conspicuous anisonucleosis (Diff–Quik, 400X).

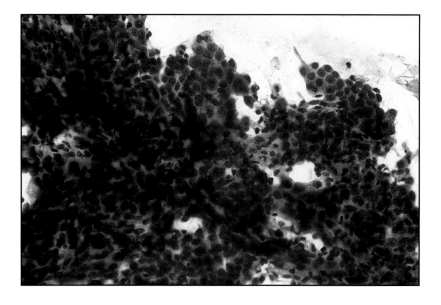

Image 8.48
Papanicolaou-stained smear of the same case shows crowded clusters of epithelial cells with overriding of the nuclei and a cribriform-like pattern (200X).

Image 8.49
Higher magnification of the same case shows focal loss of cellular cohesion, anisonucleosis, and micronucleoli, features not typically seen in radial scar (Papanicolaou, 400X).

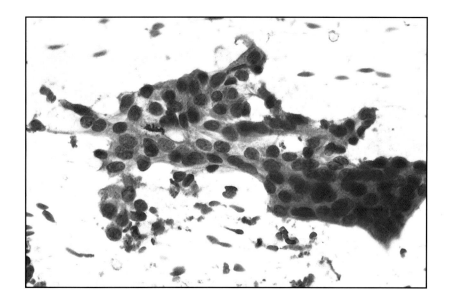

Image 8.50
Another view of the same case of radial scar: nuclear enlargement, anisonucleosis, and nucleoli with a few spindle cells featuring myoepithelial cells (Papanicolaou, 400X).

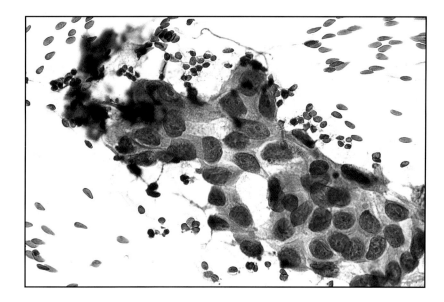

Image 8.51
A reticulated pattern of immunostaining for muscle-specific actin confirms the presence of myoepithelial cells in a histologically proven radial scar with areas of atypical hyperplasia (Immunoperoxidase, 400X).

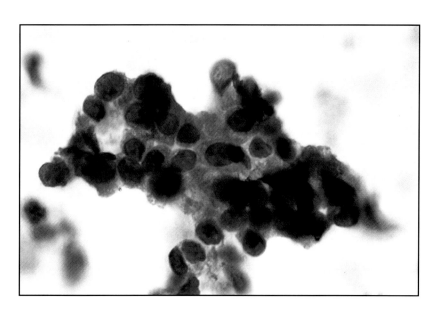

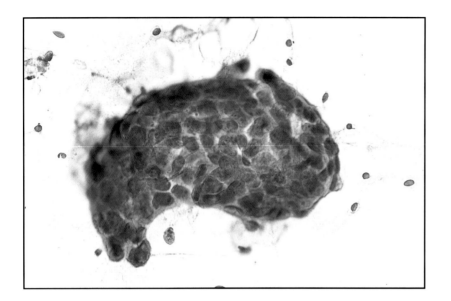

Image 8.52
The absence of myoepithelial cells within the clusters of epithelial cells and the distinctly enlarged yet uniform nuclei distinguish tubular carcinoma from fibroadenoma (Papanicolaou, 400X).

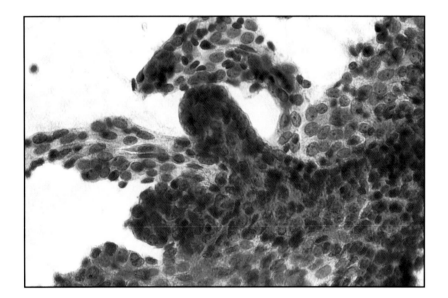

Image 8.53
Myoepithelial cells admixed with an epithelial component and small nucleoli in a fibroadenoma (Papanicolaou, 200X).

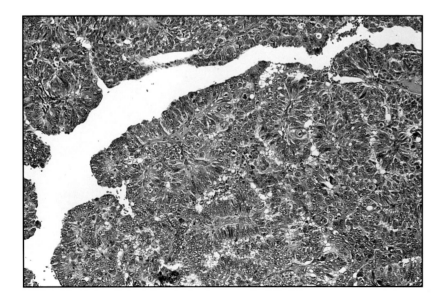

Image 8.54
Tissue section demonstrates atypical papillary structures surrounding vascular cores in papillary carcinoma (H&E, 100X).

Image 8.55
Higher magnification of the same case shows papillary fronds with a vascular core and neoplastic epithelial cells (H&E, 200X).

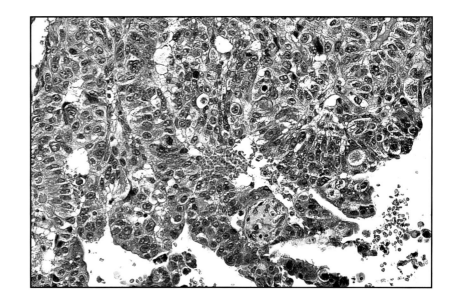

Image 8.56
Cellular smear of the same case of papillary carcinoma shows fibrovascular cores surrounded by papillary fronds (Papanicolaou, 100X).

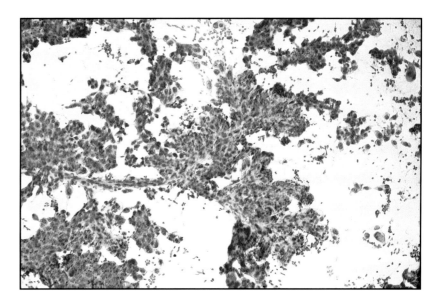

Image 8.57
Higher magnification of the same case shows a hemorrhagic background with a monotonous population of atypical epithelial cells isolated and in clusters (Papanicolaou, 200X).

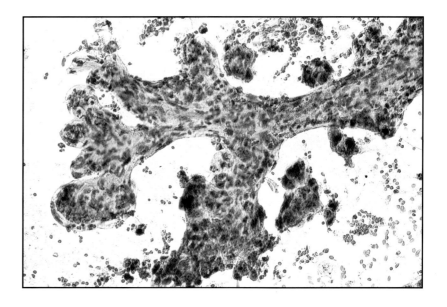

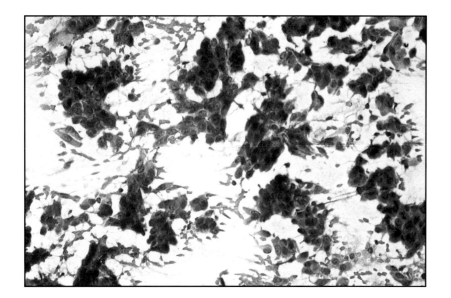

Image 8.58
Another case of papillary carcinoma, rich in cellularity with papillae of various sizes (Papanicolaou, 100X).

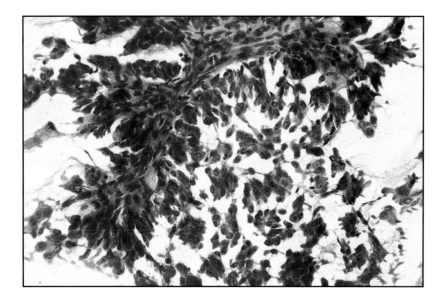

Image 8.59
Higher magnification of the same case shows a vascular core with attached papillary fronds resembling a waterfall (Papanicolaou, 200X).

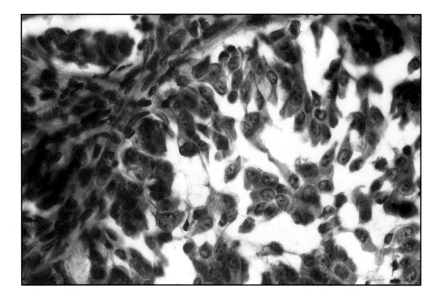

Image 8.60
Higher magnification of the same case shows papillae of various sizes and isolated atypical cells with a tall columnar appearance (Papanicolaou, 400X).

Image 8.61
Another view of papillary carcinoma: a cluster of neoplastic columnar cells with nuclear pseudoinclusions (Papanicolaou, 1000X).

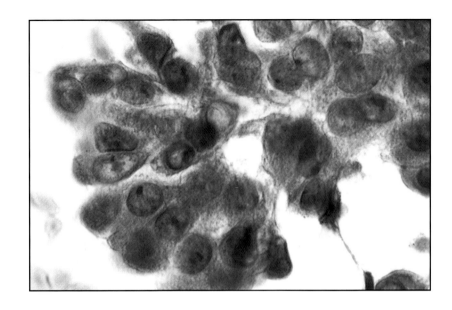

Image 8.62
Papillary carcinoma: a monotonous cell population with a few large naked nuclei in the background (Papanicolaou, 200X).

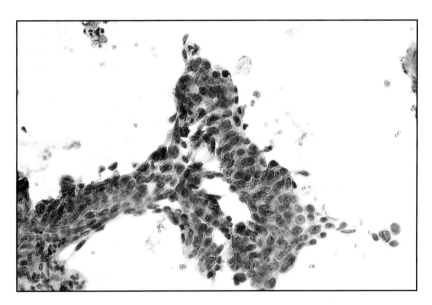

Image 8.63
In contrast to papillary carcinoma, the naked nuclei in fibroadenoma are small (Diff-Quik, 200X).

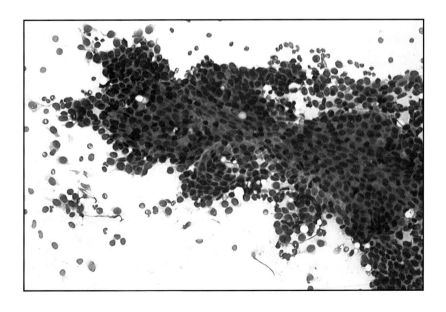

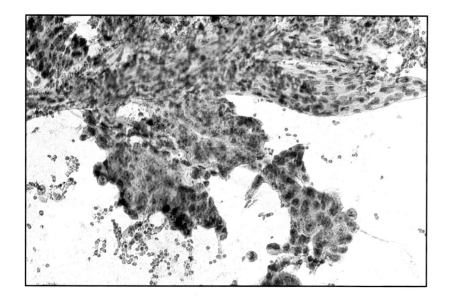

Image 8.64
Population of one cell type with a papillary configuration characteristic of papillary carcinoma (Papanicolaou, 200X).

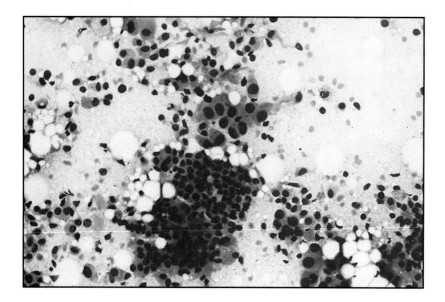

Image 8.65
Several cell types with a heterogeneous pattern, a feature that distinguishes papilloma (shown here) from papillary carcinoma (Diff-Quik, 200X).

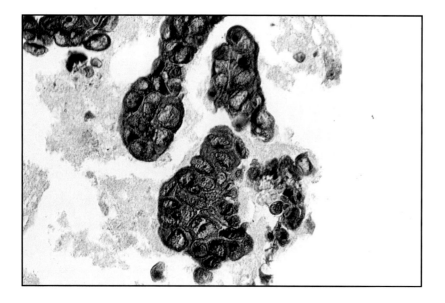

Image 8.66
Positive immunostaining for carcinoembryonic antigen is characteristic of papillary carcinoma (Immunoperoxidase, 400X).

Image 8.67
Tissue section from a case of mucinous carcinoma (H&E, 400X).

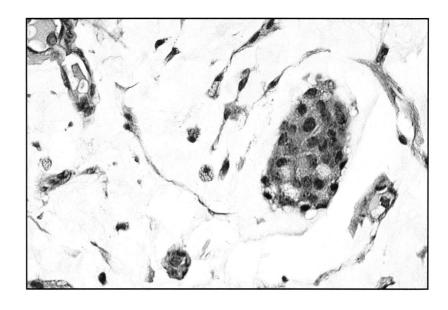

Image 8.68
Smear of colloid carcinoma with extracellular mucin and clustering of epithelial cells (Mucicarmine, 200X).

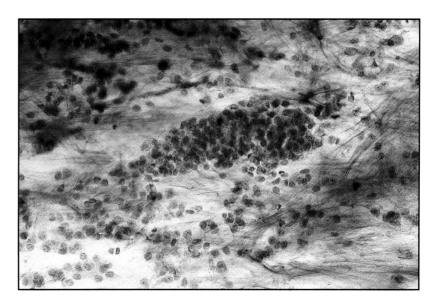

Image 8.69
Dispersed cell pattern seen in a smear of a colloid carcinoma with abundant extracellular mucin (Papanicolaou, 100X).

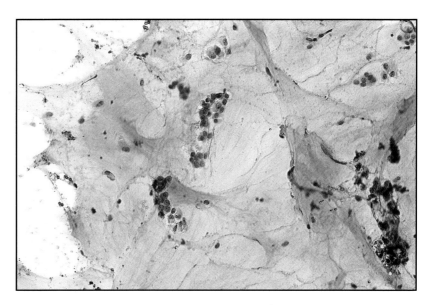

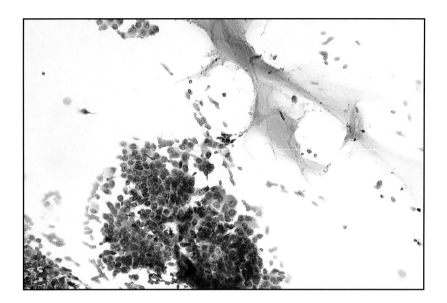

Image 8.70
Papanicolaou-stained smear of a colloid carcinoma with clusters of tightly packed epithelial cells in a mucinous background (200X).

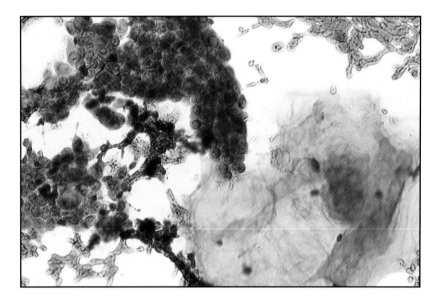

Image 8.71
Higher magnification of the same case shows a cluster of epithelial cells with minimal atypia (Papanicolaou, 400X).

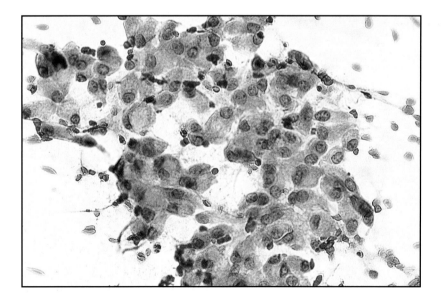

Image 8.72
Cell block preparation of colloid carcinoma with occasional signet ring formation (H&E, 400X).

Image 8.73
Smear of a mucocele-like lesion shows ductal cells scattered and in clusters with collections of mucoid material (Papanicolaou, 200X) (courtesy of Nour Sneige, MD).

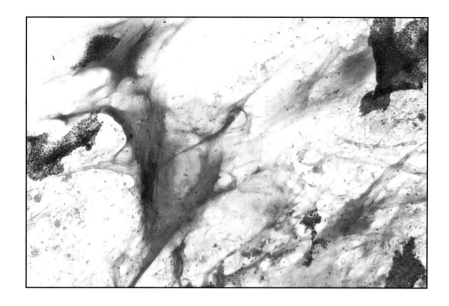

Image 8.74
Corresponding tissue sections diagnosed as mucocele (H&E, 200X) (courtesy of Nour Sneige, MD).

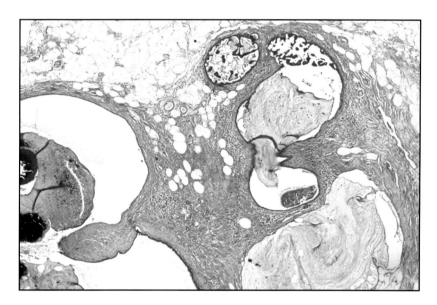

Image 8.75
Tissue section of a signet ring carcinoma: most of the neoplastic cell population exhibits a signet ring pattern (H&E, 1000X).

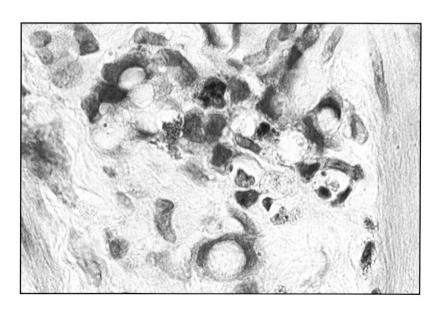

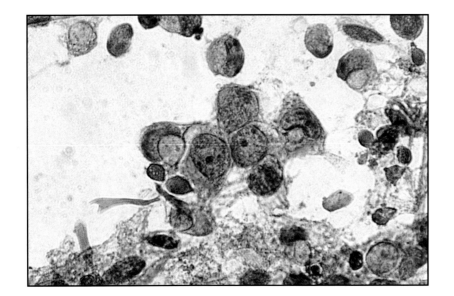

Image 8.76
Cellular aspirate of a signet ring cell carcinoma (Papanicolaou, 400X).

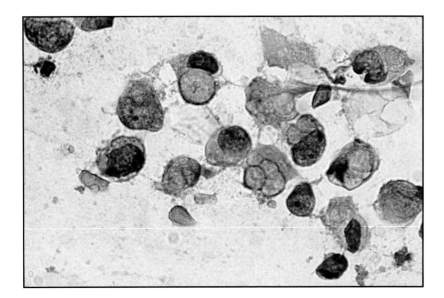

Image 8.77
Signet ring carcinoma: Dispersed cell pattern consisting of small cells with crescent-shaped nuclei compressed to the cell periphery by vacuoles (Papanicolaou, 400X).

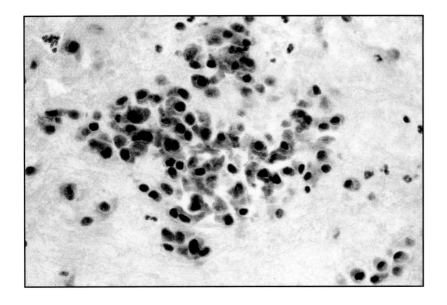

Image 8.78
Expression of gross cystic disease fluid protein–15 (GCDFP-15) in a cell-block preparation of a signet ring carcinoma (200X).

Image 8.79
Smear of secretory carcinoma displays variably sized tumor cells with moderate to abundant, granular or lacy cytoplasm with signet ring forms. The background shows erythrocytes and cellular debris (Papanicolaou, 400X).

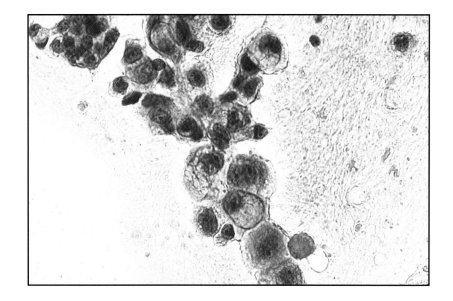

Image 8.80
In contrast to signet ring carcinoma, a tumor diathesis and multivacuolated, lacy cytoplasm are seen in secretory carcinoma (Papanicolaou, 1000X).

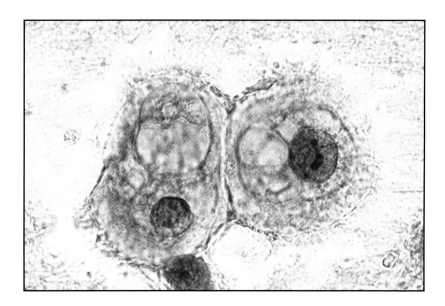

Image 8.81
The histologic appearance of medullary carcinoma is characterized by syncytial groups of highly neoplastic epithelial cells surrounded by lymphocytes and plasma cells (H&E, 200X).

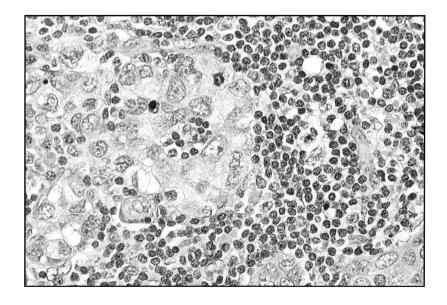

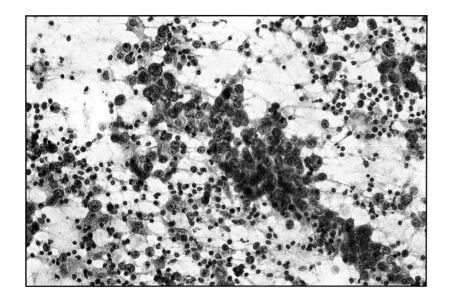

Image 8.82
Highly cellular aspirate of medullary carcinoma (H&E, 100X).

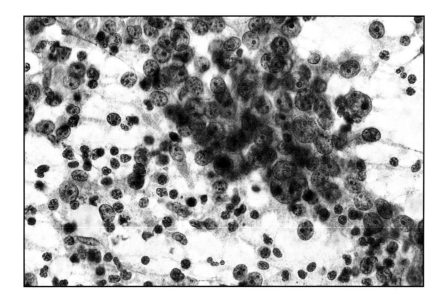

Image 8.83
Loose, syncytial cluster of neoplastic epithelial cells admixed with lymphocytes and plasma cells in an aspirate of medullary carcinoma (H&E, 200X).

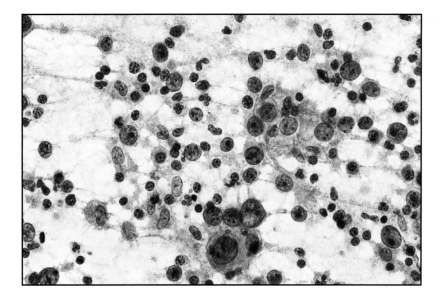

Image 8.84
Conspicuous degree of cellular pleomorphism and anisonucleosis in aspirate of medullary carcinoma (H&E, 200X).

Image 8.85
Papanicolaou-stained smear of medullary carcinoma shows similar features (400X).

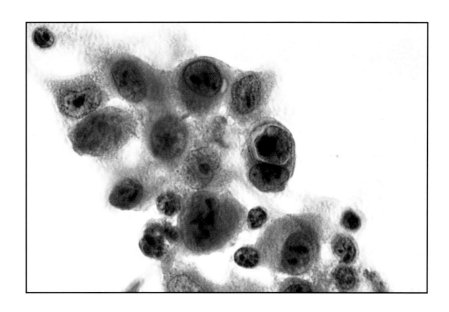

Image 8.86
Neoplastic epithelial cells admixed with lymphocytes and plasma cells in medullary carcinoma (Papanicolaou, 200X).

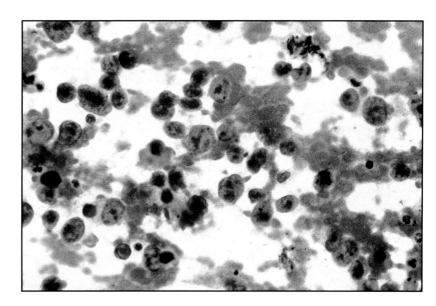

Image 8.87
Mammary carcinoma with carcinoid features: moderately cellular smear with groups of small round cells with oval nuclei and abundant cytoplasm (Papanicolaou, 200X).

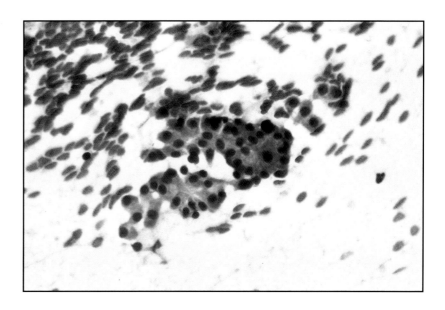

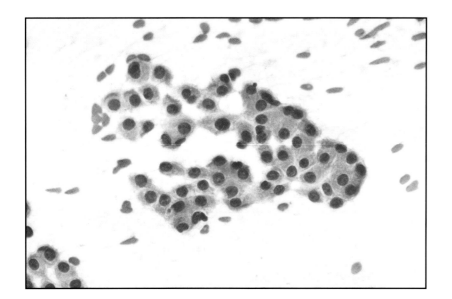

Image 8.88
The same tumor cells forming acini and glandlike structures (Papanicolaou, 200X).

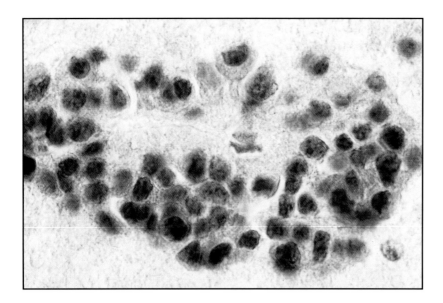

Image 8.89
Cell-block preparation of the same case demonstrates positive immuno-staining for chromogranin (400X).

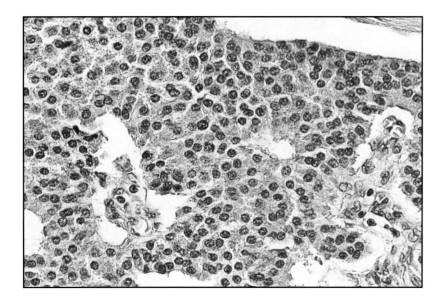

Image 8.90
Corresponding tissue section with morphologic features typical of carcinoid tumor (H&E, 200X).

Image 8.91
Cellular smear from aspirate of carcinoid tumor metastatic to the breast with a dispersed population of uniform small cells with abundant, granular cytoplasm and eccentric nuclei. The chromatin pattern is fine (Papanicolaou, 400X).

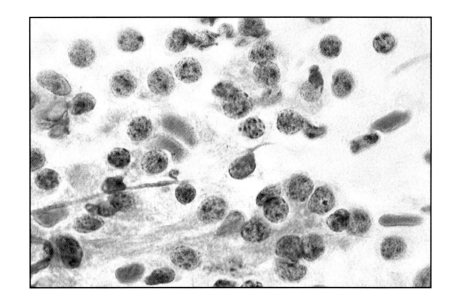

Image 8.92
Tissue section of a previously resected small intestine tumor diagnosed as carcinoid tumor (H&E, 200X).

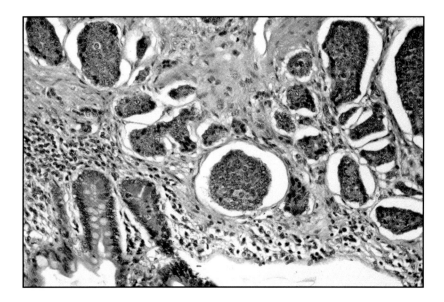

Image 8.93
Higher magnification of the same case demonstrates solid nests of uniform cells supported by a delicate, fibrovascular stroma (H&E, 400X).

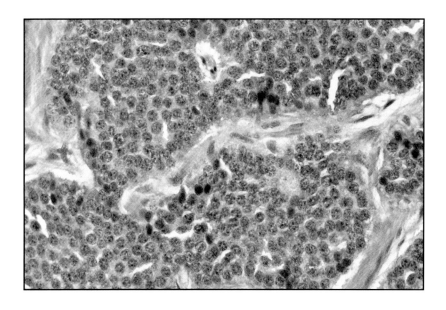

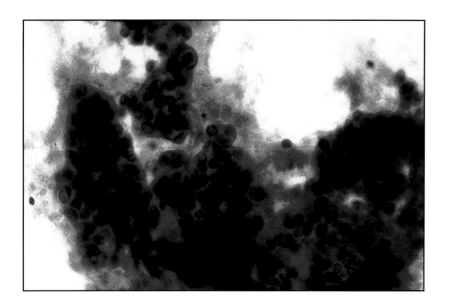

Image 8.94
Direct smear of an intracystic carcinoma reveals a hemorrhagic background containing loosely arranged atypical cells with a tendency to form papillae (H&E, 400X). Reproduced with permission from: Silverman J, Masood S, Ducatman B, et al: Can FNA biopsy separate atypical hyperplasia, carcinoma in situ and invasive carcinoma of the breast? Cytomorphologic criteria and limitations in diagnosis. *Diagn Cytopathol* 9:713–728, 1993.

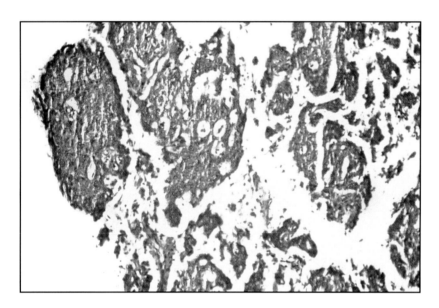

Image 8.95
Cell-block preparation of the same case displays fragments of tissue with a cribriform pattern (H&E, 200X). Reproduced with permission from: Silverman J, Masood S, Ducatman B, et al: Can FNA biopsy separate atypical hyperplasia, carcinoma in situ and invasive carcinoma of the breast? Cytomorphologic criteria and limitations in diagnosis. *Diagn Cytopathol* 9:713–728, 1993.

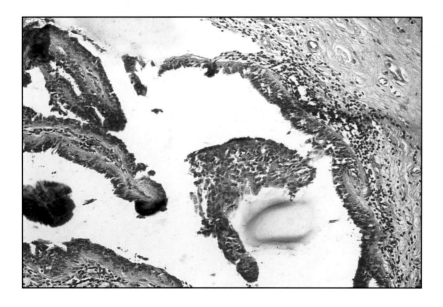

Image 8.96
Tissue section of the same case shows a cyst containing atypical papillae supported by a fibrovascular core. There is no cyst wall invasion by the tumor cells (H&E, 200X).

References

1. Rosen PP, Ashikari K, Thaler H, et al: A comparative study of some pathological features of mammary carcinoma in Tokyo, Japan, and New York. *Cancer* 39:429–434, 1977.

2. Fisher ER, Gregorio RM, Fisher B, et al: The pathology of invasive breast cancer. A syllabus derived from the findings of the National Surgical Adjunct Breast Project (protocol no. 4). *Cancer* 36:1–85, 1975.

3. Page DL, Anderson TJ: *Diagnostic Histopathology of the Breast.* New York, NY, Churchill Livingstone Inc, 1987, pp. 198–205.

4. Sakamoto G, Sugano H, Hartman WH: Comparative pathological study of breast carcinoma among American and Japanese women. In: McGuire WL, ed. *Breast Cancer: Advances in Research and Treatment,* vol 6. New York, NY, Plenum Publishing Corp, 1981, pp. 211–231.

5. McDivitt RW, Stewart FW, Berg JW: Tumors of the breast. In: *Atlas of Tumor Pathology* (2nd series, fascicle 2). Washington, DC, Armed Forces Institute of Pathology, 1968.

6. Carter D, Pipkin RD, Shepard RH, et al: Relationship of necrosis and tumor border to lymph node metastasis and 10 year survival in carcinoma of the breast. *Am J Surg Pathol* 2:39–46, 1978.

7. Giano R: Mononuclear cells in malignant and benign human breast tissue. *Arch Pathol Lab Med* 107:415–417, 1983.

8. Silverberg SG, Chitali AR: Assessment of significance of proportions of intraductal and infiltrating tumor growth in ductal carcinoma of the breast. *Cancer* 32:830–837, 1978.

9. Freedman LS, Edwards DN, McConnell EM, et al: Histological grade and other prognostic factors in relation to survival of patients with breast cancer. *Br J Cancer* 40:44–55, 1979.

10. Rosen PP, Mendez-Botet CJ, Nisselbaun JS, et al: Pathological review of breast lesions analyzed for estrogen receptor protein. *Cancer Res* 35:3187–3194, 1975.

11. Contesso G, DeRarne JC, Mouriesse H, et al: Anatomorphologic du cancer de sein et recepteurs hormonaux. *Pathol Biol* 31: 747–754, 1983.

12. McCarty KS Jr, Barton TK, Fetter BF, et al: Correlation of estrogen and progesterone receptors with histologic differentiation in mammary carcinoma. *Cancer* 46:2851–2858, 1980.

13. Helin EJ, Helle MJ, Kollioniemi OP, et al: Immunohistochemical determination of estrogen and progesterone receptors in human breast carcinoma. Correlation with histopathology and DNA flow cytometry. *Cancer* 63:1761–1767, 1989.

14. Douglas-Jones AG, Barr WT: Breast carcinoma with tumor giant cells, report of a case with fine needle aspiration cytology. *Acta Cytol* 33:1:109–114, 1989.

15. Fisher ER, Palekar AS, Gregorio RM, et al: Mucoepidermoid and squamous cell carcinomas of breast with reference to squamous metaplasia and giant cell tumors. *Am J Surg Pathol* 7:15–27, 1983.

16. Bondeson L: Aspiration cytology of breast carcinoma with multinucleated reactive stromal giant cells. *Acta Cytol* 28:313–316, 1984.

17. Cook SS, DeMay R: Adenocarcinoma of the breast with osseous metaplasia: report of a case with needle aspiration cytology. *Acta Cytol* 28:317–320, 1984.

18. Fry HJB: Osteoclastoma (myeloid sarcomas of the human female breast). *J Pathol Bacteriol* 30:529–536, 1927.

19. Dixon JM, Anderson TJ, Page DL, et al: Infiltrating lobular carcinoma of the breast: an evaluation of the incidence and consequence of bilateral disease. *Br J Surg* 70:513–516, 1983.

20. Rosen PP: The pathological classification of human mammary carcinoma: past, present and future. *Ann Clin Lab Sci* 9:144–156, 1979.

21. Zajicek J: *Aspiration Biopsy Cytology*, Part I. Basel, Switzerland, Karger, 1974.

22. Ashikari R, Huvos AG, Urban JA, et al: Infiltrating lobular carcinoma of the breast. *Cancer* 31:110–116, 1973.

23. Rosen PP, Lesser ML, Senie RT, et al: Epidemiology of breast carcinoma, IV: age and histologic tumor type. *J Surg Oncol* 19:44–51, 1982.

24. Ermier WJ, Gaffey TA, Welch JS, et al: Linitis plastica caused by metastatic lobular carcinoma of the breast. *Mayo Clin Proc* 55: 747–753, 1980.

25. Smith DB, Howell A, Harris M, et al: Carcinomatous meningitis associated with infiltrating lobular carcinoma of the breast. *Eur J Surg Oncol* 11:33–36, 1985.

26. Mohammed RJ, Lakatua DJ, Haus E, et al: Estrogen and progesterone receptors in human breast cancer. Correlation with histologic subtype and degree of differentiation. *Cancer* 58:1076–1081, 1986.

27. Harris JR, Hellman S, Henderson IC, et al: *Breast Diseases.* Philadelphia, Pa, JB Lippincott Co, 1987, pp. 181–185.

28. Fechner RE: Histologic variants of infiltrating lobular carcinoma of the breast. *Hum Pathol* 6:373–378, 1975.

29. Martinez V, Azzopardi JG: Invasive lobular carcinoma of the breast: incidence and variants. *Histopathology* 3:467–488, 1979.

30. Kline TS, Joshi LP, Neal HS: Fine needle aspiration of the breast: diagnostic pitfalls. *Cancer* 44:1458–1464, 1979.

31. Koss LG, Woyke J, Olszewski W: *Cytologic Interpretation and Histologic Bases.* New York, NY, Igaku-Shoin, 1984.

32. Kline TS: *Handbook of Fine Needle Aspiration Biopsy Cytology.* St. Louis, Mo, CV Mosby Co, 1988, pp. 199–252.

33. Kline TS, Kannan V, Kline IK: Appraisal and cytomorphological analysis of common carcinomas of the breast. *Diagn Cytopathol* 1:188–193, 1985.

34. Eusebi V, Betts CM, Haagensen DE, et al: Apocrine differentiation in lobular carcinoma of the breast: a morphologic, immunologic and ultrastructural study. *Hum Pathol* 15:134–140, 1984.

35. Eusebi V, Maghales F, Azzopardi JG: Pleomorphic lobular carcinoma of the breast. An aggressive tumor showing apocrine differentiation. *Hum Pathol* 23:655–662, 1992.

36. Dabbs DJ, Grenko KT, Silverman JF: Fine needle aspiration cytology of pleomorphic lobular carcinoma of the breast: duct carcinoma as a diagnostic pitfall. *Acta Cytol* 38:923–926, 1994.

37. Antoniades K, Spector HB: Similarities and variations among lobular carcinoma cells. *Diagn Cytopathol* 3:55–59, 1987.

38. Leach C, Howell LP: Cytodiagnosis of classic lobular carcinoma and its variants. *Acta Cytol* 36:199–202, 1992.

39. Salhany K, Page DL: Fine needle aspiration of mammary lobular carcinoma in situ and atypical lobular hyperplasia. *Am J Clin Pathol* 92:22–26, 1989.

40. Nguyen G: Fine needle aspiration cytology of lobular carcinoma of the breast: an analysis of 31 cases. *Acta Cytol* 37:820, 1992. Abstract.

41. Kristina A, Spector B: Similarities and variations among lobular carcinoma cells. *Diagn Cytopathol* 3:55–59, 1987.

42. Sneige N: Current issues in fine needle aspiration of the breast: cytologic features of in situ lobular and ductal carcinomas and clinical implications of nuclear grading. *Cytopathology Annual* 7:155-171, 1992.

43. Kline TS, Kline IK: High risk lesions. In: Kline TS. *Guides to Clinical Aspiration Biopsy*. New York, NY, Igaku-Shoin, 1989, pp. 235–248.

44. Silverman J, Masood S, Ducatman B, et al: Can FNA biopsy separate atypical hyperplasia, carcinoma in situ and invasive carcinoma of the breast? Cytomorphologic criteria and limitations in diagnosis. *Diagn Cytopathol* 9:713–728, 1993.

45. Cornil V, Rannier L: *Manuel d'Histologie Pathologique*. Paris, France, Germer-Bailliere, 1869, pp. 1167–1170.

46. Anderson JA, Carter D, Linnell F: A symposium on sclerosing duct lesions of the breast. *Pathol Annu* 21:145–179, 1986.

47. Andersson I, Andren L, Hildell J, et al: Breast cancer screening with mammography: a population-based, randomized trial with mammography as the only screening mode. *Radiology* 132:273–276, 1979.

48. Patchefsky AS, Shaver GS, Schwartz GF, et al: The pathology of breast cancer detected by mass population screening. *Cancer* 40: 1659–1670, 1977.

49. Linell F, Ljungberg O, Anderson I: Breast carcinoma: aspects of early stages, progression and related problems. *Acta Pathol Microbiol Scand (Suppl)* 272:1–233, 1980. Abstract.

50. Carstens PHB: Tubular carcinoma of the breast: a study of frequency. *Am J Clin Pathol* 70:204–210, 1978.

51. Lagios MD, Rose MR, Margolin FR: Tubular carcinoma of the breast. Association with multicentricity, bilaterality and family history of mammary carcinoma. *Am J Clin Pathol* 73:25–30, 1981.

52. Oberman HA, Fidler WJ Jr: Tubular carcinoma of the breast. *Am J Surg Pathol* 3:387–395, 1979.

53. Cooper HS, Patchefsky AS, Krall RA: Tubular carcinoma of the breast. Association with multicentricity, bilaterality and family history of mammary carcinoma. *Am J Clin Pathol* 73:25–30, 1981.

54. Tavassoli FA: *Pathology of the Breast*. Norwalk, Conn, Appleton and Lange, 1992, pp. 315–426.

55. Bondeson L, Lindholm K: Aspiration cytology of tubular breast carcinoma. *Acta Cytol* 34:15–201, 1990.

56. Silverman JF: Breast. In: Bibbo M, ed. *Comprehensive Cytopathology*. Philadelphia, Pa, WB Saunders Co, 1991, pp. 703–770.

57. Cleary PMG, Mayze JD: Recognition of tubular breast carcinoma on fine needle aspiration cytology. *Acta Cytol* 36:773, 1992. Abstract.

58. Lofgren M, Andersson I, Bondenson L, et al: X-ray guided fine needle aspiration for the cytologic diagnosis of non-palpable breast lesions. *Cancer* 61:1032–1037, 1988.

59. Gupta RK, Dowle C: Fine needle aspiration cytology of tubular carcinoma of the breast in a young woman. *Diagn Cytopathol* 7:72–74, 1991.

60. Dei Tos AP, Della-Giustina D, Martin VD, et al: Aspiration biopsy cytology of tubular carcinoma of the breast. *Diagn Cytopathol* 11:146–150, 1994.

61. de la Torre M, Lindholm K, Lindgren A: Fine needle aspiration cytology of tubular breast carcinoma and radial scar. *Acta Cytol* 38:884–890, 1994.

62. Frierson HF Jr, Iezzoni J, Covell JL: Stereotaxic fine needle aspiration cytology of radial scars. *Acta Cytol* 37:814, 1993. Abstract.

63. Hangensen CD: *Diseases of the Breast,* 3rd ed. Philadelphia, Pa, WB Saunders Co, 1986, pp. 729-757.

64. Rosen PP: Pathology of breast cancer. In: Harris JR, Hellman S, Anderson IC, Kinne DW, eds. *Breast Diseases*. Philadelphia, Pa, JB Lippincott Co, 1987, pp. 147–209.

65. Carter D: Intraductal papillary tumors of the breast. A study of 78 cases. *Cancer* 39:1689–1692, 1977.

66. Ramos CV, Doeghart C, Restrapo GL: Intracystic papillary carcinoma of the male breast. *Arch Pathol Lab Med* 109:858–861, 1985.

67. Papotti M, Gugliotta P, Eusebi V, et al: Immunohistochemical analysis of benign and malignant papillary lesions of the breast. *Am J Surg Pathol* 7:451–461, 1983.

68. Kline TS, Kannan V: Papillary carcinoma of the breast: a cytomorphologic analysis. *Arch Pathol Lab Med* 110:189–191, 1986.

69. Naran S, Simpson J, Gupta RK: Cytologic diagnosis of papillary carcinoma of the breast in needle aspirates. *Diagn Cytopathol* 4:33–37, 1988.

70. Nguyen GK, Redburn J: Aspiration cytology of papillary carcinoma of the breast. *Diagn Cytopathol* 8:511–516, 1992.

71. Baroales RH, Suhrland MJ, Stanley MW: Papillary neoplasms of the breast: fine needle aspiration findings in cystic and solid cases. *Diagn Cytopathol* 10:336–341, 1994.

72. Dei Tos AP, Della-Giustina D: Aspiration biopsy cytology of malignant papillary neoplasms. *Diagn Cytopathol* 8:580–584, 1992.

73. Kini S, Miller JM, Hamburger JI, et al: Cytopathology of papillary carcinoma of the thyroid by fine needle aspiration biopsy. *Acta Cytol* 24:511–521, 1980.

74. Azzopardi JG: *Problems in Breast Pathology.* London, England, WB Saunders Co, 1979.

75. Fisher ER, Palekar AS, Redmond C, et al: Pathologic findings from the National Surgical Adjuvant Breast Project (Protocol 4), VI. Invasive papillary cancer. *Am J Clin Pathol* 73:312–322, 1980.

76. Komaki K, Sakamoto G, Sugaro H, et al: The morphologic feature of mucous leakage appearing in low papillary carcinoma of the breast. *Hum Pathol* 22:231–236, 1991.

77. Sneige N, White VA, Katz RL: Ductal carcinoma in situ of the breast: fine needle aspiration cytology of 12 cases. *Diagn Cytopathol* 5:371–377, 1989.

78. Robinson RR: Gelatiniform cancer of the breast. *Trans Pathol Soc London* 4:275–278, 1852.

79. Lavrey M: Tumour gelatiniforme on colloide de la mammella. *Bull Soc Chir Paris* 3:345–547, 1853.

80. Lange F: Der gallertkrebs der brustdruse. *Beitr Klin Chir* 16:1–60, 1896.

81. Gaabe G: Der gallertkrebs der brustdruse. *Beitr 2 Klin Chir* 60:760–807, 1908.

82. Lebert H: Beittaege zur kenntnis des gallertkrebs. *Arch Pathol Anat* 4:192, 1852.

83. Tellem M, Nedwick A, Amenta PS, et al: Mucin producing carcinoma of the breast: tissue culture, histochemical and electron microscopic study. *Cancer* 19:573–584, 1966.

84. Geschikter CF: Gelatinous mammary cancer. *Ann Surg* 108:321–346, 1938.

85. Rasmussen BB, Rose C, Christensen IB: Prognostic factors in primary mucinous breast carcinoma. *Am J Clin Pathol* 87:155–160, 1987.

86. Clayton F: Pure mucinous carcinoma of the breast: morphologic features and prognostic correlates. *Hum Pathol* 17:34–38, 1986.

87. Silverberg SG, Kay S, Chitale AR, et al: Colloid carcinoma of the breast. *Am J Clin Pathol* 55:355–363, 1971.

88. Hull MJ, Seo FS, Battersby JS, et al: Signet ring cell carcinoma of the breast. A clinicopathologic study of 24 cases. *Am J Clin Pathol* 73:31–35, 1980.

89. Jao W, Lao IO, Chawdbury LN, et al: Ultrastructural aspects of mucinous (colloid) breast carcinoma. *Diagn Gynecol Obstet* 2:83–92, 1980.

90. Masood S, Barwick KW: Estrogen receptor expression of the less common breast carcinomas. *Am J Clin Pathol* 93:437, 1990. Abstract.

91. Toikhanen S, Eerola E, Ekfors T: Pure and mixed mucinous breast carcinomas: DNA stemline and prognosis. *J Clin Pathol* 41:300–303, 1988.

92. Palombini L, Fulciniti F, Vetrani A, et al: Mucoid carcinoma of the breast on fine needle aspiration biopsy sample: cytology and ultrastructure. *Appl Pathol* 2:70–75, 1984.

93. Wall RW, Glant MD: The cytomorphology of mucinous carcinoma of the breast by fine needle aspiration. *ASCP Cytopathology Check Sample,* C 87-12 (C-174). Chicago, Ill, American Society of Clinical Pathologists, 1987.

94. Wilkinson EJ, Franzini DA, Masood S: Cytological needle sampling of the breast: techniques and end results. In: Bland KI, Copoland EM, eds. *The Breast.* Philadephia, Pa, WB Saunders, 1990, pp. 475–498.

95. Zajdela A, Durand JC, Veith F: Aspect cytologique de quelques varietes particulieres d'epitheliomas mammaires. *Bull Cancer* 62: 227–240, 1975.

96. Rosen PP: Mucocele-like tumors of the breast. *Am J Surg Pathol* 10:646, 1986.

97. Bharagava V, Miller TR, Cohen MB: Mucocele-like tumors of the breast. Cytologic findings in two cases. *Am J Clin Pathol* 95: 875–877, 1991.

98. Fanning TV, Sneige N, Staerkel G: Mucinous breast lesions: fine needle aspiration findings. *Acta Cytol* 34:754, 1990.

99. Hamele-Bern D, Cram ML, Rosen PP: Mammary mucocele-like lesions (MLL): benign and malignant. *Mod Pathol* 8:1–18, 1995. Abstract.

100. Duane GB, Kanter MH, Branigan T, et al: A morphologic and morphometric study of cells from colloid carcinoma of the breast obtained by fine needle aspiration: distinction from other breast lesions. *Acta Cytol* 31:742–750, 1987.

101. Stanley MW, Tani EM, Skoog L: Mucinous breast carcinoma and mixed mucinous infiltrating ductal carcinoma. A comparative cytologic study. *Diagn Cytopathol* 5:34–38, 1989.

102. Hull MT, Seo IS, Battersby JS, et al: Signet ring cell carcinoma of the breast. A clinicopathologic study of 24 cases. *Am J Clin Pathol* 73:31–35, 1980.

103. Marino MJ, Livolsi VA: Signet ring carcinoma of the female breast: a clinicopathologic analysis of 24 cases. *Cancer* 48:1830–1837, 1981.

104. Saphir O: Mucinous carcinoma of the breast. *Surg Gynecol Obstet* 72:908–914, 1941.

105. Steinbrecher JS, Silverberg SO: Signet ring carcinoma. The mucinous variant of infiltrating lobular carcinoma. *Cancer* 37:828–840, 1976.

106. Raju O, Ma CK, Shaw A: Signet ring variant of lobular carcinoma of the breast: a clinicopathologic and immunohistochemical study. *Mod Pathol* 6:516–520, 1993.

107. d'Amore ESG, Maisto L, Gatteschi MB, et al: Secretory carcinoma of the breast. Report of a case with fine needle aspiration biopsy. *Acta Cytol* 30:309-312, 1986.

108. Craig JP: Secretory carcinoma of the breast in an adult. Correlation of aspiration cytology and histology on the biopsy specimen. *Acta Cytol* 29:589-592, 1985.

109. Shinagawa T, Tadokoro M, Kitamura H, et al: Secretory carcinoma of the breast: correlation of aspiration cytology and histology. *Acta Cytol* 38:909–914, 1994.

110. Oberman HA: Breast lesions in adolescent female. *Pathol Annu* 14:175–201, 1979.

111. Tavassoli FA, Norris HG: Secretory carcinoma of the breast. *Cancer* 45:2404–2413, 1980.

112. Lapey JD: Lipid-rich mammary carcinoma: diagnosis by cytology. Case report. *Acta Cytol* 21:120–122, 1977.

113. Geschikter CF: *Diseases of the Breast: Diagnosis, Pathology and Treatment,* 2nd ed. Philadelphia, Pa, JB Lippincott Co, 1945, p. 565.

114. Moore OS Jr, Foote FW Jr: The relatively favorable prognosis of medullary carcinoma of the breast. *Cancer* 2:635–642, 1949.

115. Maier WP, Roseman GP, Goldman LI, et al: A ten year study of medullary carcinoma of the breast. *Surg Obstet Gynecol* 144: 695–698, 1977.

116. Richardson RW: Medullary carcinoma of the breast. A re-evaluation of 95 cases of breast cancer with inflammatory stroma. *Cancer* 61:2503–2510, 1988.

117. Schwartz GF: Solid circumscribed carcinoma of the breast. *Ann Surg* 169:165–174, 1969.

118. Azzopardi JG: *Problems in Breast Pathology.* Philadelphia, Pa, WB Saunders Co, 1979, pp. 244–247.

119. Ridolfi RL, Rosen PP, Pott A, et al: Medullary carcinoma of the breast: a clinicopathologic study with 10 year follow-up. *Cancer* 40:1365–1385, 1977.

120. Howell LP, Kline TS: Medullary carcinoma of the breast. A rare cytologic finding in cyst fluid aspirate. *Cancer* 65:277-282, 1990.

121. Daroca PJ: Medullary carcinoma of the breast with granulomatous stroma. *Hum Pathol* 18:761–763, 1987.

122. Horsfall DJ, Telley WD, Orell SR, et al: Relationship between ploidy and hormone receptors in primary breast cancer. *Br J Cancer* 53:23–28, 1986.

123. Erhardt K, Auer G, Folin A, et al: Mammary carcinoma: comparison between histologic type, estrogen receptor and nuclear DNA content. *Am J Clin Oncol* 1:83–89, 1986.

124. Harris M, Lesrells AM: The ultrastructure of medullary, atypical medullary and non-medullary carcinoma of the breast. *Histopathology* 10:405–414, 1986.

125. McCune KH, Varma M, Spence RA: Breast lymphoma: fine needle aspiration biopsy. *Ulster Med J* 61:110–111, 1992.

126. Feyrter F, Hartman G: Uber die carcinoide wuchsform des carcinoma mammae, insbesondere das carcinoma solidum (gelatinosum) mammae. *Frankf Z Pathol* 73:221–235, 1963.

127. Azzopardi JG, Murette P, Goddeeris P, et al: "Carcinoid" tumors of the breast: the morphological spectrum of argyrophil carcinomas. *Histopathology* 6:549–569, 1982.

128. Cubilla AL, Woodruff JM: Primary carcinoid tumor of the breast: a report of eight patients. *Am J Surg Pathol* 1:283–292, 1977.

129. Kaneko H, Nojo H, Ishikawa S, et al: Norepinephrine-producing tumors of bilateral breasts. A case report. *Cancer* 41:2002–2007, 1978.

130. Taxy JB, Tischler AS, Insalaco SJ, et al: "Carcinoid" tumor of the breast: a variant of conventional breast cancer. *Hum Pathol* 12:170–179, 1981.

131. Toyoshima S: Mammary carcinoma with argyrophil cells. *Cancer* 52:2129–2138, 1983.

132. Papotti M, Macri L, Finzi G, et al: Neuroendocrine differentiation in carcinomas of the breast: a study of 51 cases. *Semin Diagn Pathol* 6:174–188, 1989.

133. Skoog L: Aspiration cytology of a male breast carcinoma with argyrophilic cells. *Acta Cytol* 31:379–381, 1987.

134. Bussalati G, Pugliotta P, Sapine A, et al: Chromogranin-reactive endocrine cells in argyrophilic carcinomas (carcinoids) and normal tissue of the breast. *Am J Pathol* 120:186–192, 1985.

135. Ni K, Ribbo M: Fine needle aspiration of mammary carcinoma with features of a carcinoid tumor. A case report with immunohisto-chemical and ultra-structural studies. *Acta Cytol* 38:73–78, 1994.

136. Hussein KA, Sanders DSA, Preece PE, et al: Argyrophil carcinoma of the breast: a cytologic, histochemical and ultrastructural study of a case. *Diagn Cytopathol* 5:217–220, 1989.

137. Lazarevic B, Rodgers JB. Aspiration cytology of carcinoid tumor of the breast. A case report. *Acta Cytol* 27:329–333, 1983.

138. Oertel YC: *Fine Needle Aspiration of the Breast*. Stoneham, Mass, Butterworth, 1987.

139. Ravinsky E, Carers DJ: Cytology of argyrophilic carcinoma of the breast. *Acta Cytol* 29:1–6, 1985.

140. Harrist TJ, Kalisher L: Breast metastasis: an unusual manifestation of a malignant carcinoid tumor. *Cancer* 40:3102–3106, 1977.

141. Lozowski MJ, Faegenburg D, Mishriki Y, et al: Carcinoid tumor metastatic to breast diagnosed by fine needle aspiration: case report and literature review. *Acta Cytol* 33:191–194, 1989.

142. Hugh JC, Jackson FI, Hanson J, et al: Primary breast lymphoma: an immunohistologic study of 20 new cases. *Cancer* 66:2602–2611, 1990.

143. Wiseman C, Liao KT: Primary lymphoma of the breast. *Cancer* 29:1705–1712, 1972.

144. Jean HJ, Akagi T, Hoshida Y, et al: Primary non-Hodgkin malignant lymphoma of the breast. *Cancer* 70:2451–2459, 1992.

145. Squires E, Betsill W: Intracystic carcinoma of the breast: a correlation of cytomorphology, gross pathology, microscopic pathology and clinical data. *Acta Cytol* 25:267–271, 1981.

146. Corkill ME, Sneige N, Fanning T, et al: Fine needle aspiration cytology and flow cytometry of intracystic papillary carcinoma of breast. *Am J Clin Pathol* 94:673–680, 1990.

CHAPTER NINE

Primary Breast Carcinoma, Special Types

Metaplastic Carcinoma

Metaplastic carcinoma is a rare variant of breast cancer that characteristically contains both epithelial and mesenchymal elements as well as a transitional form between them.[1-3] This heterogeneous neoplasm characteristically contains ductal carcinoma cells mixed with areas of spindle, squamous, chondroid, or osseous differentiation. Metaplastic carcinoma should be distinguished from other tumors with mixed epithelial and mesenchymal components, such as phyllodes tumor with coexisting carcinoma,[4,5] carcinoma with osteoclast-like giant cells,[6] and coexisting but separate carcinoma and sarcoma in the same breast.[7]

Metaplastic carcinoma has also been described as sarcomatoid carcinoma, spindle cell carcinoma, or carcinoma with sarcoma-like stroma.[8] The term carcinosarcoma has also been used interchangeably with spindle cell carcinoma, pseudosarcoma, sarcomatoid carcinoma, and matrix-producing carcinoma.[9] The term carcinosarcoma of the breast refers to a biphasic neoplasm, at least 50% of which is composed of neoplastic spindle cells with high mitotic activity; the tumor's other component is epithelial.[9]

The origin of metaplastic carcinoma remains controversial. Some authors believe that metaplastic carcinoma derives from an undifferentiated cell with the capacity to differentiate in both an epithelial and a mesenchymal direction.[10,11] Others suggest that the tumor has a myoepithelial origin.[12-14] However, metaplastic carcinomas elaborate only epithelial antigens immunocytochemically. The epithelial nature of this tumor is further supported by the identification of numerous well-developed desmosomes and tonofilaments by electron microscopy.[15]

Metaplastic carcinoma is frequently associated with an unfavorable prognosis, especially if the mesenchymal component is dominant.[8] Tumor cells may be hormone-receptor negative and aneuploid.[14–16] The cytologic diagnosis of metaplastic carcinoma may be difficult. Scantly cellular aspirates or those that show only one component may lead to false diagnoses of sarcoma or carcinoma. Thus, an extensive search for epithelial and mesenchymal components may be necessary to exclude the possibility of metaplastic carcinoma.[17–22] Repeat FNABs of unusual cases might increase the accuracy of FNAB diagnosis by improving tumor sampling.[20]

FNAB smears of metaplastic carcinoma are frequently rich in cellularity, with the tumor cell population set in a myxoid background. The myxoid material is granular or fibrillary and metachromatic. The mesenchymal cells are elongated, atypical, and pleomorphic. There are also multinucleated cells, some of which have uneven, hyperchromatic nuclei and a conspicuous number of abnormal mitotic figures. Also present, singly or in small groups, are round or oval atypical cells with the sharply demarcated cytoplasm characteristic of carcinoma. Positive immunostaining for vimentin, cytokeratin, and S-100 may be seen in both the epithelial and the sarcomatoid components (Images 9.1 through 9.8).[15–22]

Ultrastructurally, epithelial tumor cells show desmosomes, round or irregular nuclei with evenly distributed chromatin, and inconspicuous nucleoli. Some of the cells may be embedded in the basal lamina. The cytoplasm contains many organelles, including occasional dilated endoplasmic reticulum. Intracytoplasmic lumens and tonofilaments may not be present. In contrast, sarcomatoid areas have elongated, irregular nuclei with inconspicuous nucleoli and prominent, dilated, rough endoplasmic reticulum in the cytoplasm. A large number of ribosomes, polyribosomes, and Golgi apparatuses are also seen, and there is no basal lamina.[17]

The cytologic differential diagnosis includes stromal sarcoma, spindle cell proliferations, angiosarcoma, phyllodes tumor, and metastatic carcinoma.[20,23,24] Fine needle aspirates of pseudosarcomatous fasciitis and fibromatosis contain microtissue fragments and individually arranged spindle cells with a bland appearance. Ancillary studies, including electron microscopy and immunocytochemistry, are the diagnostic adjuncts most helpful in differentiating between metaplastic carcinoma and other lesions such as pure sarcoma and phyllodes tumor.

Metaplastic carcinoma with squamous components must also be differentiated from subareolar abscess.[25,26] Either lesion may show retraction or peau d'orange and epithelial atypia. However, in contrast to metaplastic carcinoma, which occurs at any site in the breast and clinically presents as a palpable mass, subareolar abscess is typically confined to the subareolar area and is often preceded by a history of multiple abscesses at the same site.

Cytomorphology of Metaplastic Carcinoma
Rich cellularity
Pleomorphic population of tumor cells with biphasic pattern
Highly atypical spindle and epithelial cells
Multinucleation
Mitosis

Squamous Cell Carcinoma

Primary squamous cell carcinomas of the breast are extremely rare, with fewer than 50 cases reported in the literature. Focal squamous differentiation can occur in ductal carcinoma. Of the 24 cases of breast carcinoma with squamous differentiation reported by Cornog et al,[27] only two were pure squamous cell carcinomas. Overall, the incidence of primary squamous cell carcinoma of the breast ranges between 0.02% and 0.075%, based on a review of two series of more than 1,000 cases.[28,29] Patients range from 29 to 72 years old, with a mean of 50 years. Lymph node metastasis may occur. While some investigators believe that the prognosis of squamous cell carcinoma is comparable to that of other infiltrating breast carcinomas, the acantholytic or poorly differentiated variant has been associated with a poor prognosis. Occasionally, squamous cell carcinoma can be hormone-receptor positive, with a diploid DNA content and high S-phase fraction. The tumor is usually large, varying in size from 2 to 23 cm. The majority are cystic.[30–33] The cyst contents vary from straw-colored green to brownish and necrotic.[31,34] Squamous cell carcinoma of the breast can be diagnosed by FNAB.[30,32,35–39] Following aspiration, the tumor either persists or rapidly recurs.[31]

Microscopically, squamous cell carcinomas are characterized by the presence of various cell types, including large cell keratinizing, acantholytic, spindle cell, or a combination of these. The cells may line a cystic lesion or present as a solid growth. Keratin pearls, intercellular bridges, keratohyaline granules, and necrosis are other features of squamous cell carcinoma. Lesions in which the spindle cell pattern predominates may cause diagnostic difficulty. The epithelial nature of such tumors must be confirmed by immunostaining for epithelial markers such as cytokeratin. In addition, the cell type, as demonstrated by the presence of tonofilaments, intercellular bridges, or both by electron microscopy, helps to establish the diagnosis of squamous cell carcinoma (Figure 9.1). As in the other squamous cell carcinomas, neoplastic

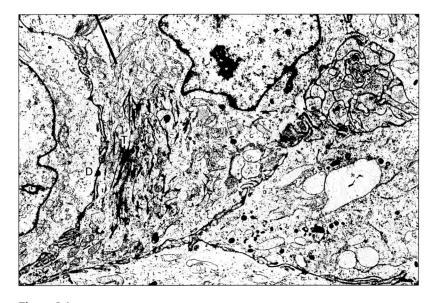

Figure 9.1
Ultrastructural features of squamous cell carcinoma of the breast: bundles of tonofilaments (T) and desmosomes (D) with intercellular bridges (arrow) (29,500X; inset, 38,000X).

epithelial cells, isolated and in sheets, may show evidence of intracytoplasmic keratinization and intercellular bridges. Inflammatory cells, including multinucleated histiocytes, are present in cystic tumors (Images 9.9 through 9.12).

The cytologic differential diagnosis includes epidermal inclusion cyst, duct cell carcinoma with a squamous component, mucoepidermoid carcinoma, and fibroadenoma with squamous metaplasia.[36,40–42] FNABs of epidermal inclusion cysts show benign squamous cells. The presence of tumor cells with glandular differentiation in addition to malignant squamous cells is characteristic of duct cell carcinoma with a focal squamous component.[43] Mucoepidermoid carcinoma can be easily differentiated from pure squamous cell carcinoma by the presence of clusters of malignant squamous cells and mucin-secreting cells.[44] Another diagnostic possibility is metastatic squamous cell carcinoma, which can be excluded by careful examination of the patient's history and clinical presentation.[35]

Cytomorphology of Squamous Cell Carcinoma
Cellular aspirate
Atypical epithelial cells isolated and in clusters
Intracytoplasmic keratinization
Intercellular bridges
Inflammatory and necrotic background

Mucoepidermoid Carcinoma

First described by Patchefsky et al[45] in 1979, mucoepidermoid carcinoma of the breast remains a rare tumor. The estimated incidence of mucoepidermoid carcinoma is approximately 0.3% of all breast cancers.[46] The tumor occurs as a palpable mass in women between the ages of 31 and 87, with a median age of 57. Clinical presentation is variable. The tumor may have been present from a few weeks to almost 20 years.[45–48]

Gross appearance varies according to the degree of squamous differentiation. The median size of the tumor is 2.5 cm. It can present as an ill-defined or a well-circumscribed lesion. Microscopically, mucoepidermoid carcinoma is composed of an intimate admixture of adenocarcinoma with squamous cell carcinoma. The proportion of each determines the degree of differentiation as well as the prognosis. Fisher et al[46] reported a favorable prognosis for cases of low-grade mucoepidermoid carcinoma. Since then, however, reported cases of high-grade lesions have been associated with a poor prognosis.[48–50]

Cytologic diagnosis of mucoepidermoid carcinoma is possible if both components are present in the aspirate.[48–50] FNAB smears of mucoepidermoid carcinoma show clusters of neoplastic epithelial cells with features of squamous differentiation and clusters of mucin-secreting cells. Presence of the characteristic mixed pattern should be sufficient to rule out a diagnosis of pure squamous cell carcinoma or mucin-producing adenocarcinoma.

Cytomorphology of Mucoepidermoid Carcinoma
Cellular smear
Atypical epithelial cells with features of squamous differentiation and
  evidence of mucin production

Adenoid Cystic Carcinoma

A rare breast tumor, adenoid cystic carcinoma constitutes less than 1% of all breast cancers.[51,52] Morphologically, it is identical to tumors that occur in salivary gland and other areas.[53] First described by Foote and Stewart[54] in 1946, adenoid cystic carcinomas of the breast occur in various age groups, usually in patients between 34 and 75 years, and have a favorable prognosis.[51,53] The tumor has been described in men.[55] Because of its favorable prognosis, adenoid cystic carcinoma is best treated by conservative surgery.[51,56,57] Adenoid cystic carcinoma shows a predilection for the subareolar region but is not associated with nipple discharge. Skin ulceration, peau d'orange, or dimpling are common clinical presentations of adenoid cystic carcinoma, particularly of tumors that are large or superficial.[51,56] The size of adenoid cystic carcinoma ranges from a few millimeters to up to 12 cm in diameter, with a median of 2.2 cm.[52]

Grossly, the lesion is well defined and displays a gray to yellow color on cut surface. Rarely, cystic areas are grossly visible. Microscopically, adenoid cystic carcinoma is an infiltrative tumor characterized by a proliferation of nests and islands of bland tumor cells in solid, cribriform, tubular, and trabecular arrangements. A basaloid population of tumor cells and a smaller population of cells with eosinophilic cytoplasm surround amorphous, eosinophilic material (ie, hyaline bodies) (Image 9.13). This basement membrane–like material shows a strong positive reaction with laminin.[57]

FNAB smears of adenoid cystic carcinoma are cellular, with clusters of small cells with scant cytoplasm; round, hyperchromatic nuclei; and occasional micronucleoli. The cells are typically arranged around cores of acellular, homogeneous material that are translucent with Papanicolaou stain and pink with May-Grünwald–Giemsa stain (Images 9.14 through 9.16).[58–61]

The differential diagnosis of adenoid cystic carcinoma includes lobular and mucinous carcinoma, so-called carcinoid tumor, small cell undifferentiated carcinoma, lymphoma, cribriform intraductal pseudoadenoid cystic carcinoma, and collagenous spherulosis.[60] Collagenous spherulosis is usually an incidental finding of microscopic dimensions, whereas adenoid cystic carcinoma forms a mass of macroscopic proportions and manifests as a palpable breast lesion. In addition, collagenous spherulosis, which is associated with the spectrum of fibrocystic change, is characterized by the presence of two cell types, epithelial and myoepithelial cells, as opposed to the monomorphic pattern of adenoid cystic carcinoma. Furthermore, the cells in collagenous spherulosis are layered and contain more cytoplasm. In scanty aspirates, the presence of extracellular metachromatic spherules may cause interpretative errors and lead to false diagnosis of adenoid cystic carcinoma. This type of extracellular material can be produced from inspissated secretory material or stromal fragments in a variety of conditions, such as fibrocystic change, fibroadenoma, or duct cell carcinoma.[62] Thus, extreme caution should be exercised in the interpretation of sparsely cellular aspirates containing extracellular matrix. Cellular monomorphism, presence of extracellular metachromatic spherules, and absence of the traditional cytologic features of malignancy are the distinguishing features of adenoid cystic carcinoma. Myospherulosis is another remote possibility that should be excluded.

Cytomorphology of Adenoid Cystic Carcinoma
Cellular aspirate with monomorphic pattern
Clusters of small cells with scanty cytoplasm, hyperchromatic nuclei, and
   rare micronucleoli
Minimal cytologic atypia
Arrangement of tumor cells around acellular and homogeneous material

Apocrine Carcinoma

Apocrine carcinoma is a rare variant of ductal carcinoma that occurs in advanced age, the peak incidence being during the sixth and seventh decades of life.[63] Controversy remains regarding the prognosis of this tumor. Although it has been suggested that patients with apocrine carcinoma may have a longer survival,[64] this hypothesis has not been substantiated in comparisons with other duct cell carcinomas.[65,66] Apocrine carcinomas originate in cells with a potential to differentiate into apocrine cells. The cells are often positive for gross cystic disease fluid protein.[67] Apocrine carcinoma occurs in both females and males and manifests as a solid or cystic mass ranging from 0.5 to 5 cm in diameter.[68,69]

Histologically, the majority of apocrine carcinomas consist of solid cords and sheets of neoplastic apocrine cells with characteristic abundant, eosinophilic cytoplasm. The granules are typically PAS-positive, diastase-resistant, Sudan black and toluidine blue–positive glycolipids. In areas where glandular differentiation occurs and lumens are present, the cells may exhibit apical cytoplasmic snouts along the luminal margin. The degree of atypia varies, and tumor cells may occasionally present with bizarre, multilobulated nuclei containing multiple nucleoli (Image 9.17).[68,69]

FNAB of apocrine carcinoma yields abundant, pleomorphic tumor cells. The cells have abundant, basophilic to eosinophilic, granular cytoplasm. The nuclei are enlarged and vesicular and are centrally or eccentrically located. The nucleoli are prominent and may be multiple (Images 9.18 through 9.20).[70] Ultrastructurally, the cells show abundant membrane-bound vesicles with a dense, homogeneous, osmophilic core; prominent mitochondria with a dense matrix; and well-developed, rough endoplasmic reticulum.[71]

Well-differentiated apocrine carcinoma must be distinguished from apocrine metaplasia and hyperplastic apocrine cells seen in proliferative breast disease. Aside from the accompanying polymorphous cell population in proliferative lesions, lack of significant hyperchromasia and anisonucleosis are cytologic features that favor a diagnosis of benign apocrine change (Images 9.21 and 9.22). Other lesions included in the differential diagnosis are lipid-rich and secretory carcinoma. Lipid-rich carcinoma is characterized by the presence of abundant, multivacuolated, lipid-rich cells with a more uniform nuclear appearance and a lack of multiple nucleoli.[72] Secretory carcinoma consists of sheets of neoplastic cells with prominent intracellular spaces, cytoplasmic vacuolization, and signet ring formation.[73]

Cytomorphology of Apocrine Carcinoma
Tumor cellularity
Atypical cells with abundant, granular cytoplasm

Large, irregular nuclei
Marked anisonucleosis
Prominent, multiple nucleoli
Inflammatory background

Inflammatory Carcinoma

Inflammatory carcinoma is a distinct clinical presentation of infiltrating duct cell carcinoma that frequently manifests as extensive dermal lymphatic involvement. Described by Lee and Tannenbaum[74] and Taylor and Metzler[75] as an aggressive breast cancer, inflammatory carcinoma represents between 1% and 2% of all breast carcinomas.[74,75] In inflammatory carcinoma, the breast is enlarged, with diffuse erythema, extensive edema, and peau d'orange. Frequently, no palpable, discrete mass is found.[74,76] Regardless of the mode of therapy, patients with inflammatory carcinoma die of the disease shortly after diagnosis.[77] Inflammatory carcinomas are often hormone-receptor negative and have a high proliferation index.[78,79]

Clinically, in the absence of a palpable mass, inflammatory carcinoma could be misinterpreted as an inflammatory process.[80] FNAB can confirm the presence of tumor cells. The neoplastic cells have cytologic features similar to those of infiltrating duct cell carcinoma. Tumor cells often display nuclear membrane irregularity, anisonucleosis, and macronucleoli. A diathesis of debris and blood is frequently present (Images 9.23 through 9.26).[81]

Cytomorphology of Inflammatory Carcinoma
Variable cellularity
Necrotic background
Neoplastic epithelial cells with features of infiltrating duct cell carcinoma

Lipid-Rich Carcinoma

First described by Aboumrad, Horn, and Fine in 1963,[82] lipid-secreting carcinoma is a rare invasive carcinoma of the breast accounting for only 1.4% to 1.6% of invasive breast lesions. Although this tumor was originally described as aggressive, the aggressive nature of the lesion remains to be established.[83–86] Clinically, patients ranging in age from 33 to 81 years present with an ill-defined mass. Occasionally the tumor may cause skin ulceration and a peau d'orange appearance.

Lipid-rich carcinomas vary in size, have irregular borders, and lack chalky streaks or umbilication. This tumor is characterized by the presence of foamy or diffusely vacuolated neoplastic cells containing a large amount of neutral lipid, which forms the bulk of the tumor (Image 9.27).[82,85–87] Van Bogaert and Maldague[84] divided lipid-rich carcinoma into three variants: histiocytoid, sebaceous, and apocrine. The sebaceous variant was characterized by greater nuclear pleomorphism and more bubbly cytoplasm than the histiocytoid. The apocrine variant had tumor cells with a hobnail appearance lining the glandular lumen. In the histiocytoid variant, the tumor cells contained abundant, foamy cytoplasm.

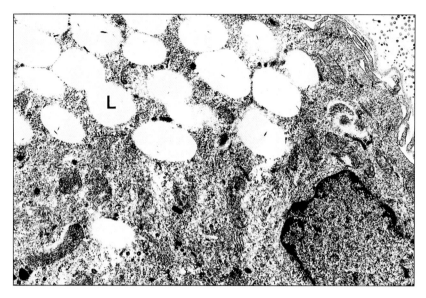

Figure 9.2
Ultrastructure features of lipid-rich carcinoma: multiple lipid droplets (L) in the cytoplasm of tumor cells (13,400X).

Insabato et al[88] reported the cytomorphology of lipid-rich breast carcinoma for the first time via fine needle aspiration biopsy of a 45-year-old woman. Microscopically, the smears were cellular, with loosely cohesive tumor cells. The cytoplasm contained small cytoplasmic vacuoles that varied in number from single, occupying most of the cytoplasm, to multiple, producing a foamy appearance. The vacuoles often were in a perinuclear area. The nuclei showed mild pleomorphism and had a distinct nuclear membrane, a coarse chromatin pattern, and small nucleoli. Nuclear vacuoles and indentations were occasionally seen. The diagnosis of lipid-rich carcinoma was verified histologically by the presence of an overwhelming number of diffusely vacuolized cells dispersed in a prominent, desmoplastic tissue within the mastectomy specimen. Our experience is limited to one case with cytomorphology similar to that described by Insabato et al[88] (Images 9.28 through 9.30). In that case we established the diagnosis by electron microscopy (Figure 9.2).

Classic infiltrating lobular carcinoma is an important differential diagnosis. However, infiltrating lobular carcinoma is composed of tumor cells that frequently have intracytoplasmic lumens that are well demarcated and contain condensed mucous globules easily recognized with special stains.[89] Ultrastructural study of infiltrating lobular carcinoma reveals the presence of intracytoplasmic lumens with microvilli. This is in contrast with the tumor cells of lipid-rich carcinoma, which contain many small and large lipid vacuoles in their cytoplasm.

Recently, an apocrine carcinoma with multivacuolated, lipid-rich giant cells was reported.[90] However, it is not clear whether it should be classified as a subgroup of lipid carcinoma or of apocrine carcinoma.

Cytomorphology of Lipid-Rich Carcinoma
Moderate cellular yield
Loosely cohesive cell arrangement

Foamy, vacuolated tumor cells containing neutral lipid
Atypical, indented nuclei with nuclear vacuoles
Small nucleoli

Secretory Carcinoma

Secretory carcinoma, also known as juvenile carcinoma, is an uncommon variant of ductal carcinoma that was first described in children by McDivitt and Stewart in 1966.[91] Since then, this tumor has been reported at all ages and also in men, and is now called secretory carcinoma regardless of the patient's age.[92,93] The behavior of this tumor seems to be age dependent. When it occurs in children, secretory carcinoma is associated with a better prognosis than the usual duct cell carcinoma, so a conservative surgical approach with local excision and a long follow-up is advocated. Secretory carcinoma in older age groups (ie, >20 years) should be treated like other infiltrating duct cell carcinomas.[91,92]

Clinically, in addition to manifesting as a mass throughout the breast, secretory carcinoma has also been seen in the subareolar region or axillary tail and may cause nipple discharge. Grossly, the lesion is firm, discrete, and well defined, with a median diameter of 3 cm. Histologically, secretory carcinoma is characterized by the presence of extensive extra- and intracellular secretory material. The tumor cells are relatively monotonous and bland in appearance. The cells have regular nuclei with inconspicuous nucleoli. The cytoplasm is abundant and granular and may contain vacuoles and droplets (Images 9.31 and 9.32). The secretory material has been found to be PAS-positive, diastase-resistant; alcian-blue positive; and only occasionally positive for mucicarmine.[92] Positive immunostaining for milk protein and carcinoembryonic antigen has also been observed.[93]

Reports on FNABs of secretory carcinoma demonstrate the existence of specific cytomorphologic features that are sufficiently characteristic to warrant a definitive preoperative diagnosis.[73,94–101] The aspirates are cellular, consisting of numerous dissociated cells, small cell groups, and stromal fragments. Tumor cells are often arranged around a fibrovascular core or in a gland-like structure consisting of a small amount of centrally located mucoid material covered by multiple layers of epithelial cells. Shinogawa et al[101] described these gland-like structures as mucous globular structures. They are generally uniform in size, with minimal cellular atypia or mitosis. When multiple, mucous globular structures resemble a bunch of grapes. The degree of nuclear atypia is variable, and the smears may contain occasional clusters of cells with cytologic features similar to those of ordinary duct cell carcinoma cells (Images 9.33 through 9.38).[96,101]

The cytologic hallmark of secretory carcinoma is the presence of prominent intracytoplasmic vacuoles containing inspissated secretory material that forms hyalin globules. This material is granular and strongly eosinophilic with Giemsa stain and homogeneous and orange or gray-green with Papanicolaou stain. Some of the cells contain multiple vacuoles and some are signet ring cells without visible secretory material. Occasionally, tumor cells are binucleated. Proteinaceous material is also seen in the background.[94–101]

The cytologic differential diagnosis includes other types of breast carcinoma in which vacuoles are seen, such as ductal, tubular, lobular, mucinous, adenoid cystic, signet ring cell, lipid-rich, and glycogen-rich carcinomas, as well as metastatic adenocarcinoma. The vacuoles in duct cell, lobular, mucinous, and signet ring carcinomas are not nearly as numerous as in secretory carcinoma and are always smaller.[102–104] In adenoid cystic carcinoma, extracellular mucin and dense pink globules are surrounded by regular epithelial cells.[105]

Lipid- and glycogen-rich carcinomas can be ruled out with staining, because the vacuoles in each type of tumor cell have specific histochemical properties.[72,106] Metastatic renal cell carcinoma shows a vascular pattern with clear cells that may be visualized easily in a fine needle aspirate.[105] Secretory carcinoma should also be differentiated from nonneoplastic entities, particularly in young women. Pregnancy and lactational changes can be detected by examining smears for evidence of a proteinaceous background, cellular cohesion, histiocytes, and multinucleation.[107]

Cytomorphology of Secretory Carcinoma
Cellular aspirate
Proteinaceous background
Variable cellular arrangement, including bunches of grapes or mucous
*   globular structures*
Prominent intracytoplasmic vacuoles
Granular cells
Signet ring cells
Variable nuclear atypia
No mitosis or necrosis

Paget's Disease

Clinically, Paget's disease appears as an eczematous or ulcerated lesion of the nipple and areola (Figure 9.3). It is associated with an underlying

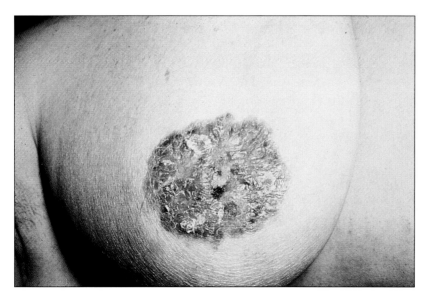

Figure 9.3
Gross appearance of Paget's disease characterized by an eczematous lesion of the nipple.

breast cancer. This lesion can be sampled by scraping or by fine needle aspiration biopsy. The smears show easily recognized malignant cells with centrally located nuclei and abundant clear cytoplasm. Tumor cells are seen in a background of keratinous material, inflammatory cells, and squamous cells. Although malignant melanoma is extremely rare in the nipple area, when present it sometimes has clinical and cytologic features similar to those of Paget's disease. Paget's disease often shows positive immunostaining for estrogen and progesterone receptors, carcinoembryonic antigen, and epithelial membrane antigen, whereas malignant melanoma shows a positive reaction with S-100 and HMB-45 protein. Reactions with mucin and periodic acid–Schiff are positive in Paget's disease and negative in melanoma (Images 9.39 through 9.43).[108]

Cytomorphology of Paget's Disease
Variable cellularity
Pleomorphic cell population
Large cells with centrally located nuclei
Clear cytoplasm
Mucin positivity

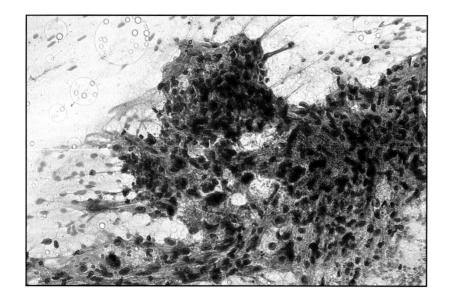

Image 9.1
Aspirate of metaplastic (sarcomatoid) carcinoma of the breast shows a group of spindle-shaped malignant cells and tumor giant cells (Papanicolaou, 200X).

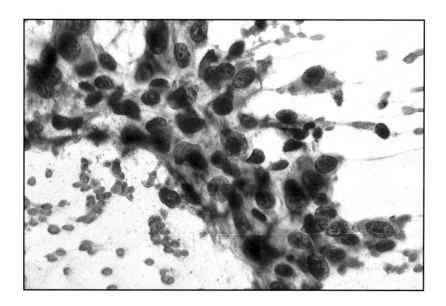

Image 9.2
Fine needle aspirate of metaplastic carcinoma consisting of pleomorphic neoplastic spindle cells (Papanicolaou, 400X).

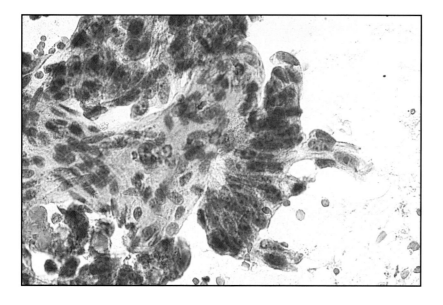

Image 9.3
Group of epithelial cells representing the carcinomatous component adjacent to sarcomatous portion in metaplastic carcinoma (Papanicolaou, 400X).

Image 9.4
Cell block preparation of metaplastic carcinoma. The tumor cells show intense positivity for vimentin (Immunoperoxidase, 200X).

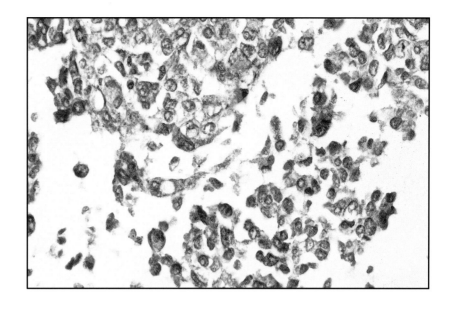

Image 9.5
Cell block preparation of metaplastic carcinoma. Clusters of tumor cells show a positive reaction for cytokeratin (Immunoperoxidase, 200X).

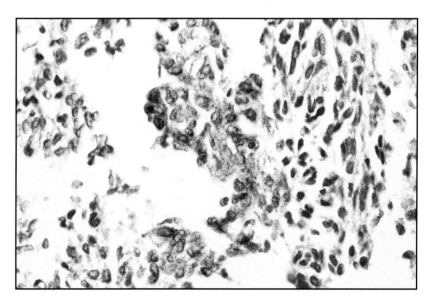

Image 9.6
Corresponding tissue section of metaplastic carcinoma displays spindle-shaped, pleomorphic tumor cells with tumor giant cells (H&E, 400X).

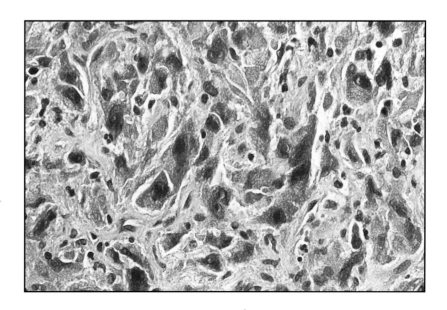

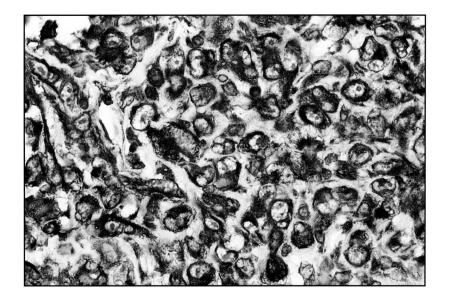

Image 9.7
Corresponding tissue section of metaplastic carcinoma shows strong positivity for vimentin (Immunoperoxidase, 400X).

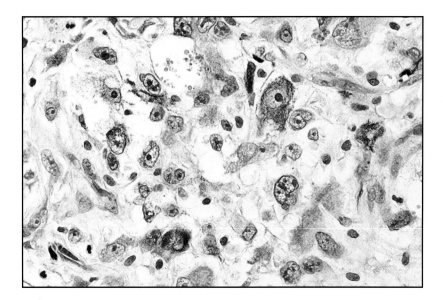

Image 9.8
Focal positive immunostaining for cytokeratin in corresponding tissue section of metaplastic carcinoma (Immunoperoxidase, 400X).

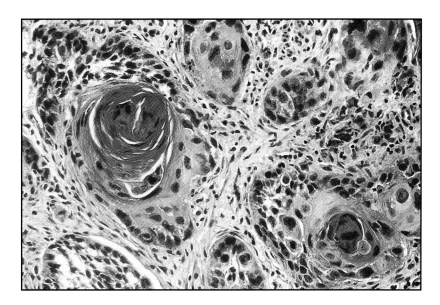

Image 9.9
Histologic appearance of squamous cell carcinoma of the breast: neoplastic epithelial cells with pearl formation and keratinization (H&E, 400X).

Image 9.10
Aspirate of squamous cell carcinoma of the breast reveals clusters of highly atypical epithelial cells in a necrotic background (Papanicolaou, 400X).

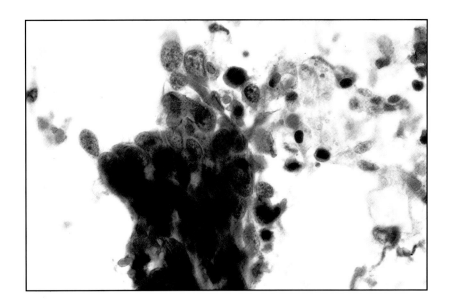

Image 9.11
Another view of the same case shows individual cell keratinization and mitosis in a necrotic background (Papanicolaou, 400X).

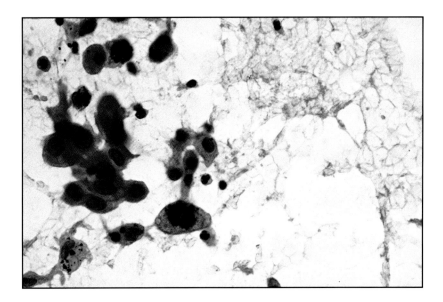

Image 9.12
Cell block preparation of the same case demonstrates a cluster of neoplastic epithelial cells with squamous differentiation (H&E, 400X).

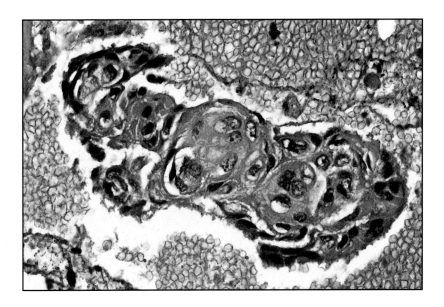

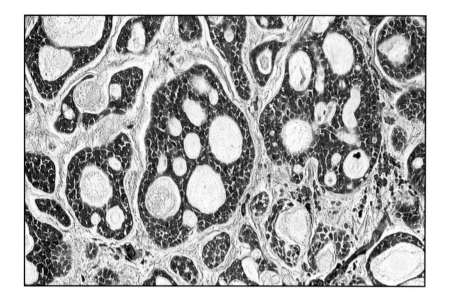

Image 9.13
Histologic appearance of adenoid cystic carcinoma of the breast: proliferation of nests and islands of uniform small cells in solid and cribriform patterns surrounding amorphous eosinophilic material (H&E, 200X).

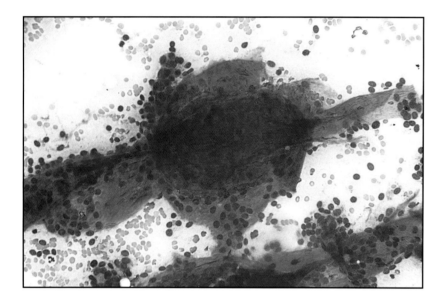

Image 9.14
Cellular aspirate of adenoid cystic carcinoma of the breast shows bland-appearing tumor cells admixed with acellular and homogeneous material (hyaline bodies) (Diff-Quik®, 200X).

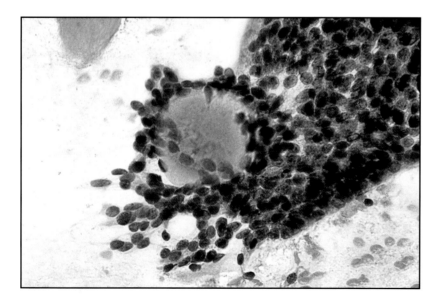

Image 9.15
Higher magnification of the same case reveals small cells with round to oval, hyperchromatic nuclei and scant cytoplasm surrounding the hyaline bodies (Papanicolaou, 400X).

Image 9.16
Oil magnification of the same case (Papanicolaou, 1000X).

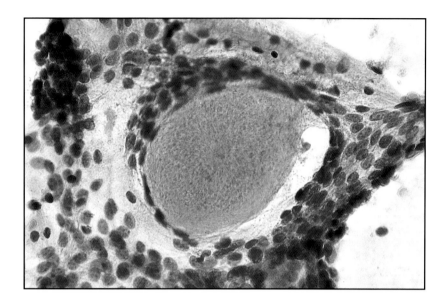

Image 9.17
Histologic appearance of apocrine carcinoma: neoplastic epithelial cells with abundant, eosinophilic cytoplasm (H&E, 200X).

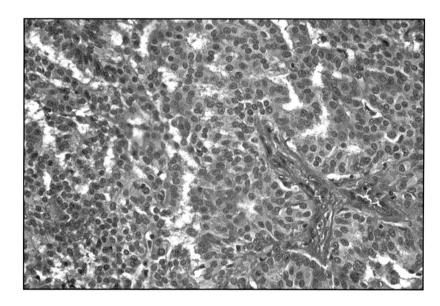

Image 9.18
Aspirate of apocrine carcinoma reveals a dispersed cell pattern and epithelial cells of various sizes (Diff-Quik, 400X).

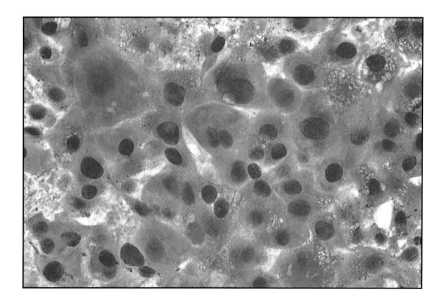

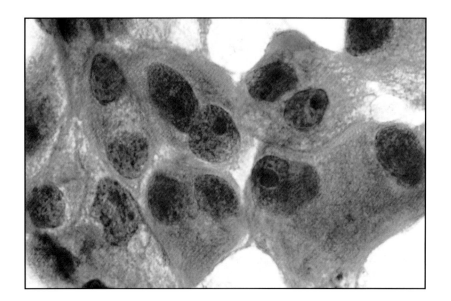

Image 9.19
Hyperchromasia and anisonucleosis in aspirate of apocrine carcinoma (Papanicolaou, 1000X).

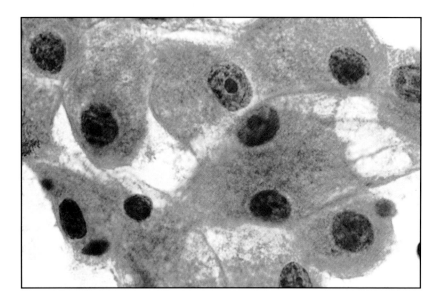

Image 9.20
Nucleoli and abundant cytoplasm in smear of apocrine carcinoma (Papanicolaou, 1000X).

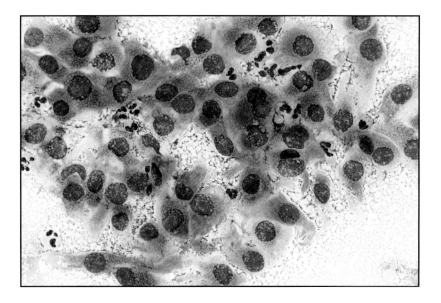

Image 9.21
Hyperplastic apocrine cells with features different from those of apocrine carcinoma. Note the uniformity of the nuclear features (Diff-Quik, 200X).

Image 9.22
Higher magnification reveals the presence of conspicuous nucleoli in a cluster of reactive apocrine cells and absence of anisonucleosis (Diff-Quik, 400X).

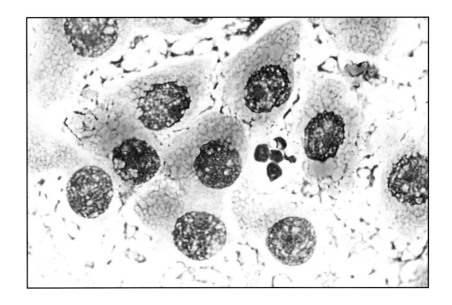

Image 9.23
Involvement of the dermal lymph nodes by inflammatory carcinoma of the breast (H&E, 200X).

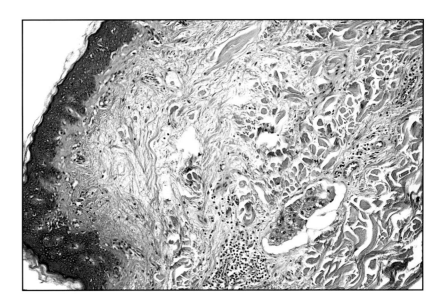

Image 9.24
Higher magnification of the same case reveals the presence of neoplastic epithelial cells in a lymphatic channel (H&E, 400X).

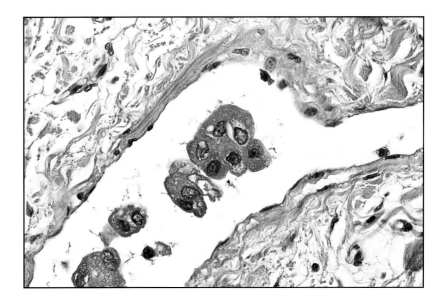

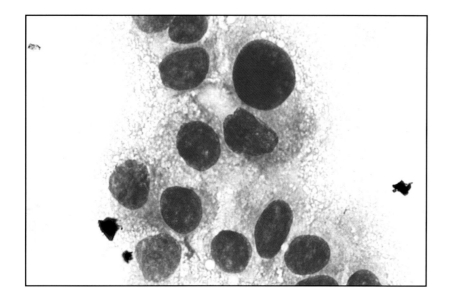

Image 9.25
Aspirate of inflammatory carcinoma shows a loosely cohesive cluster of malignant epithelial cells (Diff-Quik, 400X).

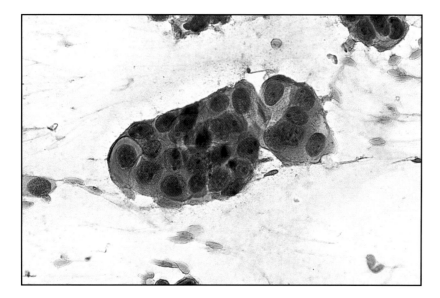

Image 9.26
Papanicolaou-stained smear of the same case with morphologic features characteristic of an infiltrating duct cell carcinoma (400X).

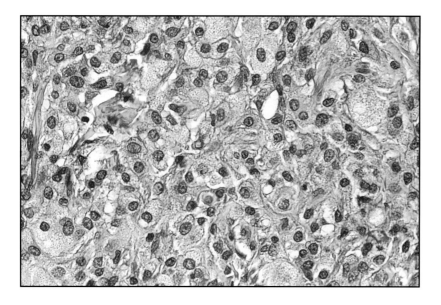

Image 9.27
Histologic appearance of lipid rich carcinoma: diffuse infiltration of vacuolated neoplastic cells within the stroma (H&E, 200X).

Image 9.28
Cellular aspirate of lipid-rich carcinoma consisting of variably sized epithelial cells isolated and in clusters (Diff-Quik, 100X).

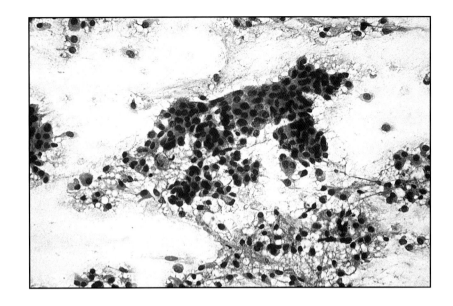

Image 9.29
Higher magnification of the same case demonstrates a pleomorphic population of tumor cells with indistinct cell borders; foamy, vacuolated cytoplasm; and nuclear atypia. The nuclei are hyperchromatic with occasional nucleoli and nuclear indentation (Diff-Quik, 400X).

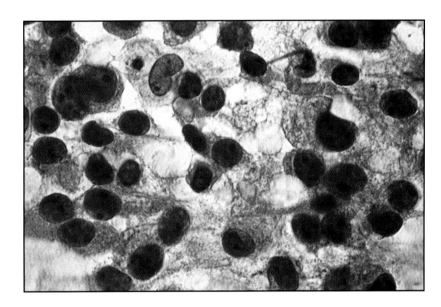

Image 9.30
Papanicolaou-stained smear of the same case shows multivacuolated tumor cells in a necrotic background (400X).

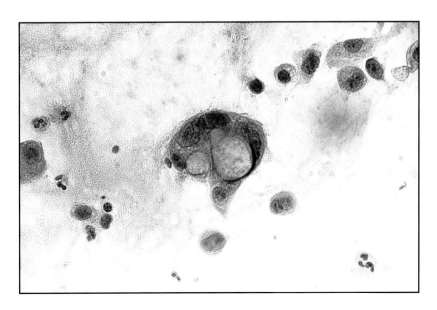

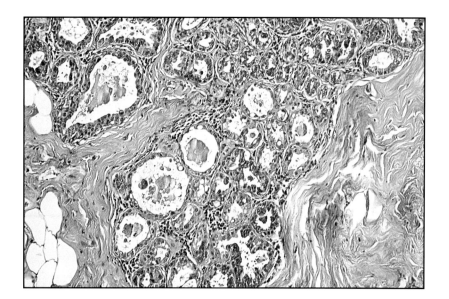

Image 9.31
Histologic appearance of secretory carcinoma: glandular type with expanded lumens and conspicuous inspissated material forming a follicular pattern (H&E, 100X).

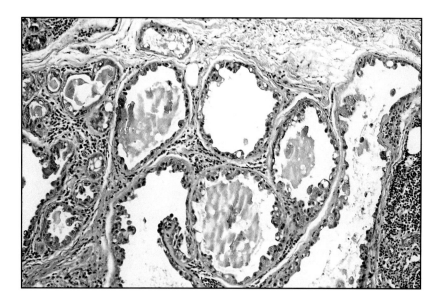

Image 9.32
Another view of secretory carcinoma demonstrating various-sized follicular-like structures with inspissated material (H&E, 200X).

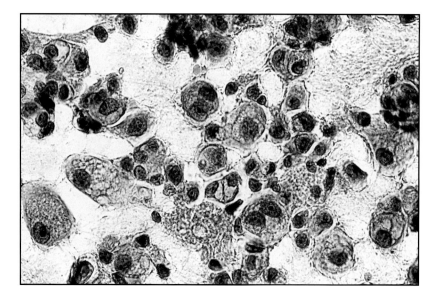

Image 9.33
Cellular aspirate of secretory carcinoma displays foamy and vacuolated cells (Papanicolaou, 200X).

Image 9.34
Bunch of grape-like structures consisting of clustered vacuolated cells containing inspissated mucoid material seen in an aspirate of secretory carcinoma (Papanicolaou, 200X).

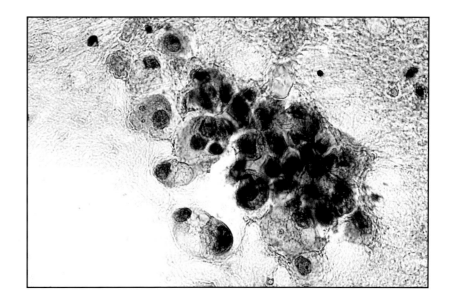

Image 9.35
Aspirate of secretory carcinoma of the breast displays loosely cohesive clusters of tumor cells with granular cytoplasm, and round to oval nuclei intermingled with signet ring cells, mucous globular structures, and intravacuolated secretions (Papanicolaou, 1000X).

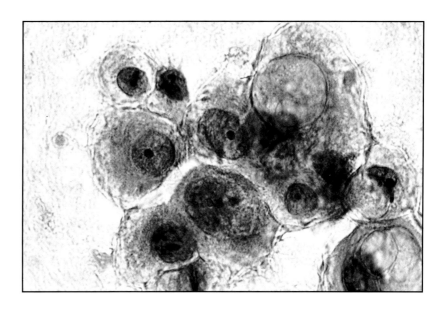

Image 9.36
Aspirate of secretory carcinoma shows vacuoles of various sizes ranging from small and single to large and multiple (Diff-Quik, 1000X).

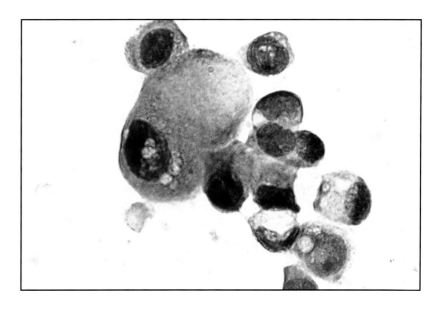

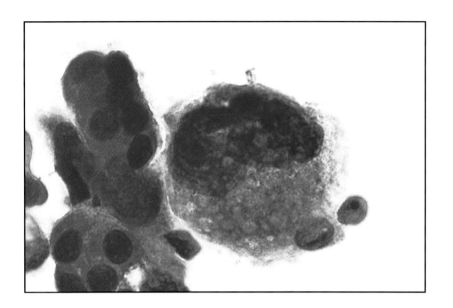

Image 9.37
Different view of the same case of secretory carcinoma shows a cluster of tumor cells. Some have a single nucleus; others are binucleated. Note the presence of multiple vacuoles in an enlarged, binucleated cell (Diff-Quik, 1000X).

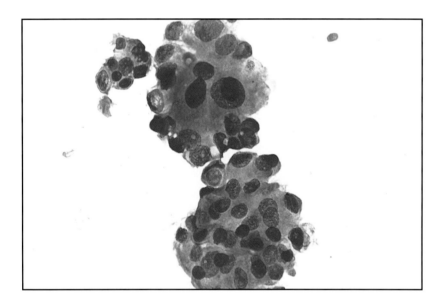

Image 9.38
Cluster of pleomorphic tumor cells similar to those seen in ordinary duct cell carcinoma, observed in an aspirate of a secretory carcinoma (Diff-Quik, 200X).

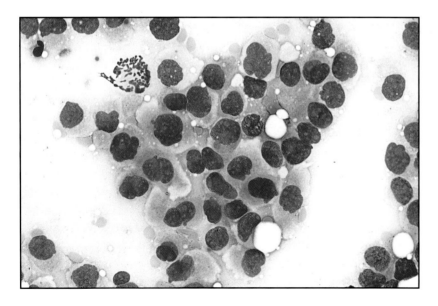

Image 9.39
Aspirate of Paget's disease shows a loosely cohesive cluster of variably sized epithelial cells (Diff-Quik, 200X).

Image 9.40
Papanicolaou-stained smear of the same case demonstrates clusters of neoplastic epithelial cells with centrally located nuclei and clear cytoplasm (400X).

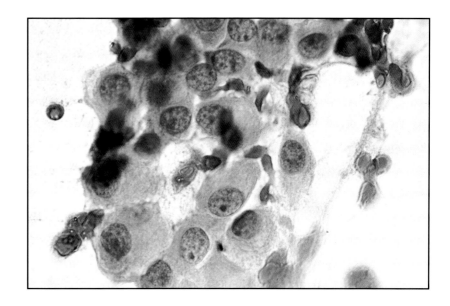

Image 9.41
Expression of estrogen receptor evidenced by nuclear staining in malignant cells seen in Paget's disease (200X).

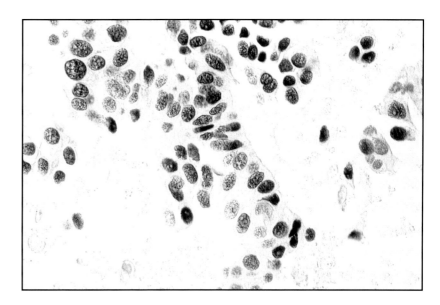

Image 9.42
Histologic appearance of Paget's disease: infiltration of malignant cells into the epidermis (H&E, 400X).

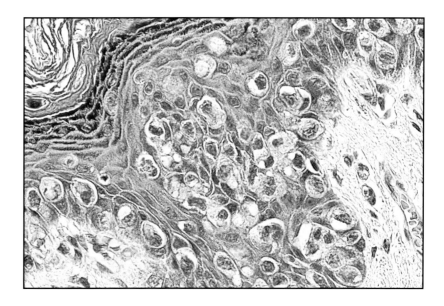

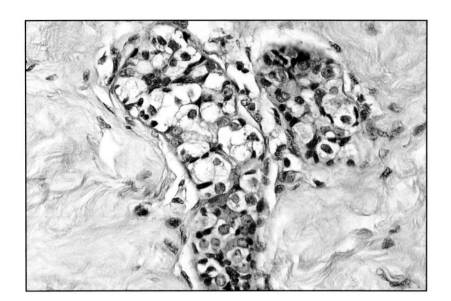

Image 9.43
Clusters of neoplastic epithelial cells in the stroma, evidence of an underlying duct cell carcinoma in Paget's disease of the breast (H&E, 400X).

References

1. Gonzalez-Licea A, Yardley JH, Hartman WH: Malignant tumor of the breast with bone formation. *Cancer* 20:1234–1247, 1967.

2. Kahn LB, Uys CJ, Dale J, et al: Carcinoma of the breast with pseudosarcomatous metaplasia. *Cancer* 53:1908–1917, 1984.

3. Oberman HA: Metaplastic carcinoma of the breast: A clinicopathologic study of 29 patients. *Am J Surg Pathol* 11:918–919, 1987.

4. Leong ASY, Meredith DJ: Tubular carcinoma developing within a recurring cystosarcoma phyllodes of the breast. *Cancer* 46:1863–1867, 1980.

5. Thiis Knudsen PJ, Gestergaard J: Cystosarcoma phyllodes with lobular and ductal carcinoma in situ. *Arch Pathol Lab Med* 111: 873–875, 1987.

6. Gupta RK, Wakefield SJ, Holloway LJ, Simpson JS: Immunocytochemical and ultrastructural study of the rare osteoclast type carcinoma of the breast in a fine needle aspirate. *Acta Cytol* 32:79–82, 1988.

7. Harris M, Persaud V: Carcinosarcoma of the breast. *J Pathol* 112: 99–105, 1974.

8. Rosai J: *Ackerman's Surgical Pathology.* St Louis, Mo, CV Mosby Co, 1989, p. 1237.

9. Wargotz ES, Norris HJ: Metaplastic carcinomas of the breast, III. Carcinosarcoma. *Cancer* 64:1490–1499, 1989.

10. Kaufmann MW, Marti JR, Gallager HS, Hoehn JL: Carcinoma of the breast with pseudo-sarcomatous metaplasia. *Cancer* 53:1908–1971, 1984.

11. Liombant-Bosch A, Peydro A: Malignant mixed osteogenic tumors of the breast. *Virchows Arch [Pathol Anat]* 366:1–14, 1975.

12. Hager J, Lederer B: Maligner mischtumor der brustdruese. *Zentralbl Allg Pathol* 121:522–525, 1977.

13. Wargotz ES, Norris HJ: Metaplastic carcinomas of the breast, I. Matrix producing carcinoma. *Hum Pathol* 20:628–635, 1989.

14. Oberman HA: Metaplastic carcinoma of the breast. A clinicopathologic study of 29 patients. *Am J Surg Pathol* 11:918–929, 1987.

15. Santeusanio G, Pascal RR, Bisceglia M, et al: Metaplastic breast carcinoma with epithelial phenotype of pseudosarcomatous components. *Arch Pathol Lab Med* 112:82–85, 1988.

16. Flint A, Oberman HA, Davenport RD: Cytophotometric measurements of metaplastic carcinoma of the breast: correlation with pathologic features and clinical behavior. *Mod Pathol* 1:193–197, 1988.

17. Jebsen PW, Hagmar BM, Nesland JM: Metaplastic breast carcinoma: A diagnostic problem in fine needle aspiration biopsy. *Acta Cytol* 35:396–402, 1991.

18. Boccato P, Briani G, d'Atri C, et al: Spindle cell and cartilaginous metaplasia in a breast carcinoma with osteoclast-like stromal cells. *Acta Cytol* 32:75–78, 1988.

19. Silverman JF, Geisinger KR, Frable WJ: Fine needle aspiration cytology of mesenchymal tumors of the breast. *Diagn Cytopathol* 4:50–58, 1988.

20. Stanley MW, Tani EM, Skoog L: Metaplastic carcinoma of the breast: fine needle aspiration cytology of seven cases. *Diagn Cytopathol* 5:22–28, 1989.

21. Kline TS, Kline IK: Metaplastic carcinoma of the breast diagnosed by aspiration biopsy cytology: report of two cases and literature review. *Diagn Cytopathol* 6:63–67, 1990.

22. Das DK, Samhan M, Bashir HM, et al: Metaplastic carcinoma of the breast in a renal transplant recipient. *Acta Cytol* 38:917–922, 1994.

23. Stanley MW, Tani EM, Horwitz CA, et al: Primary spindle cell sarcomas of the breast: diagnosis by fine needle aspiration. *Diagn Cytopathol* 4:244–249, 1988.

24. Silverman JF, Feldman PS, Cavell JL, et al: Fine needle aspiration cytology of neoplasms metastatic to the breast. *Acta Cytol* 31: 291–304, 1987.

25. Silverman JF, Lannin DR, Unverferth M, et al: Fine needle aspiration cytology of subareolar abscess of the breast: spectrum of cytomorphologic findings and potential diagnostic pitfalls. *Acta Cytol* 30:413–419, 1986.

26. Galblum LI, Oertel YC: Subareolar abscess of the breast: diagnosis by fine needle aspiration. *Am J Clin Pathol* 80:396–499, 1983.

27. Cornog JL, Mobini J, Steiger HT: Squamous carcinoma of the breast. *Am J Clin Pathol* 55:410–417, 1971.

28. Eggers JW, Chesney TM: Squamous cell carcinoma of the breast: a clinicopathological analysis of eight cases and review of the literature. *Hum Pathol* 15:526–531, 1984.

29. Dalla Palma P, Parenti A: Squamous breast cancer: report of two cases and review of the literature. *Appl Pathol* 1:14–24, 1983.

30. Hsiu JG, Hawkins AG, D'Amato NA: A case of pure squamous cell carcinoma of the breast diagnosed by fine needle aspiration biopsy. *Acta Cytol* 29:650–651, 1985.

31. LaFreniere R, Moskowitz LB, Ketchamn AS: Pure squamous cell carcinoma of the breast. *J Surg Oncol* 31:113–119, 1986.

32. Prasad N, Prasad P: A case of pure squamous cell carcinoma of the breast diagnosed by fine needle aspiration biopsy. *Indian J Pathol Microbiol* 31:71–72, 1988.

33. Shousha S, James AH, Fernandez D, et al: Squamous cell carcinoma of the breast. *Arch Pathol Lab Med* 108:893-896, 1984.

34. Li Z, Yutain L: Squamous cell carcinoma of the breast. *Am J Surg* 147:701–702, 1984.

35. Chen KTK: Fine needle aspiration cytology of squamous cell carcinoma of the breast. *Acta Cytol* 34:664–668, 1990.

36. Leiman G: Squamous carcinoma in breast aspiration cytology. *Acta Cytol* 26:201–209, 1982.

37. Macia M, Ces JA, Becerra E, et al: Pure squamous cell carcinoma of the breast: report of a case diagnosed by aspiration cytology. *Acta Cytol* 33:201–204, 1989.

38. Gubin N: A case of pure squamous cell carcinoma of the breast diagnosed by fine needle aspiration biopsy. *Acta Cytol* 29:650–651, 1985.

39. Lazarevic B, Katatikarn V, Marks RA: Primary squamous cell carcinoma of the breast: diagnosis by fine needle aspiration cytology. *Acta Cytol* 28:321–324, 1984.

40. Koward LM, Verhulst LA, Copeland CM, et al: Epidermoid cyst of the breast. *Can Med Assoc J* 131:217–219, 1984.

41. Salmi R: Epidermoid metaplasia in mammary fibroadenoma with formation of keratin cysts. *J Pathol Bacteriol* 74:221–222, 1957.

42. Shousha S: Squamous metaplasia in fibroadenoma of the breast. *Histopathology* 10:1001–1002, 1986.

43. Kevi J, Duong HD, Leffall LD Jr: High-grade mucoepidermoid carcinoma of the breast. *Arch Pathol Lab Med* 105:612–614, 1981.

44. Trapasso Rl, McCarty KS Jr, Proia AD, et al: Adenosquamous differentiation: mammary needle aspiration cytology. *Acta Cytol* 25: 196–198, 1981.

45. Patchefsky AS, Frauenhoffer CM, Krall RA, et al: Low-grade mucoepidermoid carcinoma of the breast. *Arch Pathol Lab Med* 103:196–198, 1979.

46. Fisher ER, Palelcar AS, Gregorio RM, et al: Mucoepidermoid and squamous cell carcinoma of the breast with reference to squamous metaplasia and giant cell tumors. *Am J Surg Pathol* 7:15–27, 1983.

47. Hastrup N, Sehested M: High-grade mucoepidermoid carcinoma of the breast. *Histopathology* 9:887–892, 1985.

48. Leong ASY, Williams JAR: Mucoepidermoid carcinoma of the breast: high-grade variant. *Pathology* 17:516–521, 1985.

49. Kovi J, Duong HD, Leffal HD: High-grade mucoepidermoid carcinoma of the breast. *Arch Pathol Lab Med* 105:612–614, 1981.

50. Peltinato G, Insabato L, DeChiara A, et al: High-grade mucoepidermoid carcinoma of the breast, fine needle aspiration cytology and clinicopathologic study of a case. *Acta Cytol* 33:195–200, 1989.

51. Anthony PP, James PD: Adenoid cystic carcinoma of the breast: prevalence, diagnostic criteria and histogenesis. *J Clin Pathol* 28: 647–655, 1975.

52. Cavanzo FJ, Taylor HB: Adenoid cystic carcinoma of the breast: an analysis of 21 cases. *Cancer* 24:740–745, 1969.

53. Peters GN, Wolff M: Adenoid cystic carcinoma of the breast: report of 11 new cases. Review of the literature and discussion of biological behavior. *Cancer* 52:1752–1760, 1979.

54. Foote FW Jr, Stewart FW: A histologic classification of carcinoma of the breast. *Surgery* 19:74–99, 1946.

55. Hjorth S, Magnusson PA, Blomquist P: Adenoid cystic carcinoma of the breast. Report of a case in male and review of the literature. *Acta Clin Scand* 143:155–158, 1977.

56. Galloway JR, Woolner LB, Clagget OT: Adenoid cystic carcinoma of the breast. *Surg Gynecol Obstet* 122:1289–1294, 1966.

57. Lamovex I, Us-Krasovec M, Zidar A, et al: Adenoid cystic carcinoma of the breast: a histologic, cytologic and immunohistochemical study. *Semin Diagn Pathol* 6:153–164, 1989.

58. Oertel YC, Galblum LI: Fine needle aspiration of the breast: diagnostic criteria. *Pathol Annu* 18:375–407, 1983.

59. Galed-Placid I, Garcia-Ureta E: Fine needle aspiration biopsy diagnosis of adenoid cystic carcinoma of the breast. A case report. *Acta Cytol* 36:364–366, 1992.

60. Greshang LE: Adenoid cystic carcinoma of the breast. *Arch Pathol Lab Med* 101:307–309, 1977.

61. Stanley MW, Toni EM, Rutquist LE, et al: Adenoid cystic carcinoma of the breast: diagnosis by fine needle aspiration. *Diagn Cytopathol* 9:184–187, 1993.

62. Johnson TL, Kini SH: Cytologic features of collagenous spherulosis of the breast. *Diagn Cytopathol* 7:417–419, 1991.

63. Azzopardi JG: Problems in breast pathology. In: Bennington JL, ed. *Major Problems in Pathology,* vol 11. Philadelphia, Pa, WB Saunders Co, 1979, pp. 286, 341.

64. Bonser GM, Dossett JA, Jull JW: *Human and Experimental Breast Cancer.* London, England, Pitman Medical, 1981, p. 322.

65. Eusebi V, Millis RR, Cattani MG, et al: Apocrine carcinoma of the breast. A morphologic and immunocytochemical study. *Am J Pathol* 123:532–541, 1986.

66. Abati AD, Kimmel M, Rosen PP: Apocrine mammary carcinoma. A clinicopathologic study of 72 cases. *Am J Clin Pathol* 94:371–377, 1990.

67. Mazoujian G, Bodian C, Hangensen DE Jr, et al: Expression of GCDFP-15 in breast carcinomas. Relationship to pathologic and clinical factors. *Cancer* 63:2156–2161, 1989.

68. Frable WJ, Kay S: Carcinoma of the breast. Histologic and clinical features of apocrine tumors. *Cancer* 21:756–763, 1968.

69. Bryant J: Male breast cancer: a case of apocrine carcinoma with psammoma bodies. *Hum Pathol* 12:751–753, 1981.

70. Zajdela A, Ghossein NA, Pilleran JP, et al: The experience of aspiration cytology in the diagnosis of breast cancer. Experience at the Fondation Curie. *Cancer* 35:499–506, 1975.

71. Ito F, Avai, Suzuki M, et al: Apocrine carcinoma of the breast with cytologic, histologic and electron microscopic findings: a case report. *Acta Cytol* 36:792, 1992. Abstract.

72. Lapey JD: Lipid-rich mammary carcinoma: diagnosis by cytology. Case report. *Acta Cytol* 21:120–122, 1977.

73. Canarese G: Secretory carcinoma of the breast. Report of a case with fine needle aspiration biopsy. *Acta Cytol* 30:309–312, 1986.

74. Lee BJ, Tannenbaum NE: Inflammatory carcinoma of the breast. *Surg Gynecol* 39:580–595, 1924.

75. Taylor GW, Metzler A: Inflammatory carcinoma of the breast. *Am J Cancer* 33:33–49, 1938.

76. Levine PH, Steinborn SC, Ries IG: Inflammatory breast cancer: the experience of the surveillance, epidemiology and end results (SEER) program. *J Natl Cancer Inst* 74:291–297, 1985.

77. Kokal WA, Hill LR, Porudominsky D, et al: Inflammatory breast carcinoma: a distinctive entity. *J Surg Oncol* 30:152–155, 1985.

78. Harvey HA, Lipton A, Lawrence BV, et al: Estrogen receptor status in inflammatory carcinoma. *J Surg Oncol* 21:42–44, 1982.

79. Paradiso G, Tommasi S, Brandi M, et al: Cell kinetics and hormonal receptor status in inflammatory breast carcinoma. Comparison with locally advanced disease. *Cancer* 64:1922–1927, 1989.

80. Mussbaum H, Kagan AR, Gilbert H, et al: Management of inflammatory carcinoma. *Dis Breast* 3:25–28, 1977.

81. Kline TS: Breast lesions, diagnosis by fine needle aspiration biopsy. *Am J Diagn Gynecol Obstet* 1:11–16, 1979.

82. Aboumrad MH, Horn RC, Fine G: Lipid secreting mammary carcinoma. *Cancer* 16:521–525, 1963.

83. Ramos CV, Taylor HB: Lipid rich carcinoma of the breast. A clinico-pathologic analysis of 13 examples. *Cancer* 33:812–819, 1974.

84. Van Bogaert LJ, Maldague P: Histologic variants of lipid-secreting carcinoma of the breast. *Virchows Arch [A]* 375:345-353, 1977.

85. Kurebayashi J, Izuo M, Ishida J, et al: Two cases of lipid-secreting carcinoma of the breast: case reports with an electron microscopic study. *Jpn J Clin Oncol* 18:249–254, 1988.

86. Fisher ER, Gregorio R, Kim WS, et al: Lipid invasive cancer of the breast. *Am J Clin Pathol* 68:558–561, 1977.

87. Page DL, Anderson TJ: *Diagnostic Histopathology of the Breast.* Edinburgh, Scotland, Churchill Livingstone, 1977, pp. 256-257.

88. Insabato L, Russo R, Cascone AM, et al: Fine needle aspiration cytology of lipid-secreting breast carcinoma. A case report. *Acta Cytol* 37:752–755, 1993.

89. Spriggs AL, Jerrome DW: Intracellular mucous inclusions: a feature of malignant cells in effusions in the serous cavities, particularly due to carcinoma of the breast. *J Clin Pathol* 28:929–936, 1975.

90. Duggan MA, Young GK, Hwang WS: Fine needle aspiration of an apocrine breast carcinoma with multivacuolated, lipid-rich giant cells. *Diagn Cytopathol* 4:62–66, 1988.

91. McDivitt RW, Stewart FW: Breast carcinoma in children. *JAMA* 195:388–390, 1966.

92. Tavassoli FA, Norris HJ: Secretory carcinoma of the breast. *Cancer* 45:2404–2413, 1980.

93. Roth JA, Disconfani C, O'Malley M: Secretory breast carcinoma in a man. *Am J Surg Pathol* 12:150–154, 1988.

94. Pohar-Marinsek Z, Goloub R: Secretory breast carcinoma in a man diagnosed by fine needle aspiration biopsy, a case report. *Acta Cytol* 38:446–450, 1994.

95. Dominguez F, Riera JR, Jung P, et al: Secretory carcinoma of the breast, report of a case with diagnosis by fine needle aspiration. *Acta Cytol* 36:507–510, 1992.

96. Craig JP: Secretory carcinoma of the breast in an adult: correlation of aspiration cytology and histology on the biopsy specimen. *Acta Cytol* 29:589–592, 1985.

97. d'Amato ESG, Maisto L, Golleschi MB, et al: Secretory carcinoma of the breast: report of a case with fine needle aspiration biopsy. *Acta Cytol* 30:309–312, 1985.

98. Gupta RR, Lallu SD, Fauch R, et al: Needle aspiration cytology, immunocytochemistry and electron microscopy in a rare case of secretory carcinoma of the breast in an elderly woman. *Diagn Cytopathol* 8:388–391, 1992.

99. Shinogawa T, Tadokoro M, Takeuchi E, et al: Aspiration biopsy cytology of secretory carcinoma of the breast, a case report. *Acta Cytol* 36:189–193, 1992.

100. Nguyen GK, Neifer R: Aspiration biopsy cytology of secretory carcinoma of the breast. *Diagn Cytopathol* 3:234–237, 1987.

101. Shinogawa T, Tadokoro M, Kilamura H, et al: Secretory carcinoma of the breast: correlation of aspiration cytology and histology. *Acta Cytol* 38:909–914, 1994.

102. Batifora H: Intracytoplasmic lumina in breast carcinoma: a helpful histopathologic feature. *Arch Pathol* 99:614-617, 1975.

103. Lennart B, Karin L: Aspiration cytology of tubular carcinoma. *Acta Cytol* 34:15–20, 1990.

104. Merino MY, Livolsi VA: Signet ring carcinoma of the female breast. *Cancer* 48:1830–1837, 1981.

105. Oertel YC: Fine needle aspiration of the breast in adults. *Am J Surg Pathol* 4:465–470, 1980.

106. Fisher ER, Tavares J, Bulatoo IS, et al: Glycogen-rich clear cell breast cancer with comments concerning other clear cell variants. *Hum Pathol* 16:1085–1090, 1985.

107. Bottles K, Taylor RN: Diagnosis of breast masses in pregnant and lactating women by aspiration cytology. *Obstet Gynecol* 66:765–785, 1985.

108. Wilkinson EJ, Franzini DA, Masood S: Cytological needle sampling of the breast: techniques and end results. In: Bland K, Copland E, eds. *The Breast.* Philadelphia, Pa, WB Saunders Co, 1990, pp. 475–478.

CHAPTER TEN

Sarcomas of the Breast

Malignant mesenchymal tumors, which include phyllodes tumor and angiosarcoma, constitute less than 1% of all malignant lesions of the breast.[1,2] Except for pure spindle cell sarcomas, which arise from the specialized breast stroma, breast sarcomas are classified histogenetically as low-, intermediate-, or high-grade lesions. Classification is based on the number of mitotic figures, cellularity, pleomorphism, and presence or absence of necrosis.[3] Sarcomas metastasize through the blood stream, with the lung as the most common site of metastasis. Lymph node metastasis is extremely rare. Low-grade lesions and lesions occurring in older patients may require only wide local excision. Mastectomy with adjuvant chemotherapy is the recommended treatment for high-grade sarcomas.[4,5]

Phyllodes Tumor (Cystosarcoma Phyllodes)

Phyllodes tumor is a distinctive breast tumor composed of benign epithelial elements and a cellular spindle cell stroma.[6,7] The microscopic pattern of this tumor does not always reflect its biologic behavior.[8] The majority of phyllodes tumors are not clinically malignant, and yet cystosarcoma phyllodes has remained the standard designation for this lesion. The term phyllodes tumor, proposed by the World Health Organization, is preferable, because it avoids the deceptive implication of malignancy.[9] First described in 1838, phyllodes tumors are now divided histopathologically into benign, borderline, and malignant subgroups.[8,10–13] Phyllodes tumors constitute 0.3% of all breast tumors.[10] The average age of patients affected by the tumor is 45, which is about 20 years older than the average age of patients with fibroadenoma. Phyllodes tumors also rarely occur in men and children.[8,13–15]

The prognostic significance of morphologic features in separating benign from malignant lesions remains controversial. Tumor size, tumor margin, number of mitoses, and atypia of stromal cells are the parameters most useful in assessing the behavior of phyllodes tumors. Despite the existence of these parameters, however, there are cases in which histologically benign tumors have metastasized, while only 12% of malignant phyllodes tumors metastasize.[8,13,16] Metastasis occurs through the blood stream and has been reported in almost all organ sites. Recurrences develop in approximately 30% of patients with cystosarcoma, often within 2 years of the initial diagnosis.[13]

Clinically, phyllodes tumor manifests as a palpable mass and may grow rapidly to a large size.[17] Axillary lymph node enlargement due to reactive changes has been reported in 17% of patients with phyllodes tumor.[8] Grossly, phyllodes tumors present a highly variable picture; however, in the majority of the cases the tumor is a solid, fleshy mass with cystic areas (Figure 10.1).

Histologically, phyllodes tumor is characterized by a benign epithelial component surrounded by a cellular spindle cell stroma (Image 10.1). The tumor forms leaf-like processes that protrude into cystic spaces, distinguishing it from cellular fibroadenoma. The biphasic pattern seen in phyllodes tumor is similar to that seen in fibroadenoma, but in phyllodes tumor the stroma is often more cellular and hyperplastic. The stroma in phyllodes tumor may contain multinucleated cells with focal areas of lipoid, chondroid, chondroid and osseous, rhabdomyoblastic, and smooth muscle differentiation.[8] In aggressive phyllodes tumors, the stromal component is often fibrosarcomatous in appearance. However, other types of sarcoma, such as liposarcoma, osteosarcoma, rhabdomyosarcoma, hemangiopericytoma, and malignant fibrous histiocytoma, can occur.[13,18,19] Mastectomy remains the standard treatment for some cases of phyllodes tumor, although a more conservative approach, ie, wide local excision, is now being advocated.[8]

As in fibroadenoma, both in situ and invasive carcinomas may occur within phyllodes tumor.[13,17,20,21] Phyllodes tumors are generally positive for progesterone receptors.[22] Ploidy study by El-Naggar et al[23] showed that DNA content is a significant predictor of clinical outcome.

The cytologic features of phyllodes tumors have already been reported.[24–32] Generally, aspirates of phyllodes tumors are rich in cellularity and demonstrate a distinct biphasic pattern. The smears contain uniform populations of epithelial cells that form large, folded sheets and have oval, naked nuclei in the background. The second component of the aspirate consists of stromal fragments in which there are a conspicuous number of spindle cells. These cells are enmeshed in material that stains metachromatically with modified Wright-Giemsa stains. Isolated mesenchymal cells are also present. Foam cells, macrophages, and multinucleated giant cells frequently accompany phyllodes tumor (Images 10.2 through 10.5).

Cytologically, benign phyllodes tumors can resemble fibroadenoma. It was originally believed that the distinction between these two entities could be based primarily on assessments of the cellularity of the stromal fragments, because stromal fragments in phyllodes tumor seemed to be more cellular than stromal fragments in fibroadenoma. However, in a recent

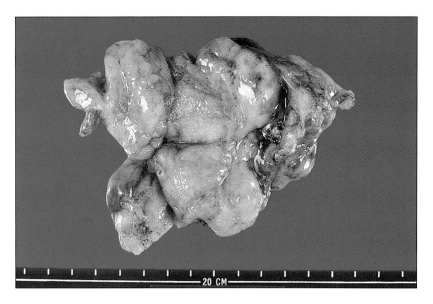

Figure 10.1

Gross image of a phyllodes tumor. The lesion is large, with a solid, fleshy appearance and small cystic areas.

study by Shimizu et al,[32] stromal hypocellularity was observed in both benign phyllodes tumor and fibroadenoma. There was no statistically significant difference in the size of stromal nuclei, the folding of epithelial sheets, or the number of foam macrophages. In contrast, the spindle cells in phyllodes tumors were enmeshed in pink-staining acid mucopolysaccharide–containing stroma, which is best demonstrated with metachromatic stains (Images 10.6 and 10.7).[33]

The main cytologic features of borderline and malignant phyllodes tumor have been defined as an abundance of stromal fragments, hypercellularity, and variation in the size and shape of the stromal nuclei.[29,34,35] The separation between the borderline and malignant subgroups of phyllodes tumors is based on the degree of stromal overgrowth, the atypicality of the stromal cells, and the number of mitoses.[28,29,32] In borderline phyllodes tumor, stromal cells have the features of fibroblasts with moderate atypia: ie, they have indented nuclei and a fine chromatin network (Images 10.8 and 10.9). In malignant phyllodes tumor, however, the nuclei of fibrous stromal cells are large, hyperchromatic, and irregularly shaped. Thus, pleomorphic polygonal or vacuolated stromal cells with increased N/C ratios are a cytologic feature of malignant phyllodes tumor (Images 10.10 and 10.11).[32,34]

Blood vessels traversing the stroma, previously suggested as a characteristic feature of malignancy in phyllodes tumor, have also been reported in benign phyllodes tumors.[29] Features that are not helpful in distinguishing between borderline and malignant phyllodes tumors are the presence or absence of foamy macrophages, multinucleated histiocytes, and apocrine metaplasia.[29] Varying degrees of epithelial proliferation can be seen in phyllodes tumors. In addition to epithelial atypia, the conspicuous degree of proliferative change seen in benign, borderline, and malignant phyllodes tumors can lead to a false-positive diagnosis of invasive breast carcinoma (Images 10.12 and 10.13).[24,25,28,31,36]

Preoperative diagnosis of borderline and malignant phyllodes tumor by FNAB is possible when both clinical and cytologic features are taken into account. Borderline and malignant phyllodes tumors are characterized by hypercellular stromal fragments; isolated stromal cells with nuclear pleomorphism; and large, folded epithelial sheets. However, cytologic distinction between benign phyllodes tumors and fibroadenoma is not practical. Cytologic features such as the pattern of cell distribution, cellularity of stromal tissue fragments, and uniformity of stromal cells are not reliable differentiating features.[32] Clinical information such as rapid growth and tumor size larger than 4 cm should alert the pathologist that phyllodes tumors is a diagnostic possibility. Multiple aspirations of the lesion should be performed, and an immediate microscopic interpretation should be made available. It is also advisable to perform frozen sections in cases in which phyllodes tumor is the suspected diagnosis.

Cytomorphology of Phyllodes Tumor

High cellularity
Biphasic pattern similar to that of fibroadenoma
Cellular stromal components with spindle cells of various sizes and shapes
Variable cytologic atypia and mitotic activity
Macrophages, multinucleated giant cells, and naked nuclei

Malignant Fibrous Histiocytoma

Malignant fibrous histiocytoma (MFH), a rare tumor, can manifest as a primary breast neoplasm, as a component of phyllodes tumor, or as a metastatic lesion.[9,37] Among the reported primary lesions are a few that occurred following radiation therapy for breast carcinoma.[38] Malignant fibrous histiocytoma is a cellular tumor composed of giant cells and pleomorphic, spindle-shaped fibroblastic cells, mixed with round histiocytes and a variable number of inflammatory cells. Other histologic variants of MFH are the monomorphic, storiform, and myxoid patterns.[39,40]

Reports on the cytomorphologic features of MFH of the breast are rare.[38,41] In a case reported by Luzzatto et al,[38] the smears revealed few cellular elements in a background of erythrocytes and cellular debris. The cells were pleomorphic, round, or spindle-shaped, with large nuclei; an uneven, granular chromatin pattern; and conspicuous nucleoli. The cells had abundant cytoplasm and contained large vacuoles. Several multinucleated cells were present, some of which showed evidence of erythrophagocytosis. Similar cytologic findings were described in three cases of MFH reported by Silverman et al.[41]

Our experience with malignant fibrous histiocytoma is limited to one case that occurred in a 16-year-old black girl. Fine needle aspiration smears demonstrated pleomorphic spindle cells isolated and in clusters intermingled with many multinucleated giant cells. The histiocytic cells had indistinct cell borders and contained intracytoplasmic vacuoles, phagocytic debris, and scattered granules. The multinucleated giant cells were arranged singly or in loose clusters. The tumor cells were positive for α_1–antichymotrypsin (Figure 10.2 and Images 10.14 through 10.22).

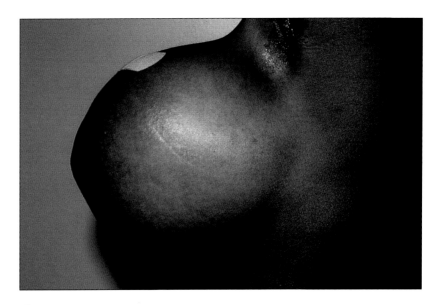

Figure 10.2
Malignant fibrous histiocytoma that presented as a large mass occupying the entire breast of a 16-year-old black girl.

Electron microscopic study may be helpful in the preoperative differential diagnosis of malignant fibrous histiocytoma,[42] which includes a rare breast carcinoma with osteoclast-like giant cells.[43] In addition to its diagnostic value, FNAB can effectively be utilized in the follow-up of patients with surgically excised breast carcinomas subjected to radiotherapy. The possibility of postradiation malignant fibrous histiocytoma makes follow-up of such patients particularly important.

Cytomorphology of Malignant Fibrous Histiocytoma
High cellularity
Pleomorphic cell population
Neoplastic spindle cells
Bizarre tumor giant cells
Mitoses

Hemangiopericytoma

Hemangiopericytoma, a very rare vascular tumor formed mainly of pericytes, was first described by Stout and Murray[44] in 1942. The most frequent locations of this tumor are in the lower extremities, the pelvic fossa, and retroperitoneum. Hemangiopericytoma in the breast is unusual.

The cytomorphology of hemangiopericytoma involving stomach, lung, and retroperitoneum has been described.[45–47] Only one case of hemangiopericytoma occurring in a male breast studied by FNAB has been reported.[48] The patient was a 40-year-old man who presented with a 10 × 10 cm mass in the left breast that appeared as a soft, radiopaque lesion in the mammogram. The FNAB smear showed fragments of tissue with knob-like formations of atypical cells and capillaries lined by plump endothelial cells. The cells had scant cytoplasm and spindle- to oval-shaped nuclei with a fine chromatin pattern. The endothelial cells were positive for vimentin and factor VIII. Spindle cells did not react to factor VIII.

In our experience, the cytologic features of hemangiopericytoma are not specific and may mimic a variety of benign and malignant spindle cell lesions of the breast (Images 10.23 through 10.25). The differential diagnosis includes angiosarcoma, malignant fibrous histiocytoma, fibrosarcoma, synovial sarcoma, and malignant schwannoma.[47] In angiosarcoma, the capillaries are lined by malignant endothelial cells that express factor VIII. Malignant fibrous histiocytomas show clusters of multinucleated cells and spindle cells reactive to α_1-antitrypsin and α_1-antichymotrypsin. Malignant schwannoma shows a positive reaction with S-100. Overall, the diagnosis of hemangiopericytoma is based on morphologic as well as immunologic characteristics, with reactivity to actin and vimentin but not to desmin or myoglobin.

Cytomorphology of Hemangiopericytoma
Moderate cellularity
Plump endothelial cells
Uniform spindle cells

Angiosarcoma

The cytomorphology of angiosarcoma, an extremely rare lesion, has rarely been described.[49–51] Characteristically, the aspirated material is cellular and shows solid to papillary, projectile, tuft-like growths of spindle, round, oval, or polygonal cells with pleomorphism, indented nuclei, hyperchromasia, irregular nuclear membranes, nucleoli, and distended cytoplasms within blood vessels. These features indicate endothelial-type tufting. Gland-like and microacinar structures are seen scattered in a necrotic background (Images 10.26 through 10.28).

Characterized by pronounced cellularity, malignant spindle cells, and endothelial-type components, angiosarcoma can mimic a variety of uncommon tumors and tumor-like conditions. These include phyllodes tumor, stromal sarcoma, metaplastic carcinoma, squamous cell carcinoma with sarcomatoid features, myoepithelioma, fibromatosis, cellular fibroadenoma, nodular fasciitis, fibrosarcoma, and reactive spindle cell proliferative lesions. Positive immunostaining for vimentin and factor VIII strongly supports a diagnosis of angiosarcoma.[51–53] Negative staining for other markers such as cytokeratin, epithelial membrane antigen, and desmin is also useful in establishing a diagnosis of angiosarcoma.

Cytomorphology of Angiosarcoma
Rich cellularity
Solid to papillary projectile-like growth
Pleomorphic cell population of atypical spindle, round, oval, and polygonal cells
Gland-like and acinar structures
Necrotic background

Stromal Sarcoma

First reported by Berg et al[54] in 1962, stromal sarcomas arise from the stroma surrounding the ductal epithelium. This unique origin excludes all other identifiable sarcomas (leiomyosarcoma, liposarcoma, myxoliposarcoma, fibrosarcoma, and malignant fibrous histiocytoma).[55,56] Cytomorphologic description of stromal sarcoma of the breast is limited to a case report by Rupp et al.[57] The cytologic specimens were moderately cellular, with cells arranged singly or in small clusters. The tumor cells had oval to spindle-shaped nuclei and were lobulated. The nuclei had a variable chromatin pattern and prominent nucleoli. The cytoplasm had a foamy appearance and contained an eccentrically placed nucleus. Mitoses were rare. Electron microscopic study revealed the presence of intercellular amorphous material and collagen. Lipid droplets; a variable number of microfilaments; and prominent, dilated, rough endoplasmic reticulum were seen in the cytoplasm. Lysosomes, mitochondria, occasional Golgi bodies, and centriole pairs were seen. The nuclei showed irregular indentation and chromatin condensation. Irregular cytoplasmic borders and pinocytotic vesicle formation were also noted. The ultrastructural findings were compatible with a primitive mesenchymal origin, probably a primitive fibroblastic origin.[56] These ultrastructural features may also be seen in malignant fibrous histiocytoma. However, malignant fibrous histiocytoma appears much more pleomorphic, with markedly atypical spindle cells and bizarre multinucleated cells.[58]

Stromal sarcomas should also be distinguished from breast carcinomas with an anaplastic or pseudosarcomatous pattern. This distinction has significant clinical implications, because the prognosis for spindle cell carcinoma and infiltrating duct cell carcinoma differs from that for stromal sarcoma. Immunoperoxidase staining for epithelial markers such as epithelial membrane antigen substantiates the diagnosis.[59] Preoperative diagnosis by FNAB may help to avoid incisional biopsies, minimizing the subsequent risk of tumor spread and the need for wider surgical margins.[60–62]

Cytomorphology of Stromal Sarcoma
Moderate cellularity
Cells dispersed and in clusters
Lobulated, oval to spindle-shaped nuclei
Conspicuous nucleoli
Foamy cytoplasm
Rare mitoses

Other Sarcomas

A variety of other soft tissue sarcomas can occur in the breast, including osteogenic sarcoma and rhabdomyosarcoma.[63–65] Cytologically, the features are similar to those seen in sarcomas occurring in other sites in the body. The FNAB smears generally demonstrate high cellularity with a pleomorphic population of spindle cells. The cells are atypical with bizarre forms present. Vacuolization and evidence of phagocytosis and multinucleation may be seen. Necrosis and mitosis are common findings. The differential diagnosis includes metaplastic carcinoma and carcinoma with multinucleated giant cells. Immunocytochemistry and electron microscopic study may help in separating sarcoma from other tumors and in classifying the sarcomatous lesion.

Image 10.1
Phyllodes tumor characterized by a biphasic pattern consisting of an epithelial component and cellular stroma (H&E, 200X).

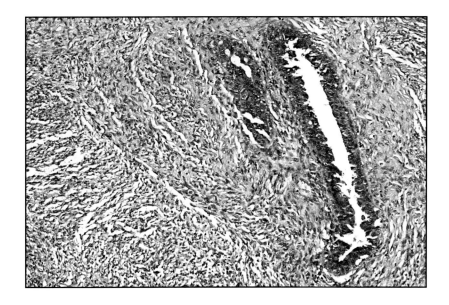

Image 10.2
Richly cellular smear of phyllodes tumor displays a biphasic pattern similar to that seen in fibroadenoma (Papanicolaou, 200X).

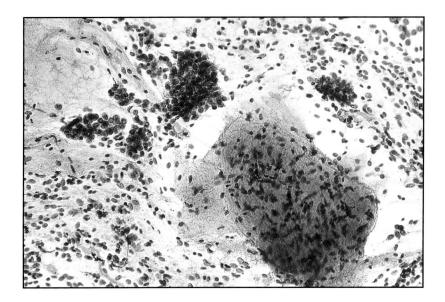

Image 10.3
Another view of the same case demonstrates a cellular stromal component and abundant, naked nuclei (Papanicolaou, 200X).

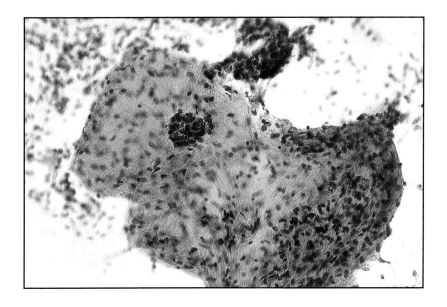

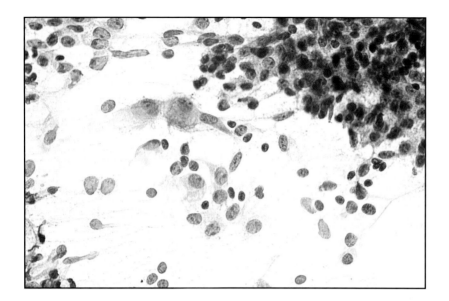

Image 10.4
Aspirate of phyllodes tumor reveals a cellular background with many isolated mesenchymal cells mixed with naked nuclei. The stromal cells are uniform with no atypia (Papanicolaou, 400X).

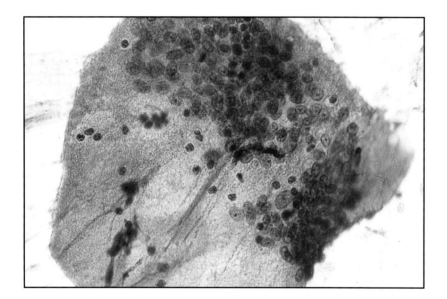

Image 10.5
Multinucleated giant cells in an aspirate of phyllodes tumor (Papanicolaou, 400X).

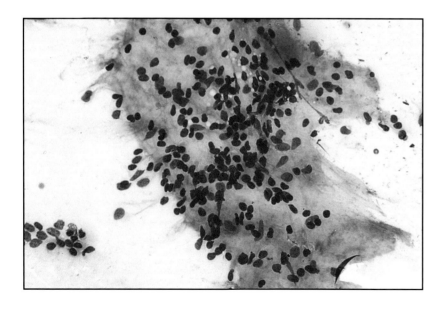

Image 10.6
Spindle cells in phyllodes tumor embedded in pink-staining acid mucopolysaccharide–containing stroma, best demonstrated by metachromatic stain (Diff-Quik®, 200X).

Image 10.7
The stromal component in phyllodes tumor is hypocellular, similar to that in fibroadenoma (Diff–Quik, 200X).

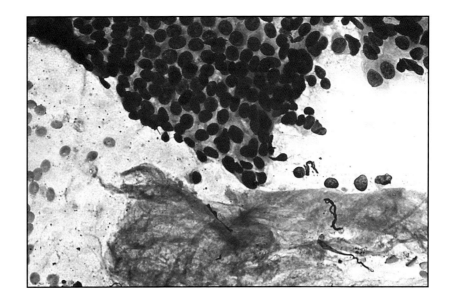

Image 10.8
Cellular aspirate of borderline phyllodes tumor with features indistinguishable from those of a cellular fibroadenoma or low-grade carcinoma (Papanicolaou, 100X).

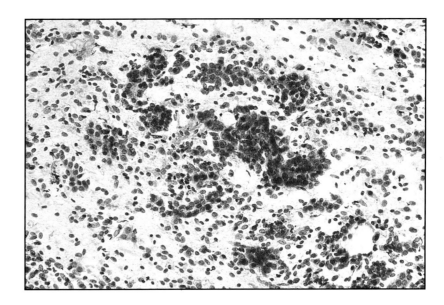

Image 10.9
Another view of the same case demonstrates a conspicuous number of stromal cells in a background typical of borderline phyllodes tumor (Papanicolaou, 200X).

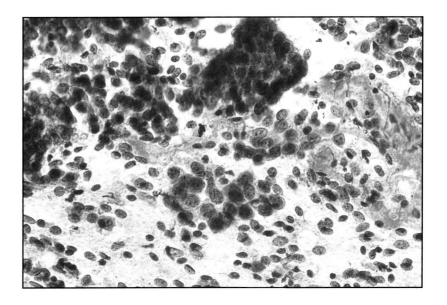

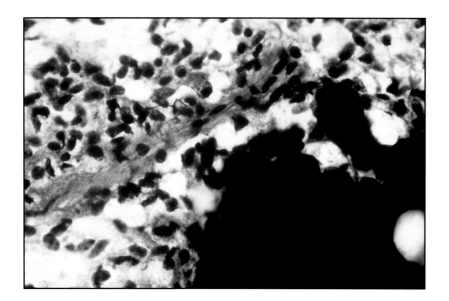

Image 10.10
Aspirate of malignant phyllodes tumor reveals the presence of an epithelial component and atypical spindle-shaped stromal cells (Papanicolaou, 200X).

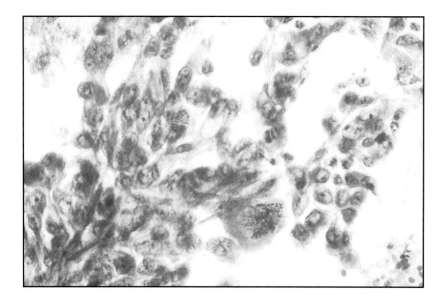

Image 10.11
Higher magnification of the same case reveals pleomorphism, mitoses, and anisonucleosis (Papanicolaou, 400X).

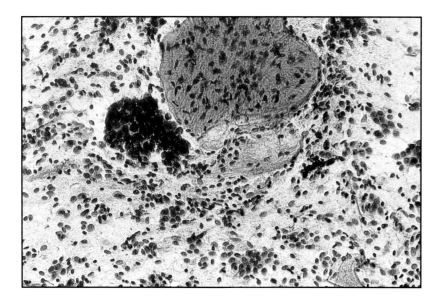

Image 10.12
As in fibroadenoma, areas of atypical hyperplasia can be seen in phyllodes tumor (Papanicolaou, 200X).

Image 10.13
Higher magnification of the same phyllodes tumor shown in Image 10.12 demonstrates a cluster of epithelial cells with overriding of the nuclei, hyperchromasia, and a cribriform-like pattern featuring atypical hyperplasia (Papanicolaou, 400X).

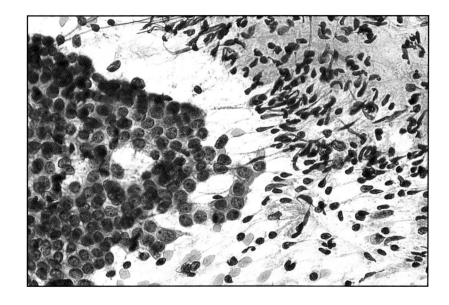

Image 10.14
Aspirate of malignant fibrous histiocytoma displays marked cellularity (Papanicolaou, 200X).

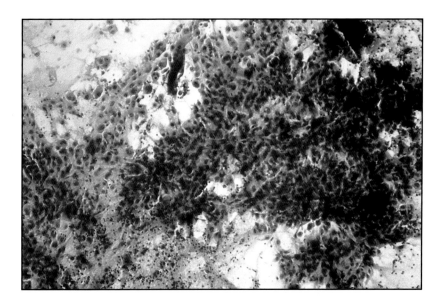

Image 10.15
Another view of the same case featuring loosely arranged atypical cells and scattered, multinucleated giant cells (Papanicolaou, 200X).

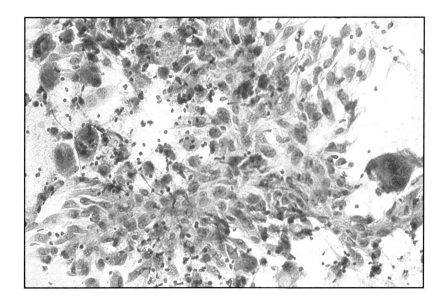

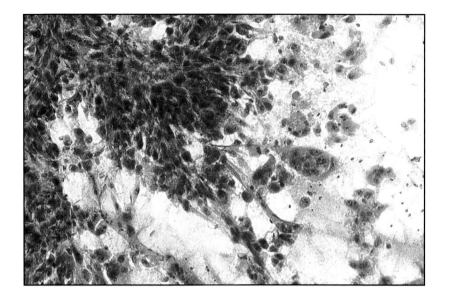

Image 10.16
Pleomorphic population of spindle cells and multinucleated cells in aspirate of the same case of malignant fibrous histiocytoma (Papanicolaou, 200X).

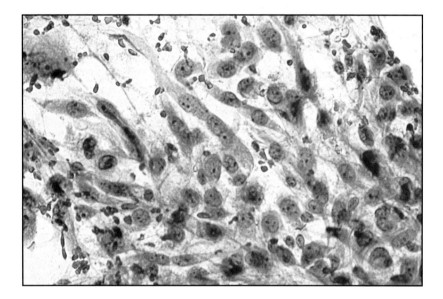

Image 10.17
Higher magnification of the same case reveals marked pleomorphism and nuclear atypia of the spindle cells (Papanicolaou, 200X).

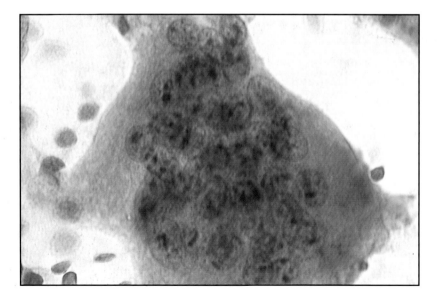

Image 10.18
Bizarre multinucleated cells, a feature of malignant fibrous histiocytoma (Papanicolaou, 400X).

Image 10.19
Abnormal mitoses and nuclear atypia in the same case of malignant fibrous histiocytoma (Papanicolaou, 400X).

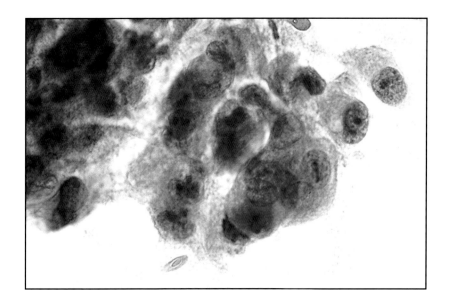

Image 10.20
Cell-block preparation of malignant fibrous histiocytoma is positive for α_1-antichymotrypsin (Immunoperoxidase, 400X).

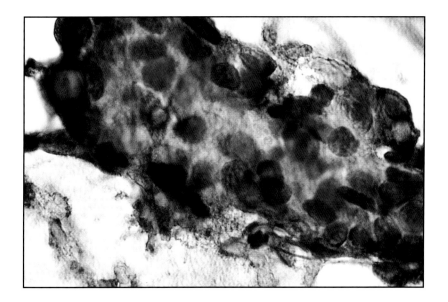

Image 10.21
Corresponding tissue section demonstrates the histologic features of malignant fibrous histiocytoma (H&E, 1000X).

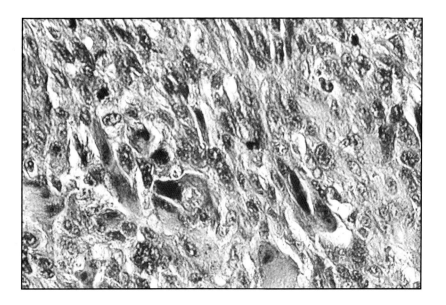

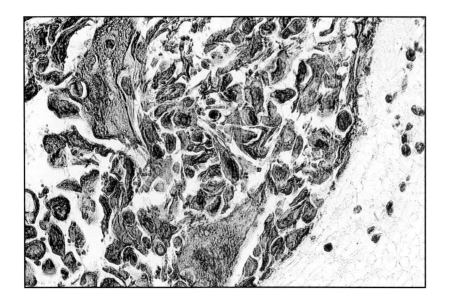

Image 10.22
Like the fine needle aspirate of this malignant fibrous histiocytoma, the resected specimen is also positive for α_1-antichymotrypsin (Immunoperoxidase, 400X).

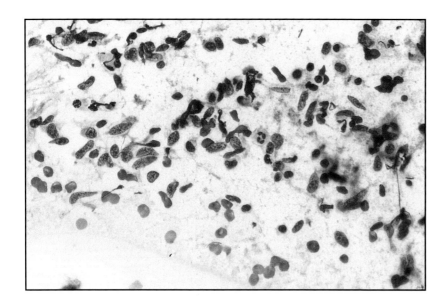

Image 10.23
Cellular aspirate of hemangiopericytoma features spindle cells isolated and in clusters in a hemorrhagic background (Papanicolaou, 100X).

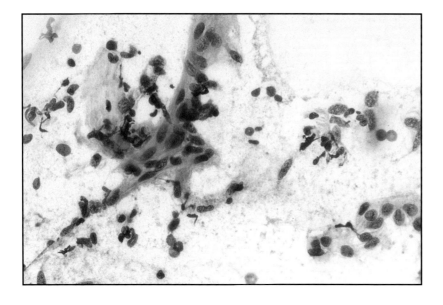

Image 10.24
Higher magnification of the same case demonstrates blood vessels surrounded by spindle cells with scant cytoplasm and a few oval-shaped cells with modest cytoplasm, probably endothelial cells (Papanicolaou, 200X).

Image 10.25
Corresponding tissue section demonstrates the histologic features of hemangiopericytoma (H&E, 200X).

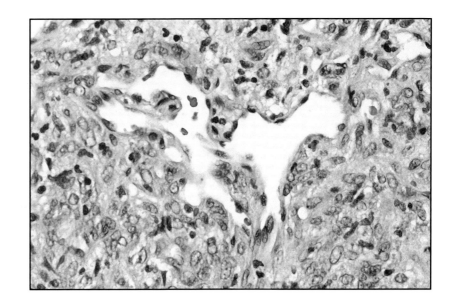

Image 10.26
Aspirate of angiosarcoma demonstrates atypical plump and spindle-shaped cells forming cleft-like projections within blood vessels in a hemorrhagic background (Papanicolaou, 200X).

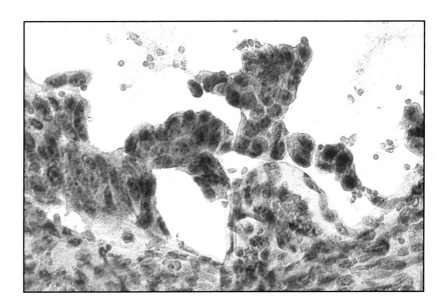

Image 10.27
Another view of the same case demonstrates similar features (Papanicolaou, 400X).

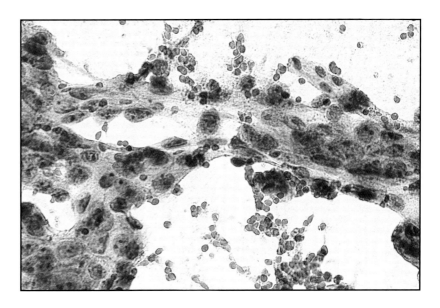

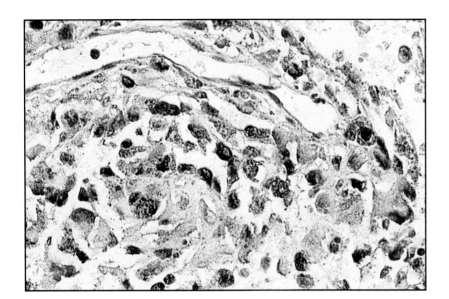

Image 10.28
Positive immunostaining for factor VIII in a cell block preparation of angiosarcoma (Immunoperoxidase, 400X).

References

1. Oberman HA: Sarcomas of the breast. *Cancer* 18:1233–1243, 1965.

2. Hill PR, Stout AP: Sarcoma of the breast. *Arch Surg* 44:1233–1243, 1965.

3. Costa J, Wesley RA, Glastein E, et al: The grading of soft tissue sarcomas. Result of a clinicopathologic correlation in a series of 163 cases. *Cancer* 53:530–541, 1984.

4. Callery CD, Rosen PP, Kinne DW: Sarcomas of the breast. A study of 32 patients with reappraisal and classification and therapy. *Ann Surg* 201:527–532, 1985.

5. Norris HJ, Taylor HB: Sarcoma and related mesenchymal tumors of the breast. *Cancer* 22:22–28, 1968.

6. Cumin W: The general view of the disease of the mamma, with cases of some of the more important affections of the gland. *Edinb Med* 27:225–240, 1982.

7. Chelius MJ: *Neue Jahrbuech der Teutschen. Medicin und Chirurgrie.* Heidelberg, Germany, Naegele und Puchelt, pp. 517-521, 1827.

8. Norris HJ, Taylor HB: Relationship of histologic features to behavior of cystosarcoma phyllodes. Analysis of ninety-four cases. *Cancer* 20:2090–2099, 1967.

9. Tavassoli FA: *Pathology of the Breast,* Norwalk, Conn, Appleton & Lange, 1992, pp 442–467.

10. Cooper WG Jr, Ackerman LV: Cystosarcoma phyllodes with a consideration of its more malignant variant. *Surg Gynecol Obstet* 77:279–283, 1943.

11. Hart WR, Bauer RC, Oberman HA: Cystosarcoma phyllodes: a clinicopathologic study of twenty-six hypercellular periductal stromal tumors of the breast. *Am J Clin Pathol* 70:211–216, 1978.

12. Page DL, Anderson JJ: *Diagnostic Histopathology of the Breast.* Edinburgh, Scotland, Churchill Livingstone, 1987, pp 341-350.

13. Pietruzka M, Barnes L: Cystosarcoma phyllodes. A clinicopathologic analysis of 42 cases. *Cancer* 41:1974-1983, 1978.

14. Ariel I: Skeletal metastasis in cystosarcoma phyllodes. *Arch Surg* 82:275-280, 1961.

15. Azzopardi JG: Problems in breast pathology. In: Bennington JL, ed. *Major Problems in Pathology,* vol 2. London, England, WB Saunders Co, 1979, pp. 346–378.

16. Ackerman LV, Taylor HB: Seminar on lesions of the breast. In: *Proceedings of the American Society of Clinical Pathologists.* Chicago, Ill, American Society of Clinical Pathologists, 1956.

17. Treves N, Sunderland DA: Cystosarcoma phyllodes of the breast: a malignant and a benign tumor. *Cancer* 4:1286–1332, 1951.

18. Aronson W: Malignant cystosarcoma phyllodes with liposarcoma. *Wis Med J* 65:184–187, 1966.

19. Mentzel T, Kosmehl H, Katenkamp D: Metastasizing phyllodes tumor with malignant fibrous histiocytoma-like areas. *Histopathology* 19:557–560, 1991.

20. Rosen PP, Urban JA: Coexistent mammary carcinoma and cystosarcoma phyllodes. *Breast* 1:9–15, 1975.

21. Ross DE: Malignancy occurring in cystosarcoma phyllodes. *Am J Surg* 88:243–247, 1954.

22. Rao BR, Muyer JS, Fry G: Most cystosarcoma phyllodes and fibroadenomas have progesterone receptors but lack estrogen receptor-stromal localization of progesterone receptors. *Cancer* 47:2016–2921, 1981.

23. El-Naggar AK, Ro JY, McLemore D, et al: DNA content and proliferative activity of cystosarcoma phyllodes of the breast. Potential prognostic significance. *Am J Clin Pathol* 93:980–985, 1990.

24. Kline TS: *Handbook of Fine Needle Aspiration Biopsy Cytology,* 2nd ed. Edinburgh, Scotland, Churchill Livingstone, 1988, pp. 232-234.

25. Simi U, Morrelti D, Iacconi P, et al: Fine needle aspiration cytopathology of phyllodes tumor: differential diagnosis with fibroadenomas. *Acta Cytol* 32:63–66, 1988.

26. Stawicki ME, Hsui JG: Malignant cystosarcoma phyllodes. A case report with cytologic presentation. *Acta Cytol* 23:61–64, 1979.

27. Stanley MW, Tani EM, Rutquist LE, et al: Cystosarcoma phyllodes of the breast: a cytologic and clinicopathologic study of 23 cases. *Diagn Cytopathol* 5:29–34, 1989.

28. Silverman JF, Geisinger KR, Frable WJ: Fine needle aspiration cytology of mesenchymal tumors of the breast. *Diagn Cytopathol* 4:50–58, 1988.

29. Rao CR, Narasimhamurthy NK, Jaganathan G, et al: Cystosarcoma phyllodes. Diagnosis by fine needle aspiration cytology. *Acta Cytol* 36:203–207, 1992.

30. Koss LG, Woylke S, Olszewski W: *Aspiration Biopsy: Cytologic Interpretation and Histologic Bases.* New York, NY, Igaku-Shoin, 1984, pp. 53–104.

31. Dusenberry D, Frable WJ: Fine needle aspiration cytology of phyllodes tumor: potential diagnosis pitfalls. *Acta Cytol* 36:215–221, 1992.

32. Shimizu K, Masana N, Yamada T, et al: Cytologic evaluation of phyllodes tumors as compared to fibroadenomas of the breast. *Acta Cytol* 38:891–897, 1994.

33. Linsk JA, Franzen S: *Clinical Aspiration Cytology,* 6th ed. Philadelphia, Pa, JB Lippincott Co, 1980, pp. 132–133.

34. Ramzy I: *Clinical Cytopathology and Aspiration Biopsy: Fundamental Principles and Practice.* Norwalk, Conn, Appleton & Lange, 1990, p. 339.

35. Griogioni WF, Santini D, Grassigli A, et al: A clinicopathologic study of cystosarcoma phyllodes: twenty case reports. *Arch Anat Cytol Pathol* 30:303–306, 1982.

36. Yamada T, Hara K, Satoh T, et al: Cell morphologies and their histopathologic backgrounds in cases with false positive reports in respect to mammary aspiration biopsy cytology. *J Jpn Soc Clin Cytol* 26:939–951, 1987.

37. Langham MR Jr: Malignant fibrous histiocytoma of the breast. A case report and review of the literature. *Cancer* 54:558–563, 1984.

38. Luzzatto R, Grossman S, Scholl JC, et al: Postradiation pleomorphic malignant fibrous histiocytoma of the breast. *Acta Cytol* 30:48–40, 1986.

39. Hajdu SI, Hajdu EO: *Cytopathology of Sarcomas and Other Non-Epithelial Tumors.* Philadelphia, Pa, WB Saunders Co, 1976, pp. 216-220.

40. Weiss SW, Enzinger FM: Myxoid variant of malignant fibrous histiocytoma. *Cancer* 39:1672–1685, 1977.

41. Silverman JF, Geisinger KR, Frable WJ: Fine needle aspiration cytology of mesenchymal tumors of the breast. *Diagn Cytopathol* 4:50–58, 1988.

42. Lindholm K, Nordgren H, Akerman M: Electron microscopy of fine needle aspiration biopsy from a malignant fibrous histiocytoma. *Acta Cytol* 23:394–401, 1979.

43. Sugaro I, Nagao K, Kondo Y, et al: Cytologic and ultrastructural studies of a rare breast carcinoma with osteoclast-like giant cells. *Cancer* 52:74–78, 1983.

44. Stout AP, Murray MR: Hemangiopericytoma: a vascular tumor featuring Zimmermann's pericytes. *Ann Surg* 116:26–33, 1942.

45. DeGaetani CF, Trentini GP: Gastric angioendothelioma: a cytologic evaluation. *Acta Cytol* 21:306–309, 1977.

46. Nguyen GK, Neifer R: The cells of benign and malignant hemangiopericytomas in aspiration biopsy. *Diagn Cytopathol* 1:327–332, 1985.

47. Nickels J, Koivuniemi A: Cytology of malignant hemangiopericytoma. *Acta Cytol* 23:119–124, 1979.

48. Jimenez-Ayala M, Diez-Nau MD, Larrad A, et al: Hemangiopericytoma in a male breast. Report of a case with cytologic, histologic and immunochemical studies. *Acta Cytol* 35:234–238, 1991.

49. Masin G, Masin F: Cytology of angiosarcoma of the breast: a case report. *Acta Cytol* 22:162–164, 1978 .

50. Stanley MW, Tani GM, Horwitz CA, et al: Primary spindle cell sarcomas of the breast. Diagnosis of fine needle aspiration. *Diagn Cytopathol* 4:244–249, 1988.

51. Gupta RK, Naran S, Dowle C: Needle aspiration cytology and immunocytochemical study in a case of angiosarcoma of the breast. *Diagn Cytopathol* 7:363–365, 1991.

52. Guarda LA, Ordonez NG, Smith JL, et al: Immunoperoxidase localization of factor VIII in angiosarcoma. *Arch Pathol Lab Med* 106:515–520, 1982.

53. Mukai K, Rosai J: Factor VIII related antigen: an endothelial marker. In: DeLellis RA, ed. *Diagnostic Immunohistochemistry.* New York, NY: Masson Publishing USA Inc, 1984, pp. 253–261.

54. Berg JW, DeCross JJ, Fracchia AA, et al: Stromal sarcoma of the breast: a unified approach to connective tissue sarcomas other than cystosarcoma phyllodes. *Cancer* 15:418–424, 1962.

55. Callery CD, Rosen PP, Kinne DW: Sarcoma of the breast. A study of 32 patients with reappraisal of classification and therapy. *Ann Surg* 201:527–532, 1985.

56. Tang PH, Petrelli M, Robecheck PJ: Stromal sarcoma of the breast: a light and electron microscopic study. *Cancer* 43:209–217, 1979.

57. Rupp M, Hafiz MA, Khalluf E, et al: Fine needle aspiration in stromal sarcoma of the breast. Light and electron microscopic findings with histologic correlation. *Acta Cytol* 32:72–74, 1988.

58. Ketai K, Goldblatt PJ: Malignant fibrous histiocytoma: cytologic, light microscope and ultrastructural studies. *Acta Cytol* 26:507–511, 1982.

59. Gal R, Gukovsky-Oren S, Lehman JM, et al: Cytodiagnosis of a spindle-cell tumor of the breast using antisera to epithelial membrane antigen. *Acta Cytol* 31:317–321, 1987.

60. Kindblom LG, Walaas L, Widehn S: Ultrastructural studies in the preoperative cytologic diagnosis of soft tissue tumors. *Semin Diagn Pathol* 3:317–344, 1986.

61. Rydholm A, Akerman M, Idvall I, et al: Aspiration cytology of soft tissue tumors. A prospective study of its influence on choice of surgical procedure. *Int Orthop* 6:209–214, 1982.

62. Akerman M, Idvall I, Rydholm A: Cytodiagnosis of soft tissue tumors and tumor-like conditions by means of fine needle biopsy. *Arch Orthop Trauma Surg* 96:61–67, 1980.

63. Metens HH, Langnickel D, Staedtler F: Primary osteogenic sarcoma of the breast. *Acta Cytol* 26:512–516, 1982.

64. Pettinato G, Manivel JC, Petrella G, et al: Primary osteogenic metaplastic carcinoma of the breast. Immunocytochemical identification in fine needle aspirates. *Acta Cytol* 33:620–626, 1989.

65. Torres V, Ferrer R: Cytology of fine needle aspiration biopsy of primary breast rhabdomyosarcoma in an adolescent girl. *Acta Cytol* 29: 430–434, 1985.

CHAPTER ELEVEN

Lymphoproliferative Disorders

Lymphoma

Lymphoproliferative disorders rarely involve the breast, manifesting either as a primary lesion or as part of a generalized process. The frequency of primary breast lymphoma is variable, ranging from 0.12% to 0.53% of all malignant breast tumors.[1-4]

Primary lymphoma may originate from a migratory lymphocyte or arise within an intramammary lymph node. It occurs in patients of all ages, ranging from 9 to 88 years, with a median of 50 years. The majority of patients present with a unilateral, palpable mass.[4] Patients with primary lymphoma complain of pain and may suffer from night sweats, fever, and weight loss. The lesion may be multiple and can cause skin changes similar to those seen with breast carcinomas. Axillary lymph node involvement is seen in 30% to 40% of patients with primary breast lymphoma.[5] Mammographically, lymphoma presents as a relatively circumscribed mass, focal or diffuse densities, or discrete nodules with irregular margins and no evidence of calcification or retraction.[6]

Grossly, the tumors seen in primary breast lymphoma are well defined, fleshy, and tan to gray, with an average size of 2 to 3 cm. Microscopically, the histologic features of primary breast lymphoma are similar to those of primary nodal involvement. Tumors occurring in pregnant and lactating women correspond to Burkitt's-type lymphoma.[2,7] Morphologic distinction between primary lymphoma and secondary involvement is impossible. Lymphomas of the breast are frequently B-cell or diffuse, large cell type.[8] The tumors are hormone receptor positive.[2,9]

315

The prognosis of primary lymphoma of the breast depends on the stage of the disease and the histologic type of the tumor. For example, lymphoblastic-type lymphoma of the breast progresses rapidly to leukemia and requires aggressive chemotherapy.[10] While some investigators believe that primary breast lymphomas have a poor prognosis,[11,12] there are some who believe that the prognosis for these tumors is comparable with that for other localized extranodal lymphomas.[3,13] The recommended treatment for primary breast lymphoma is debulking surgery followed by a combination chemotherapy with and without radiation therapy.[1]

Fine needle aspiration biopsy (FNAB) has proven valuable in the initial diagnosis of lymphomatous processes.[14,15] FNAB may be a suitable alternative for patients with clinical conditions for which surgical biopsy is not possible or for patients who present with recurrent disease. The majority of cases reported in the literature are examples of secondary involvement; examples of primary lymphoma of the breast are rare.[16–18]

The cytomorphology of breast lymphoma varies depending on the histologic subtype of the lesion. Based on reports in the literature and our own experience, FNAB smears of lymphomas are hypercellular and contain a monotonous or pleomorphic population of atypical lymphoid cells mixed with fragments of stroma, fat, and a few benign ductal epithelial cells (Images 11.1 and 11.2). The diagnosis is usually established immunophenotypically, using flow cytometry or immunocytochemistry (Figure 11.1).

The presence of atypical lymphoid cells in a patient with a history of lymphoma may indicate a recurrent process or disease progression. In the absence of a clinical history of lymphoma, however, the presence of lym-

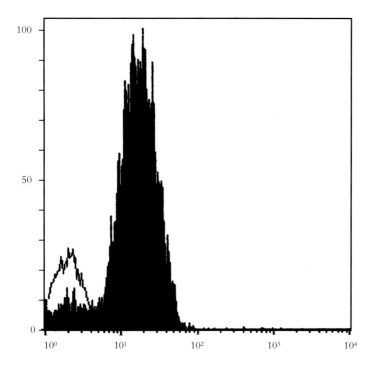

Figure 11.1
Flow cytometric analysis of a case of malignant lymphoma demonstrating a monoclonal pattern.

phoid cells in the smears may create diagnostic difficulty. Included in the cytologic differential diagnosis are chronic mastitis, fat necrosis, medullary carcinoma, anaplastic duct cell carcinoma with lymphocytic infiltrate, mammary carcinoma with neuroendocrine differentiation, and metastatic small cell carcinoma. Atypical lymphocytic infiltrate in the breast, Rosai-Dorfman disease, and an intramammary lymph node can also yield a cellular aspirate consisting of lymphoid aggregates (Images 11.3 through 11.6).

In addition to the presence of a polymorphic cell population and evidence of phagocytosis, demonstration of polyclonality by immunocytochemistry or flow cytometry is necessary to exclude a diagnosis of malignant lymphoma. The availability of immediate microscopic interpretation and processing for flow cytometric immunophenotyping is effective in correctly diagnosing lymphoproliferative disorders of the breast. A false-negative diagnosis of chronic mastitis or fat necrosis may delay appropriate treatment. False diagnosis of carcinoma rather than lymphoma may result in unnecessary surgery.

Cytomorphology of Lymphoma
High celluarity
Variable cell pattern
Monotonous or pleomorphic population of atypical lymphoid cells
Lympoglandular bodies

Hodgkin's Disease

Hodgkin's disease only rarely involves the breast. In a comprehensive review of 2,365 patients with Hodgkin's disease, Meis et al[19] reported only four cases of recurrent Hodgkin's disease of the breast. Recurrent Hodgkin's disease in the breast or chest wall is probably caused by spread along the intramammary or internal mammary lymph nodes or via direct mediastinal extension to the chest wall. Patients with Hodgkin's disease who undergo radiotherapy and/or chemotherapy have an increased risk of breast carcinoma.[20–22] Therefore, it is important to distinguish between a recurrence, a second primary malignancy, and benign breast disease in a patient treated for Hodgkin's disease.

The cytologic features of Hodgkin's disease in breast aspirates are similar to those of Hodgkin's disease found in other sites.[23,24] The aspirates are often highly cellular, with a polymorphic cell population that includes mature lymphocytes, neutrophils, and eosinophils. Intermingled with these cells are scattered giant cells with indented, bilobulated, or multilobulated nuclei containing prominent, cyanophilic nucleoli. The characteristic mirror image nuclei of Reed-Sternberg cells may also be seen (Images 11.7 through 11.9). In the absence of typical Reed-Sternberg cells, the diagnosis of Hodgkin's disease can be made when the background elements include lymphocytes, neutrophils, histiocytes, plasma cells, granulomas, necrosis, and metachromatic material.[23,24] Immunoperoxidase staining of cytologic preparations, including destained or Papanicolaou–stained smears, can demonstrate the presence of Leu M1 antigen in tumor cells and confirm a diagnosis of Hodgkin's disease,[25] obviating the need for expensive and more invasive surgical biopsy procedures.

Cytomorphology of Hodgkin's Disease
High cellularity
Polymorphic population of lymphocytes, plasma cells, and eosinophils
Reed-Sternberg cells

Granulocytic Sarcoma (Chloroma)

A rare manifestation of granulocytic leukemia, granulocytic sarcoma or chloroma is an uncommon localized tumor composed of immature myeloid cells occurring in an extramedullary site.[26] This tumor often develops during the course of myeloid leukemia. However, rarely, it may precede evidence of leukemia on peripheral blood or bone marrow studies by months or even years. The tumor may involve any tissue or organ.[27–29] It is unusual for granulocytic sarcoma to involve the breast, as was shown in an extensive autopsy study performed on patients with myelogenous leukemia.[30] In the few reported cases of leukemia involving breast, the granulocytic sarcoma mimicked a primary breast tumor both clinically and mammographically.[31–34]

The cytomorphologic features of granulocytic sarcoma have been described in vaginal smears and in malignant effusions.[35,36] There are also cases of granulocytic sarcoma of the breast diagnosed by fine needle aspiration biopsy.[33,34] The smears contain a variety of cells, varying from immature, nongranular cells to myelocytes. The undifferentiated cells have a round to oval nucleus; fine, dispersed chromatin; a distinct nuclear membrane; a small, eosinophilic nucleolus; and a rim of pale cytoplasm (Images 11.10 through 11.15). Other cells have bean-shaped or irregularly shaped nuclei with nuclear infolding. Some cells have eosinophilic granules in their cytoplasm. We agree with Pettinato et al[34] that the presence of eosinophilic myelocytes is the feature most helpful in the recognition of granulocytic sarcoma.

Ancillary studies such as special stains, immunocytochemistry, and electron microscopy may facilitate the diagnosis of granulocytic sarcoma.[27,34,36,37] Antilysozymal immunoperoxidase staining to determine the myeloid origin of cells is also helpful.[27] The differential diagnosis includes myeloid metaplasia and poorly differentiated lymphoma. Myelofibrosis often leads to extramedullary myeloid metaplasia, causing a breast mass to form.[38] Myeloid metaplasia is characterized by a variety of hematopoietic cells, including megakaryocytes, which are not present in granulocytic leukemia. Lymphoma of the breast is characterized by a monomorphic population of lymphoid cells that show no evidence of myeloid differentiation (ie, no eosinophilic myelocytes).[39]

Occasionally, granulocytic sarcoma does not progress to leukemia. Surgical removal of the lesion cures approximately 25% of cases.[40] A high index of suspicion for granulocytic sarcoma when examining an aspirate from a nonepithelial breast lesion and a search for eosinophilic myelocytes are the keys to diagnosis.

Cytomorphology of Chloroma
Variable cellularity
Spectrum of immature myeloid cells
Conspicuous number of eosinophilic myelocytes

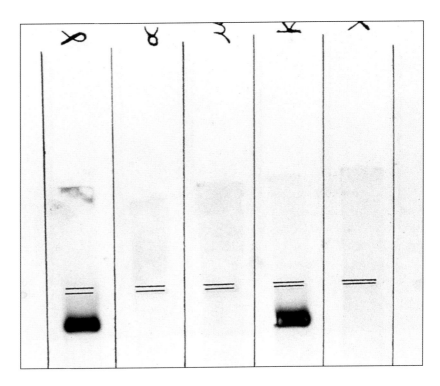

Figure 11.2
Serum protein immunoelectrophoretic pattern of a plasmacytoma reveals IgG and kappa light chains.

Plasmacytoma

Extramedullary plasmacytoma, an extremely rare occurrence in breast, is an unusual presentation of myeloma.[41,42] It has also been reported in patients with no evidence of systemic disease.[43] However, such patients should be followed with serologic and immunologic studies for early detection of multiple myeloma. Our experience is limited to one FNAB diagnosis of localized plasmacytoma in breast. The predominant cytologic features were plasma cells isolated and in aggregates, atypia, and binucleated cells. Immunostains on cell block preparations showed evidence of monoclonality (Images 11.16 through 11.19). The patient developed multiple myeloma 7 months after the diagnosis of plasmacytoma by FNAB (Figure 11.2 and Image 11.20).

Other conditions to be considered in the differential diagnosis are lesions characterized by tumor cells with eccentric nuclei, such as colloid carcinoma and the small cell variant of infiltrating duct cell carcinoma that occurs in older women. The presence of mucin in a background of colloid carcinoma and the coarse chromatin pattern seen in infiltrating duct cell carcinoma may facilitate correct diagnosis. Confirmation of monoclonality by immunocytochemistry also eliminates other possibilities.

Cytomorphology of Plasmacytoma
Cellular aspirate
Mature and atypical plasma cells
Binucleation

Sinus Histiocytosis With Massive Lymphadenopathy (Rosai-Dorfman Disease)

Sinus histiocytosis with massive lymphadenopathy, or Rosai-Dorfman disease (RDD), occurs mostly in children but may present at any age. Approximately one third of patients with RDD have extranodal manifestation.[44] Only a few cases have occurred in breast. The patients were young and black, and other sites were involved as well.[44] An aspirate from one patient with RDD who presented with a palpable breast lesion and had no evidence of a lymphoproliferative disorder contained a polymorphic population of lymphoid cells with frequent plasma cells and lymphohistiocytic aggregates.[45] The histiocytes had abundant cytoplasm with vesicular nuclei, prominent nucleoli, and slight atypia. The diagnosis of RDD was suggested by FNAB and confirmed by histologic findings. A diagnosis of RDD as a localized lesion in the breast should alert the clinician to the possibility of systemic involvement.

Cytomorphology of Rosai–Dorfman Disease
Cellular aspirate
Polymorphic population of lymphocytes
Plasma cells and histiocytes

Image 11.1
Aspirate of an intermediate-grade
malignant lymphoma, mixed small
cleaved and large cell, demonstrates a
mixed pattern of small and large lymphocytes (Diff-Quik®, 200X).

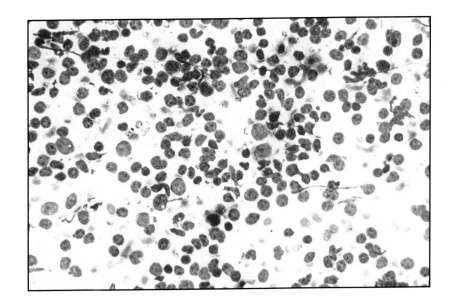

Image 11.2
Papanicolaou-stained smear of the
same case displays an admixture of
small cleaved cells, large cleaved cells,
and large noncleaved cells (400X).

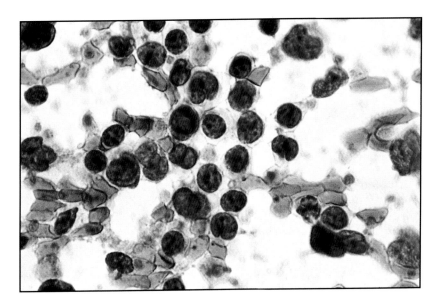

Image 11.3
Aspirate of an intramammary lymph
node reveals a polymorphous population of lymphoid cells (Diff-Quik,
200X).

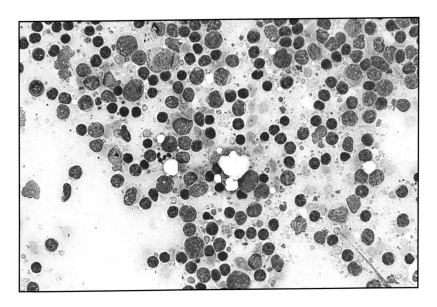

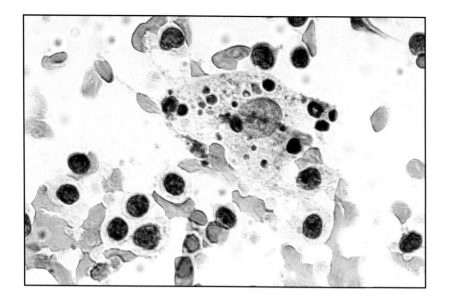

Image 11.4
In the same aspirate of intramammary lymph node, the presence of tingible bodies in a macrophage is evidence of phagocytosis and reactive hyperplasia (Papanicolaou, 1000X).

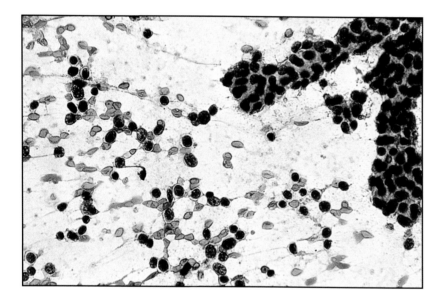

Image 11.5
Papanicolaou-stained smear of the same case demonstrates lymphoid cells and clusters of epithelial cells (200X).

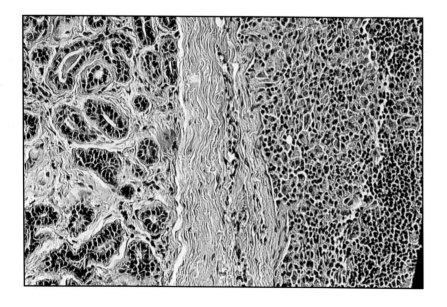

Image 11.6
Tissue section of the corresponding surgically excised lesion demonstrates a reactive lymph node with adjacent breast tissue (H&E, 200X).

Image 11.7
Breast aspirate smear of recurrent Hodgkin's disease reveals a polymorphous population of lymphocytes, plasma cells, and the presence of characteristic Reed-Sternberg cells (Diff-Quik, 200X).

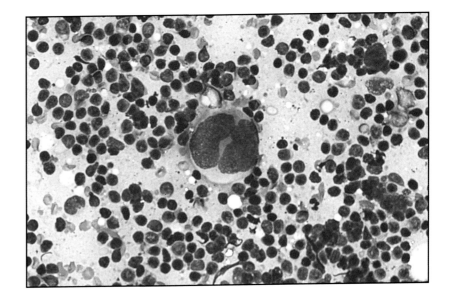

Image 11.8
Higher magnification of the same case reveals the characteristic mirror-image nuclei of Reed-Sternberg cells (Diff-Quik, 1000X).

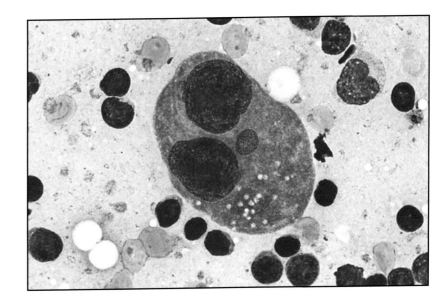

Image 11.9
Tissue section of previously surgically excised lymph node from the same patient. The histologic diagnosis was Hodgkin's disease (H&E, 200X).

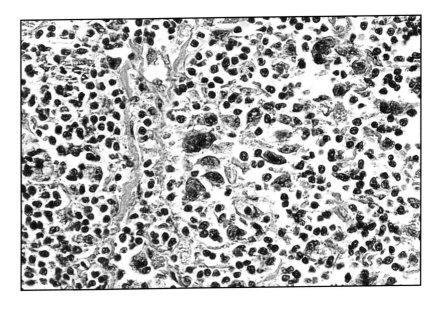

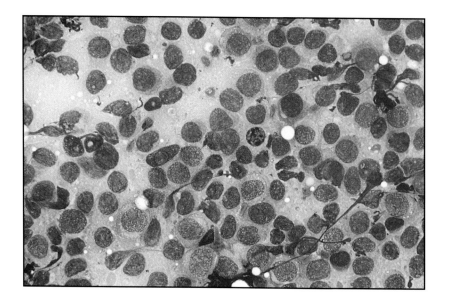

Image 11.10
Aspirate of granulocytic sarcoma involving breast is highly cellular, with abundant immature cells (Diff-Quik, 200X).

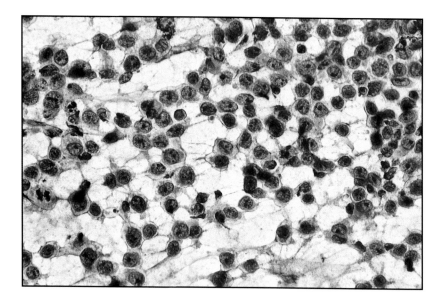

Image 11.11
Papanicolaou-stained smear of the same case shows a population of undifferentiated cells (200X).

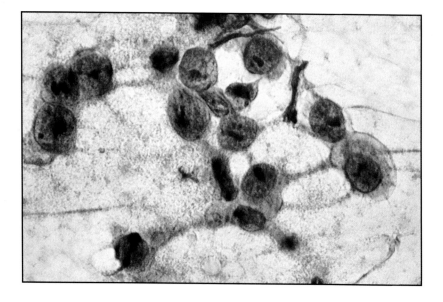

Image 11.12
Immature myeloid cells with a high N/C ratio (Papanicolaou, 400X).

Image 11.13
Higher magnification of the same case of granulocytic sarcoma reveals many cells with round to oval nuclei; fine, dispersed chromatin; a distinct nuclear membrane; small, eosinophilic nucleoli; and a rim of pale cytoplasm (Diff-Quik, 1000X).

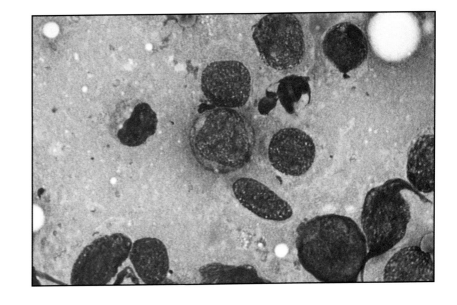

Image 11.14
Tissue section of bone marrow from the same patient shows leukemic infiltration (H&E, 100X).

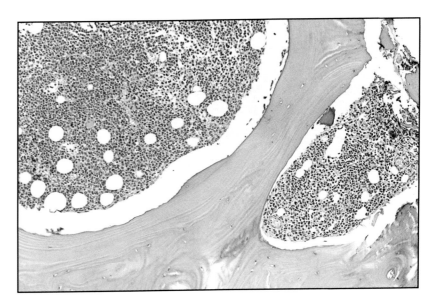

Image 11.15
Higher magnification of the same case shows undifferentiated myeloid cells replacing the bone marrow (H&E, 200X).

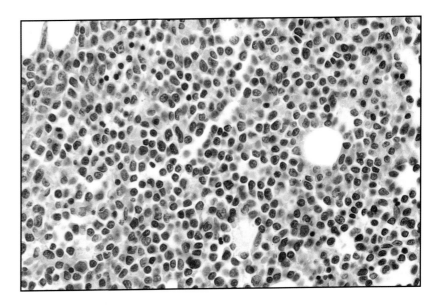

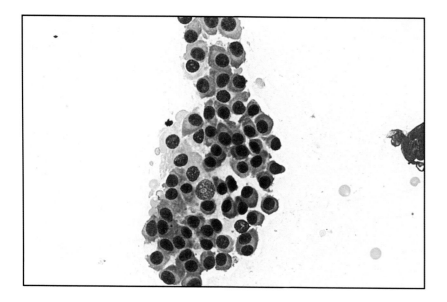

Image 11.16
Aspirate of plasmacytoma reveals a loose aggregate of rather uniform cells with the cytologic features of plasma cells (Diff-Quik, 200X).

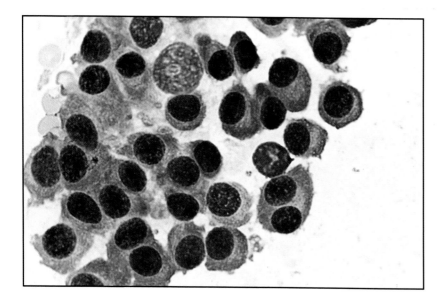

Image 11.17
Higher magnification of the same case reveals cells of different sizes and plasma cells with binucleation (Diff-Quik, 400X).

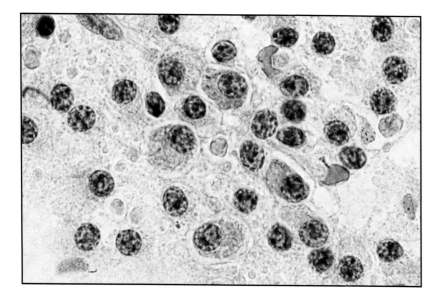

Image 11.18
Papanicolaou-stained smear of the same case demonstrates the characteristic nuclear features of plasma cells (400X).

Image 11.19
Expression of kappa light chain in a cell block preparation of plasmacytoma (Immunoperoxidase, 1000X).

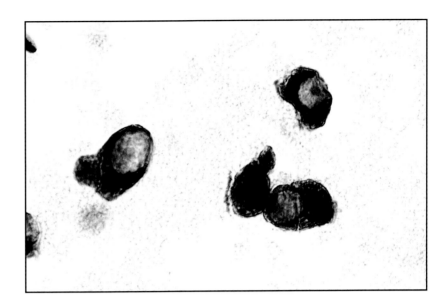

Image 11.20
Corresponding surgically excised lesion in the same case diagnosed as plasma-cytoma (H&E, 200X).

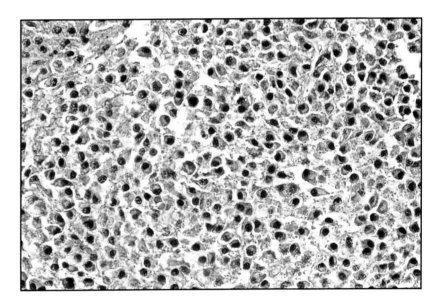

References

1. Giardini R, Piccolo C, Rilke F: Primary non-Hodgkin's lymphomas of the female breast. *Cancer* 69:725–735, 1992.

2. DeLeon DM, Villafria L, Crisostomo CI: Nonsystemic reticulum cell sarcoma of the breast. A case report. *Philippines J Surg* 16:149–151, 1961.

3. Dixon JM, Lumsden AB, Krajewski A, et al: Primary lymphoma of the breast. *Br J Surg* 74:214–217, 1987.

4. Hugh JC, Jackson FL, Hanson J, et al: Primary breast lymphoma. An immunohistologic study of 20 new cases. *Cancer* 66:2602-2611, 1990.

5. Haagensen CD: *Disease of the Breast,* 3rd ed. Philadelphia, Pa, WB Saunders Co, 1986, pp. 346–349.

6. Paulus DD: Lymphoma of the breast. *Radiol Clin North Am* 28:833–840, 1990.

7. Shepherd JJ, Wright DH: Burkitt's lymphoma presenting as bilateral swelling of the breast in females of child-bearing age. *Br J Surg* 54:776–780, 1967.

8. Cohen PL, Brooks JJ: Lymphomas of the breast. A clinicopathologic and immunohistochemical study of primary and secondary cases. *Cancer* 67:1359–1369, 1991.

9. Stark JJ, Lloyd JW, Schellhammer PF: Estrogen receptor activity in a case of Hodgkin's disease. *Ann Intern Med* 95:186–187, 1981.

10. Carbone A, Volpe R, Tirelli V, et al: Primary lymphoblastic lymphoma of the breast. *Clin Oncol* 8:367–373, 1982.

11. Oberman HA: Primary lymphoreticular neoplasm of the breast. *Surg Gynecol Obstet* 123:1047–1051, 1966.

12. Lattes R: Sarcomas of the breast. *JAMA* 201:121–122, 1967.

13. Brustein S, Filippa DA, Kimmel M, et al: Malignant lymphoma of the breast: a study of 53 patients. *Ann Surg* 205:144–150, 1987.

14. Carter TR, Feldman PS, Innes DJ Jr, et al: The role of fine needle aspiration cytology in the diagnosis of lymphoma. *Acta Cytol* 32:848–853, 1988.

15. Pontifex AH, Klimo P: Application of aspiration biopsy cytology to lymphomas. *Cancer* 53:553–556, 1984.

16. McCune KH, Varma M, Spence RAJ: Breast lymphoma: fine needle aspiration biopsy. *Ulster Med J* 61:110-111, 1992.

17. Sneige N, Zachariah S, Fanning TV, et al: Fine needle aspiration cytology of metastatic neoplasms in the breast. *Am J Clin Pathol* 92:27–35, 1989.

18. Silverman JF, Feldman PS, Covell JL, et al: Fine needle aspiration cytology of neoplasms metastatic to the breast. *Acta Cytol* 31:291–304, 1987.

19. Meis JM, Butler JJ, Osborne BM: Hodgkin's disease involving the breast and chest wall. *Cancer* 57:1859–1865, 1986.

20. Carey RW, Linjgood RM, Wood WM, et al: Breast cancer developing in four women cured of Hodgkin's disease. *Cancer* 54:2234–2235, 1984.

21. Janjan NA, Wilson JF, Gillin M, et al: Mammary carcinoma developing after radiotherapy and chemotherapy for Hodgkin's disease. *Cancer* 61:252–254, 1988.

22. Li FP, Corkery J, Canellos G, et al: Breast cancer after Hodgkin's disease in two sisters. *Cancer* 47:200–202, 1981.

23. Frable WJ, Kardos TF: Fine needle aspiration biopsy: applications in the diagnosis of lymphoproliferative diseases. *Am J Surg Pathol* 12(suppl 1):62–72, 1988.

24. Kardos TF, Vinson JH, Behm FG, et al: Hodgkin's disease. Diagnosis by fine needle aspiration biopsy: analysis of cytologic criteria from a selected series. *Am J Clin Pathol* 86:286–291, 1986.

25. Corrigan C, Sewell C, Martin A: Recurrent Hodgkin's disease in the breast: diagnosis of a case by fine needle aspiration and immunocytochemistry. *Acta Cytol* 34:669–672, 1990.

26. Rappaport H: Tumors of the hematopoietic system. In: *Atlas of Tumor Pathology* (1st series, fascicle 8). Washington, DC, Armed Forces Institute of Pathology, 1966, pp. 239–285.

27. Neiman RS, Barcos M, Berard C, et al: Granulocytic sarcoma: A clinicopathologic study of 61 biopsied cases. *Cancer* 48:1426–1437, 1981.

28. Kranse JR: Granulocytic sarcoma preceding acute leukemia: a report of six cases. *Cancer* 44:1017–1021, 1979.

29. Sears HF, Reid J: Granulocytic sarcoma: local presentation of a systemic disease. *Cancer* 37:1808–1813, 1976.

30. Liu PI, Ishimaru T, McGregor DH, et al: Autopsy study of granulocytic sarcoma (chloroma) in patients with myelogenous leukemia. *Cancer* 31:948–955, 1973.

31. Geelhood GW, Graff KS, Duttera MJ Jr: Acute leukemia presenting as a breast mass. *JAMA* 223:1488–1489, 1973.

32. Blackwell B: Acute leukemia presenting as a lump on the breast. *Br J Surg* 50:769–770, 1981.

33. Frable WJ: Thin-needle aspiration biopsy. In: Bennington JL, ed. *Major Problems in Pathology*. Philadelphia, Pa, WB Saunders Co, 61:1983, pp. 61–64.

34. Pettinato G, DeChiara A, Insabato L, et al: Fine needle aspiration biopsy of a granulocytic sarcoma (chloroma) of the breast. *Acta Cytol* 32:67–71, 1988.

35. Spahr J, Behm FG, Schneider V: Preleukemic granulocytic sarcoma of cervix and vagina: Initial manifestation by cytology. *Acta Cytol* 26:155–160, 1982.

36. Yam LT: Granulocytic sarcoma with pleural involvement: identification of neoplastic cells with cytochemistry. *Acta Cytol* 29:63–66, 1985.

37. McCarthy KS Jr, Wortman J, Daly J, et al: Chloroma (granulocytic sarcoma) without evidence of leukemia: facilitated light microscopic diagnosis. *Blood* 56:104–108, 1980.

38. Brooks JJ, Krugman DT, Damjanov I: Myeloid metaplasia presenting as a breast mass. *Am J Pathol* 4:281–285, 1980.

39. Mambo NC, Burke JS, Butler JJ: Primary malignant lymphoma of the breast. *Cancer* 39:2033–2040, 1977.

40. Meis JM, Butler JJ, Osborne ND: Granulocytic sarcoma in non-leukemic patients. *Lab Invest* 54:42, 1986. Abstract.

41. Cutler C: Plasma cell tumor of the breast with metastases. *Ann Surg* 100:392–395, 1934.

42. Merino MJ: Plasmacytoma of the breast. *Arch Pathol Lab Med* 108:676–678, 1984.

43. Ben Yehuda A, Steiner-Saltz D, Libson E, et al: Plasmacytoma of the breast. Unusual presentation of myeloma: report of two cases and review of the literature. *Blut* 58:169–170, 1989.

44. Foucar E, Rosai J, Dorfman R: Sinus histiocytosis with massive lymphadenopathy (Rosai-Dorfman disease). Review of the entity. *Semin Diagn Pathol* 7:19–73, 1990.

45. Perez-Guillerma M, Sola-Perez J, Rodriquez-Bermejo M: Malakoplakia and Rosai-Dorman disease: two entities of histiocytic origin infrequently localized in the female breast. The cytologic aspect in aspirates via fine needle aspiration cytology. *Diagn Cytopathol* 9:698–704, 1993.

CHAPTER TWELVE

Metastatic Carcinoma

Unlike metastases from the contralateral breast, the incidence of metastatic tumors from extramammary sites is extremely low and accounts for only 0.4% to 2.0% of clinically observed breast malignancies.[1–5] In autopsy studies the incidence varies from 1.4% to 6.6% of patients with malignant breast tumors.[1,2,6] In the largest series, reported by Hajdu and Urban[1] at Memorial Hospital in New York, metastatic tumors of the breast accounted for 1.2% of all breast malignancies, with 44 women and 7 men affected. As in other studies, the most common extramammary primaries in women were, in order of decreasing frequency, melanoma, lymphoma, lung carcinoma, ovarian carcinoma, and soft tissue sarcoma, followed by gastrointestinal and genitourinary primaries. Numerous studies have shown that the prostate is the most common extramammary site in men.[2,3,4,6–16]

The clinical presentation of metastatic carcinoma is similar to that of primary cancer; however, nipple retraction and discharge are not observed. The lesion is usually well defined, firm, and often movable.[1,15,17] Axillary lymph node involvement is seen only when the metastatic tumor is in the axillary tail of the breast or when lymphoma or leukemic processes involve breast and lymph nodes simultaneously. Metastatic breast tumors have a variable mammographic apppearance, ranging from an appearance similar to that of benign breast lesions such as cysts, fibroadenomas, or proliferative breast disease to an appearance similar to that of malignancies such as medullary carcinoma.[6] A discrete nodule located eccentrically in subcutaneous fat, occasional rapid growth, and lack of microcalcification are other significant features.[3,6,14]

The prognosis for patients with metastatic breast tumor is often poor, with 80% of patients dying within 1 year of diagnosis.[1,4] Patients with malignant lymphoproliferative disorders respond to chemotherapy and live longer.[13] Overall, the average age of patients with metastatic breast tumor is younger, usually under 50, compared with the average age of patients with primary breast cancer.[17] This may be due to the better blood supply in younger age groups, which may predispose the breast to be a site of metastasis.[17]

Histologically, metastatic breast tumors can simulate primary breast cancer, leading to mastectomy.[1,14,18,19] Necrosis, calcification, and in situ lesions are not typical histologic findings in metastatic breast carcinoma. Metastatic tumors are characteristically well demarcated and show evidence of periductal infiltration. Cytomorphologic differentiation between primary and metastatic breast disease is also difficult. Poorly differentiated adenocarcinoma, in particular, is easily confused with ductal carcinoma. Nonetheless, when combined with appropriate clinical history and the use of ancillary studies, fine needle aspiration biopsy (FNAB) is an effective tool in substantiating a diagnosis of tumor metastatic to the breast.[20–32] However, some investigators still believe that FNAB is of limited value in differentiating between primary and metastatic breast tumors and that surgical biopsy is necessary for definitive diagnosis.[4]

Increasing interest in the use of FNAB in the evaluation of breast lesions has provided us with ample opportunity to enhance our skills in interpreting the cytomorphology of breast lesions, including metastatic breast tumors. We have found that when combined with specific tumor markers and ultrastructural studies, FNAB is helpful in the majority of cases. Accurate diagnosis of metastatic breast tumor by FNAB may avoid unnecessary mastectomy and guide further therapy.

Aspirates of metastatic breast tumors are often cellular, with a pattern varying from dispersed single cells to cell clusters with microtissue fragments. Meticulous attention should be given to the size, shape, nuclear characteristics, and cytoplasmic features of the tumor cells. The cellular background is often clean; however, depending on the nature of the lesion, lymphoglandular bodies and extracellular mucoid or myxoid substances can be seen. Classification of metastatic tumors is based on the pattern of cell distribution and individual cell morphology.

Adenocarcinomas, melanomas, Hodgkin's disease, large cell lymphoma (B-cell lineage and Ki-1 lymphoma), and pleomorphic sarcomas such as malignant fibrous histiocytoma often manifest as a pleomorphic large cell tumor with multilobulate cells. Melanomas, lymphomas, leukemia, and carcinoid tumors are malignancies with a dispersed cell pattern. Melanomas, lymphomas (especially immunoblastic sarcoma), some adenocarcinomas, and carcinoid tumors may also have a plasmacytoid appearance.

Of the various histochemical stains, mucicarmine stain is most helpful. Although mucin positivity cannot be used to distinguish between primary and metastatic breast lesions, when associated with a history of extramammary primary malignancy, negative staining can exclude the possibility of metastasis from sites such as kidney, prostate, and thyroid.

Immunocytochemistry can be combined with clinical presentation and cytomorphology in making a differential diagnosis. As a rule, a single immunocytochemical stain is not sufficient. It is best to select a simple panel of antibodies, since pertinent negative stains are as important as the pertinent positive stains.

We have encountered 24 cases of metastatic breast tumors. The cases in order of frequency were malignant melanoma, renal cell carcinoma, lung carcinoma, genitourinary malignancies, gastrointestinal tumors, hepatocellular carcinoma, leukemia, lymphoma in women, and prostate cancer in men. In three cases, renal cell carcinoma was unsuspected clinically. Similar findings have also been reported by other investigators. A series of 20 cases of metastatic breast tumor reported by Sneige et al[27] included malignant melanoma, lung carcinoma, ovarian serous carcinoma, lymphoma, carcinoma, transitional cell carcinoma, plasma cell myeloma, and rhabdomyosarcoma. Similarly, Silverman et al[20] reported 18 cases of metastatic breast tumors that included lung carcinomas, malignant melanomas, ovarian malignancies, fallopian tube and endometrial carcinoma, transitional cell carcinoma of the bladder, prostate carcinoma, granulocytic sarcoma, lymphoma, mycosis fungoides, hepatoma, and neuroblastoma of the retroperitoneum. Scattered reports of tumors that metastasized to breast from other sites are also available.[23,28,30–32]

It is generally agreed that the clinical history; review of the previous microscopic slides; and use of special stains, electron microscopy, immunocytochemistry, and flow cytometry are effective in correctly diagnosing metastatic tumors. Depending on the cytologic differential diagnosis, the panels of antibodies used for a suspected metastatic breast lesion include cytokeratin, epithelial membrane antigen, leukocyte common antigens, neuron specific enolase, S-100, HMB-45, muscle specific actin, desmin, and vimentin. Estrogen and progesterone receptor immunocytochemical assays may also be used to distinguish between primary and metastatic breast tumors.[33–35]

Metastatic tumors often have cytomorphologic features different from the usual cytomorphologic features seen in primary breast carcinoma. A good example is malignant melanoma, which is quite cellular, with a dispersed pattern of isolated and occasionally binucleate cells. The cells have round to oval, eccentric nuclei with regular nuclear membranes and prominent nucleoli. In some cells intranuclear vacuoles are present (Images 12.1 through 12.4). Occasionally, malignant melanomas can have atypical spindle cells, recognition of which requires immunocytochemical and/or electron microscopic study (Figure 12.1 and Images 12.5 and 12.6). Metastatic renal carcinomas often have monomorphic cells isolated or in clusters, with granular or vacuolated cytoplasm and regular nuclei with distinct, round nucleoli. The epithelial cells contain lipid, which can be demonstrated by oil red O stain (Images 12.7 through 12.10).

Aspirates of small cell (oat cell) carcinoma of the lung are cellular and consist of small malignant cells with a high N/C ratio. The nuclei are oval to angulated with a characteristic salt-and-pepper chromatin pattern and no visible nucleoli. Tumor cells show positive immunostaining for neuron-specific enolase, chromogranin, and S-100. Electron microscopic study reveals the presence of neurosecretory granules (Figure 12.2 and Images 12.11 through 12.13).

Metastatic adenocarcinoma of the lung has features similar to those of other mucin-producing adenocarcinomas, and differentiation from primary breast carcinoma may be difficult (Images 12.14 through 12.17). Clinical history and chest x-ray are the most important tools in differentiation. In contrast, aspirates of metastatic squamous cell carcinoma, which is associated with a history of lung cancer, present minimal diagnostic challenge, particularly since primary squamous cell carcinoma of the breast is extremely rare (Images 12.18 through 12.21).

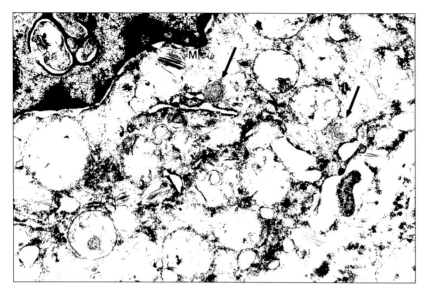

Figure 12.1
Characteristic ultrastructural features of metastatic malignant melanoma: early stage melanosomes (M) with identifiable internal lamellar pattern and later stage melanosomes (arrows) (34,200X).

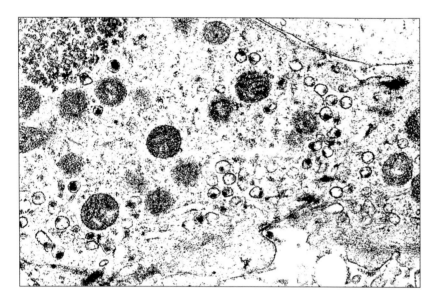

Figure 12.2
Ultrastructural feature of small cell carcinoma with neurosecretory granules (22,000X).

In the absence of a history of primary malignancy, breast aspirates with the cytomorphologic features of mucin-producing carcinoma with a signet ring pattern may create diagnostic difficulty. In our experience, the ultrastructural features of the aspirated tumor cells may assist in the distinction between primary breast carcinoma and metastases from the gastrointestinal tract (Figures 12.3 and 12.4 and Images 12.22 through 12.25).

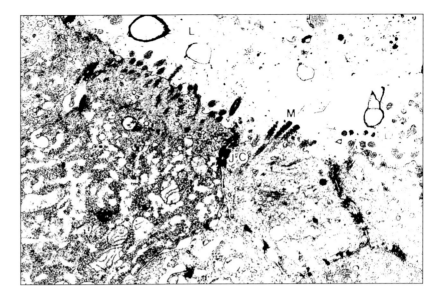

Figure 12.3
Ultrastructural features of the adenocarcinoma seen in the breast aspirate shown in Images 12.22 through 12.24. The cells of this tumor, which metastasized from the colon, form glands with a central lumen (L) showing numerous microvilli (M) and junctional complexes (JC) (14,900X).

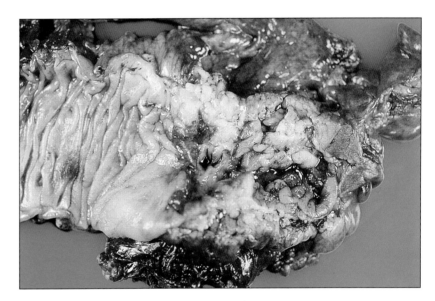

Figure 12.4
Macroscopic appearance of previously resected colon cancer of the same patient.

Hepatocellular carcinoma may also metastasize to the breast. Smears are richly cellular, with cells isolated or in clusters. The tumor cells have a high N/C ratio; abundant, granular cytoplasm; and vesicular nuclei. The chromatin is coarse, and the nucleoli can be conspicuous. Binucleation may occur, and often bile pigments are seen in intercellular, gland-like spaces. Intranuclear invagination may also be seen. Cell block preparations show tumor cells arranged in trabeculae, solid clusters, and gland-like configurations. Tumor cells show positive immunostaining for cytokeratin and alpha-fetoprotein (Images 12.26 through 12.28).

Recognition of hepatocellular carcinoma based on cytomorphologic features alone is challenging. The cytologic differential diagnosis includes primary apocrine carcinoma or epithelioid angiosarcoma, metastatic malignant melanoma, and secondary deposits of other adenocarcinomas.[16,27,36] The presence of intranuclear inclusions is nonspecific and may be observed in other pathologic conditions.[37] As previously mentioned, ancillary studies are the most effective tools in the differential diagnosis (Figure 12.5).

Sarcomas rarely metastasize to the breast and are characterized by an atypical spindle cell pattern distinct from that seen in primary breast carcinoma. Immunocytochemistry and electron microscopic studies are essential to correct diagnosis (Images 12.29 and 12.30, Figure 12.6).

Fine needle aspirates of metastatic prostate carcinoma are cellular and contain isolated cells of irregular shapes and sizes. The degree of pleomorphism and nuclear change vary depending on the degree of tumor differentiation. Often the cells display gland-like structures. Immunocytochemical staining for prostate-specific antigen is the most helpful diagnostic adjunct (Images 12.31 through 12.36). Differentiation between primary male breast carcinoma and metastasis from the prostate is important. If the lesion is a metastatic deposit from a carcinoma of the prostate, the prognosis is poor, with an average life expectancy of only 4 months. In contrast, if the lesion is a primary carcinoma of the breast, mastectomy can be performed with a far better prognosis.[38]

The cytomorphologic features of other conditions that may metastasize to the breast, such as lymphoma, leukemia, plasmacytoma, and carcinoid tumor, are similar to those of the original tumor and have already been discussed in other sections. Occasionally, unusual tumors such as choriocarcinoma may metastasize to the breast and manifest as isolated and

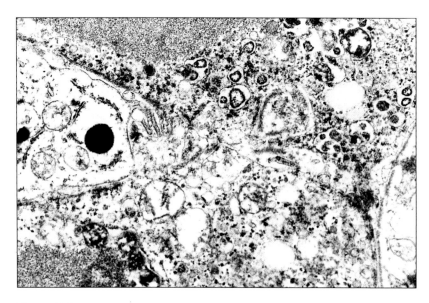

Figure 12.5
Photomicrograph of glycogen granules and bile canaliculi commonly seen in hepatocellular carcinoma (25,700X).

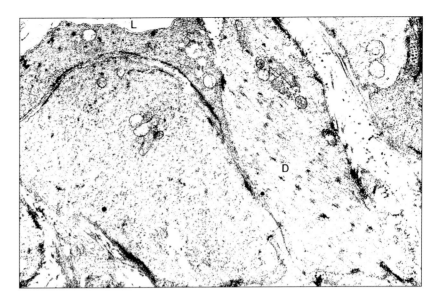

Figure 12.6
Electron microscopy of fine needle aspirate of metastatic leiomyosarcoma shown in Images 12.29 and 12.30 reveals neoplastic cells with prominent basal lamina (L), numerous thin filaments, and dense bodies (D) (18,700X).

syncytial groups of highly neoplastic cells of various sizes, displaying binucleation, multinucleation, and intracytoplasmic vacuolization. However, unusual tumors such as choriocarcinoma are not usually a diagnostic possiblity unless the patient has a positive clinical history.[28]

Breast lesions can also metastasize to many areas and create diagnostic dilemmas. It should be emphasized that a clinical history of malignancy does not necessarily exclude the possibility of a second primary cancer arising in the breast. For example, one of our patients who had a history of squamous cell carcinoma of the tongue presented with a well-defined breast lesion. An aspirate of the lesion contained neoplastic epithelial cells with no differentiating features. The tumor cells displayed nuclear atypia in both direct smears and cell block preparations. Based on the patient's history of malignancy and negative immunostaining for hormone receptors, the tumor was diagnosed as cancer, most likely a metastasis; however, the distinction between a primary and secondary lesion could not be made and surgical biopsy was recommended. Surgical excision of the breast lesion demonstrated a colloid carcinoma. Tissue section of the lesion was negative for hormone receptors, which is not a typical pattern of hormone receptor expression in colloid carcinoma. Nevertheless, when we stained the original cell block of the aspirated material for mucin, we found abundant extracellular mucin, a feature that might have pointed us to a diagnosis of colloid carcinoma initially (Images 12.37 through 12.40). Hormone receptors may play an important role in the differentiation between primary and secondary tumors and in the identification of primary tumors of unknown origin. Examples are illustrated in Images 12.41 through 12.49 and Figures 12.7 and 12.8. Based on reports in the literature and our own experience, recognition of metastatic breast lesions requires careful evaluation of any case with atypical clinical, mammographic, or cytologic features not commonly seen in primary breast malignancies.

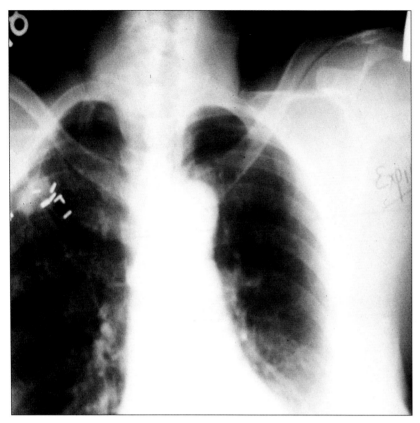

Figure 12.7
Chest x-ray of a patient with a history of primary breast cancer presenting with a solitary lung lesion. Reproduced with permission from: Masood S: Prognostic and diagnostic implications of estrogen and progesterone receptor assays in cytology. *Diagn Cytopathol* 10:263–267, 1994.

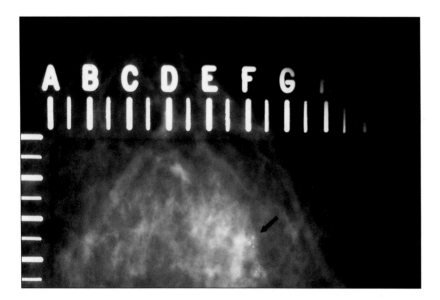

Figure 12.8
Upon further workup, the patient with metastatic bone lesion was found to have an abnormal mammogram (arrow) with clustered microcalcifications. Reproduced with permission from: Masood S: Prognostic and diagnostic implications of estrogen and progesterone receptor assays in cytology. *Diagn Cytopathol* 10:263–267, 1994.

Image 12.1
Aspirate of a metastatic malignant melanoma reveals a dispersed cell pattern. Isolated cells and a few binucleated cells are also seen (Papanicolaou, 200X).

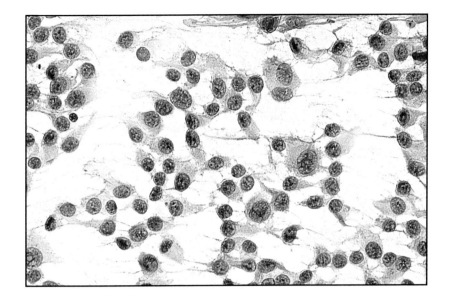

Image 12.2
Higher magnification of the same case reveals an intranuclear vacuole (Papanicolaou, 400X).

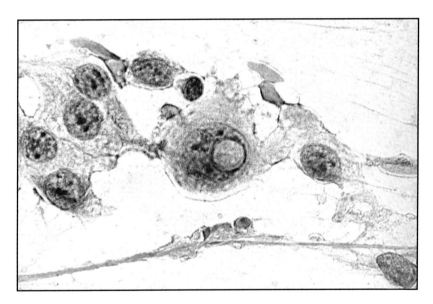

Image 12.3
Cell block preparation of the same case shows a positive reaction with HMB-45, a typical immunostaining pattern in malignant melanoma (400X).

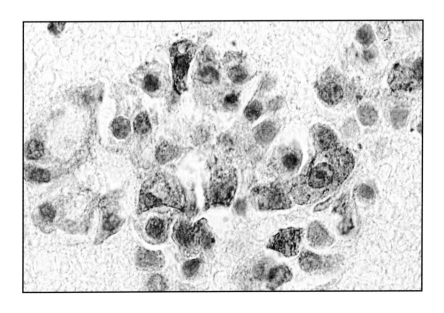

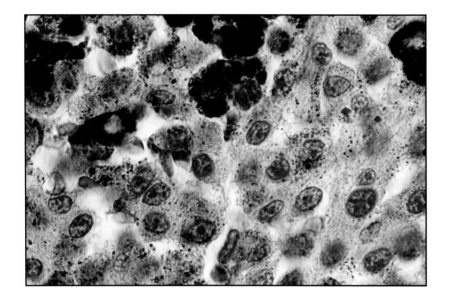

Image 12.4
Corresponding tissue section from a pigmented skin lesion of the same patient. The lesion was previously diagnosed as a primary malignant melanoma. (H&E, 400X).

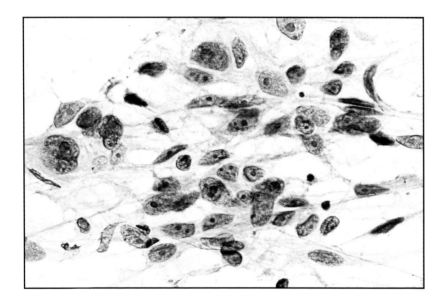

Image 12.5
Direct smear of an aspirate of metastatic malignant melanoma shows a dispersed cell pattern and conspicuous pleomorphism (Papanicolaou, 200X).

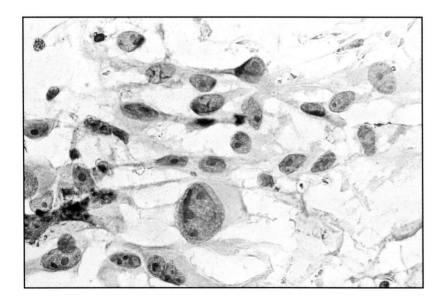

Image 12.6
Higher magnification reveals a spindle cell pattern and conspicuous, multiple nucleoli (Papanicolaou, 400X).

Image 12.7
Direct smear of metastatic renal cell carcinoma reveals a monomorphic cell population with eccentric nuclei and vacuolated cytoplasm (Diff-Quik®, 400X).

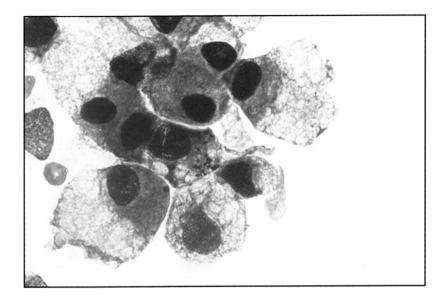

Image 12.8
Papanicolaou-stained smear of the same case shows round cells with a regular nuclear membrane and distinct nucleoli (400X).

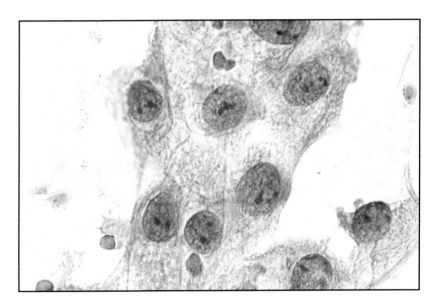

Image 12.9
Presence of oil droplets in the epithelial cells of metastatic renal cell carcinoma (Oil red O, 400X).

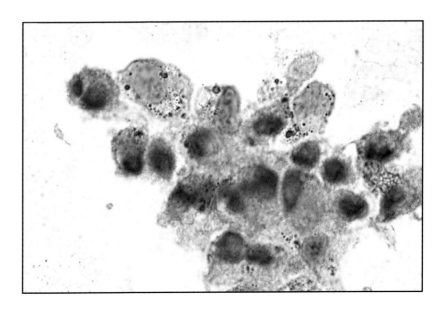

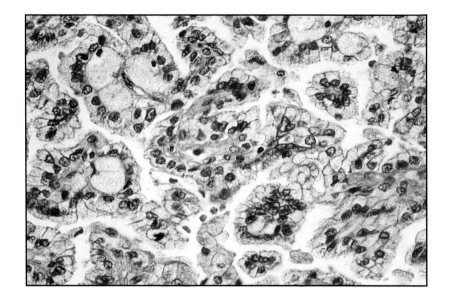

Image 12.10
Corresponding tissue section of the surgically excised lesion from the same case demonstrates histologic features of renal cell carcinoma (H&E, 200X).

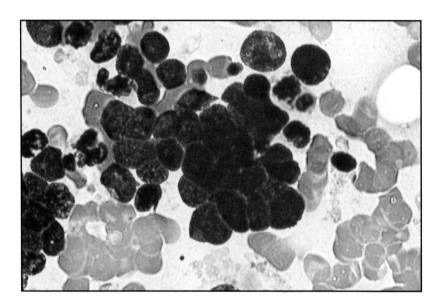

Image 12.11
Aspirate of metastatic small cell carcinoma reveals clusters of small malignant cells with conspicuous pleomorphism and anisonucleosis (Diff-Quik, 400X).

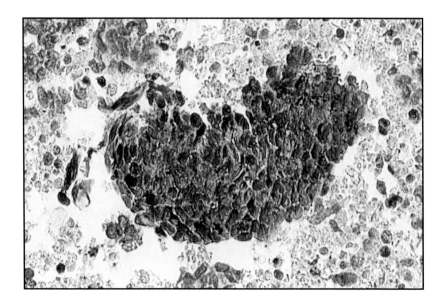

Image 12.12
Cell block preparation of metastatic small cell carcinoma demonstrates positive immunostaining for neuron-specific enolase (Immunoperoxidase, 200X).

Image 12.13
Tissue section of primary lung lesion from the same patient. The lesion was diagnosed as oat cell carcinoma (H&E, 400X).

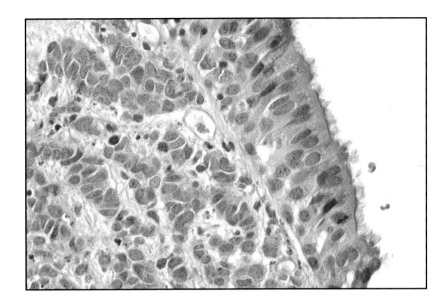

Image 12.14
Aspirate of metastatic adenocarcinoma reveals a cluster of highly neoplastic epithelial cells characterized by pleo-morphism, conspicuous nuclei, and anisonucleosis (Diff-Quik, 1000X)

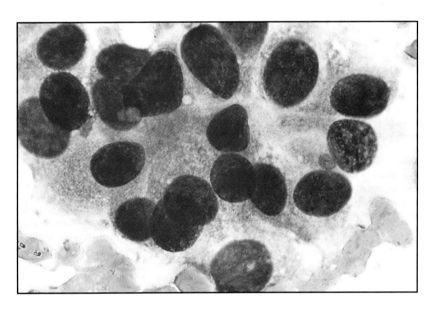

Image 12.15
Cell block preparation of the same case shows a positive reaction with mucin (Mucicarmine, 400X).

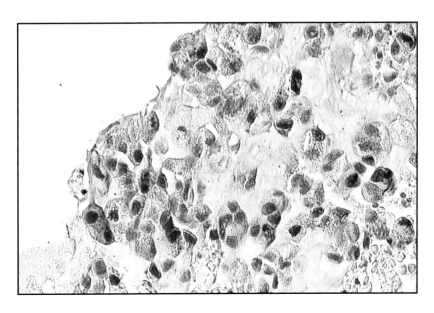

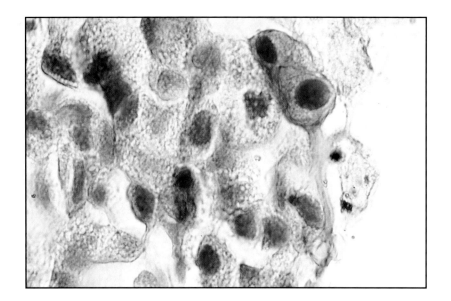

Image 12.16
Higher magnification of the same case of metastatic adenocarcinoma reveals clusters of mucin-positive tumor cells (Mucicarmine, 1000X).

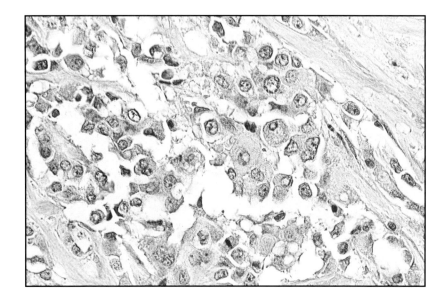

Image 12.17
Corresponding tissue section of the previously resected lung lesion of the same patient diagnosed with poorly differentiated adenocarcinoma (H&E, 400X).

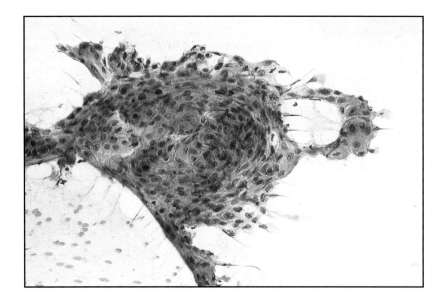

Image 12.18
Aspirate of metastatic squamous cell carcinoma reveals clusters of cohesive epithelial cells with evidence of keratinization (Papanicolaou, 200X).

Image 12.19
Another view of the same case of metastatic squamous cell carcinoma reveals clustering of epithelial cells and pearl formation (Papanicolaou, 200X).

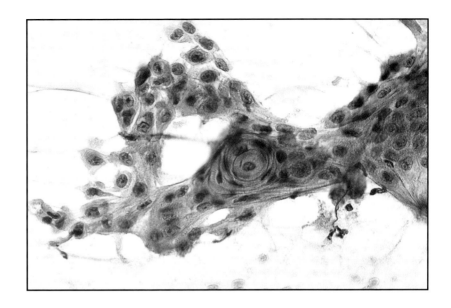

Image 12.20
Corresponding tissue section of the previously diagnosed well-differentiated squamous cell carcinoma of the lung (H&E, 200X).

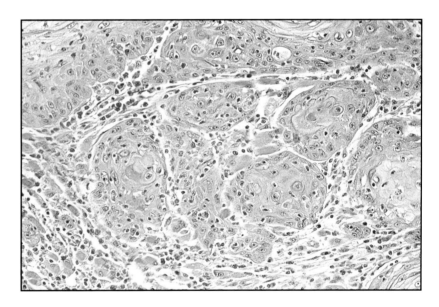

Image 12.21
Higher magnification of the same case demonstrates conspicuous keratinization and pearl formation (H&E, 400X).

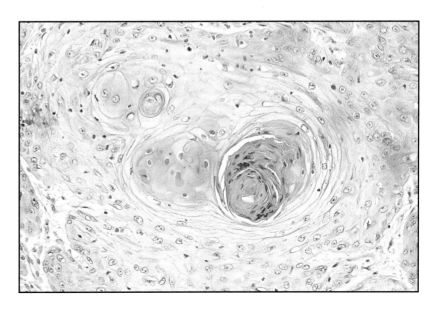

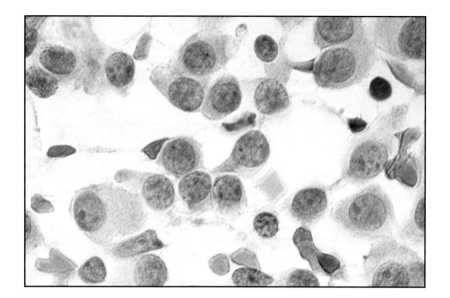

Image 12.22
Aspirate of a localized breast lesion displays a dispersed cell pattern with uniform-appearing epithelial cells (Papanicolaou, 400X).

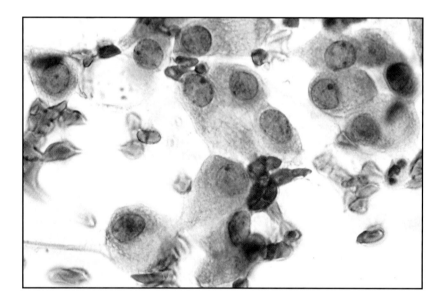

Image 12.23
Another view of the same case: round to oval-shaped cells with eccentric, uniform nuclei and granular to vacuolated cytoplasm (Papanicolaou, 400X).

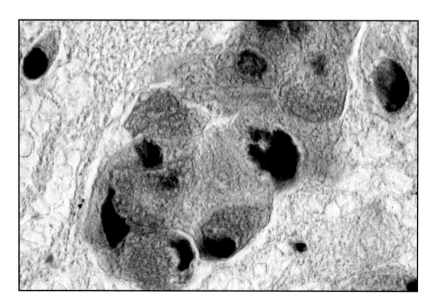

Image 12.24
Tumor cells of the same case show mucin positivity, a feature of mucin-producing adenocarcinoma that is indistinguishable from primary breast carcinoma (Mucicarmine, 1000X). The metastatic nature of this lesion was confirmed by electron microscopy (Figure 12.3) and review of previous pathology (Figure 12.4 and Image 12.25).

Image 12.25
Microscopic appearance of previously diagnosed signet ring carcinoma of the colon (H&E, 400X). This is the same case shown in Figures 12.3 and 12.4 and Images 12.22 through 12.24.

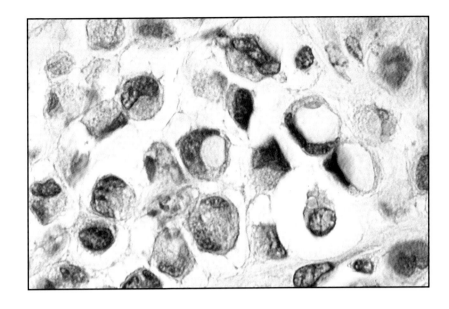

Image 12.26
Aspirate of metastatic hepatocellular carcinoma reveals a pleomorphic population of tumor cells isolated and in clusters, with an increased N/C ratio, abundant cytoplasm with vesicular nuclei, and intranuclear inclusions (Papanicolaou, 200X).

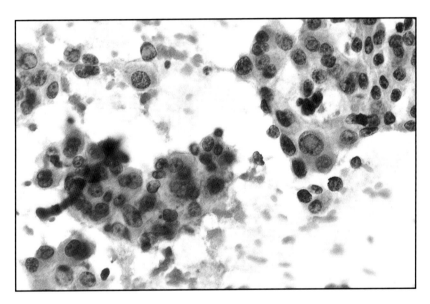

Image 12.27
Cell block preparation shows tumor cells in nests and cords with an obvious intercellular bile plug (H&E, 200X).

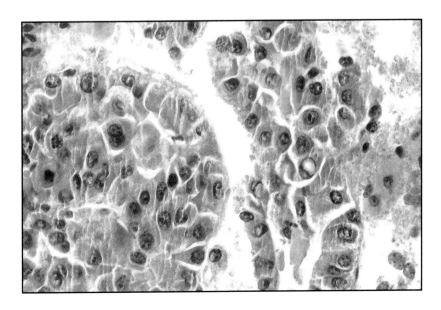

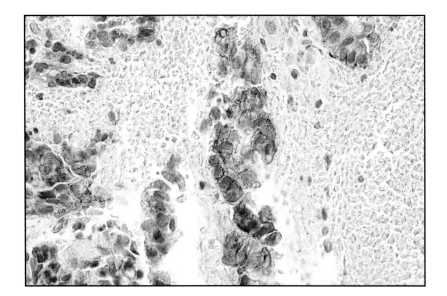

Image 12.28
Positive immunostaining for alpha-fetoprotein in cell block preparation of metastatic hepatocellular carcinoma (Immunoperoxidase, 200X).

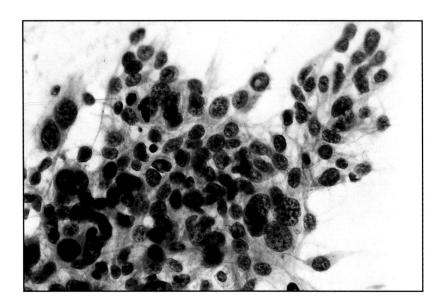

Image 12.29
Aspirate of metastatic leiomyosarcoma shows a highly pleomorphic cluster of spindle cells with many tumor giant cells, features unlike those seen in ordinary primary breast carcinoma (Papanicolaou, 400X).

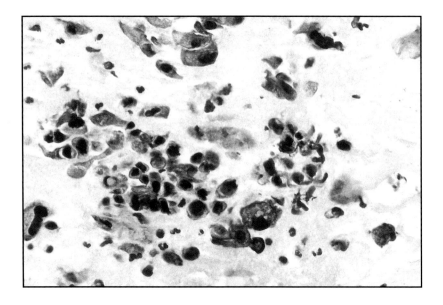

Image 12.30
Cell block preparation shows a positive immunostaining reaction with desmin, suggesting the smooth muscle origin of the tumor (Immunoperoxidase, 200X).

Image 12.31
Aspirate of prostate carcinoma metastatic to the breast reveals a loosely cohesive, rather monomorphic tumor cell population (Diff-Quik, 200X).

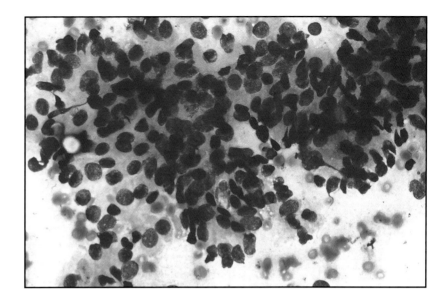

Image 12.32
Higher magnification of the same case reveals the gland-like appearance of the tumor cells (Diff-Quik, 400X).

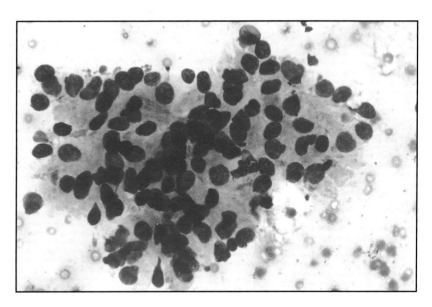

Image 12.33
Papanicolaou stain of the same aspirate reveals a uniform small cell population with round, regular nuclei and inconspicuous nucleoli (Immunoperoxidase, 200X).

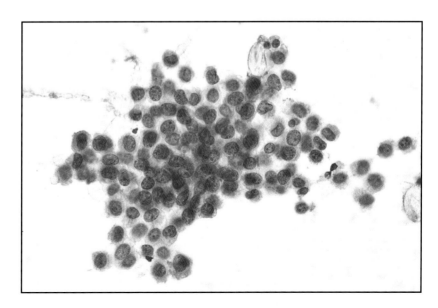

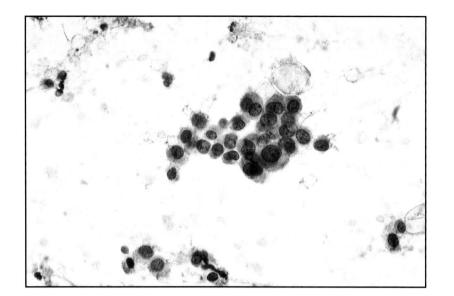

Image 12.34
Another view of the same aspirate reveals evidence of anisonucleosis (Papanicolaou, 200X).

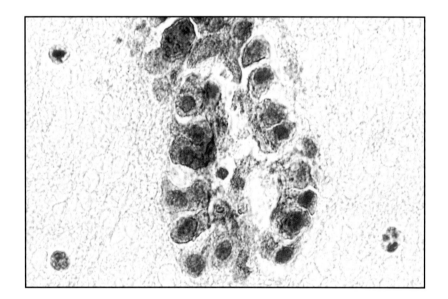

Image 12.35
Cell block preparation obtained from the same aspirate exhibits a positive reaction with prostate specific antigen, confirming the metastatic origin of the tumor cells (Immunoperoxidase, 400X).

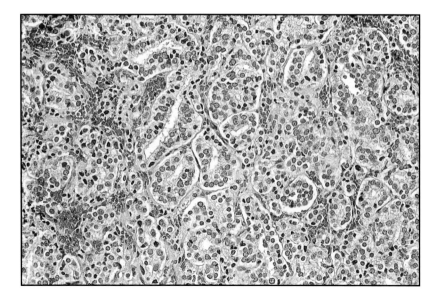

Image 12.36
Corresponding tissue section of the previously resected prostate carcinoma from the same patient (H&E, 200X).

Image 12.37
Aspirate of a well-defined breast lesion in a patient with a history of squamous cell carcinoma of the tongue. The aspirate reveals pleomorphic neoplastic epithelial cells isolated and in clusters with prominent nucleoli and modest cytoplasm (Papanicolaou, 400X).

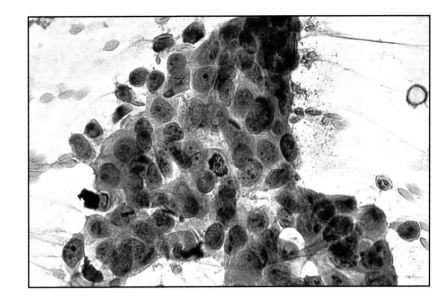

Image 12.38
Cell block preparation of the same case reveals similar features difficult to distinguish from those of primary breast carcinoma (H&E, 200X).

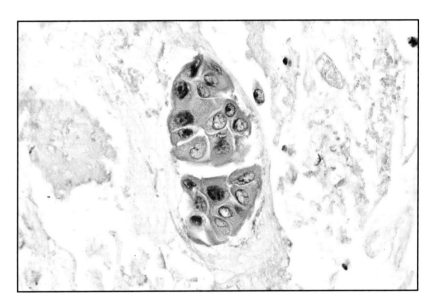

Image 12.39
Corresponding tissue section of surgically excised lesion from the same case. The lesion was diagnosed as primary colloid carcinoma of the breast (H&E, 200X).

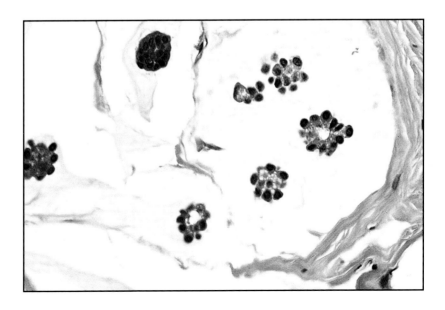

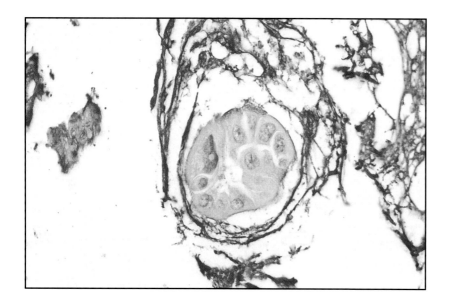

Image 12.40
Positive mucin staining in this cell block preparation could have helped to differentiate this tumor from squamous cell carcinoma metastatic to the breast (Mucicarmine, 200X).

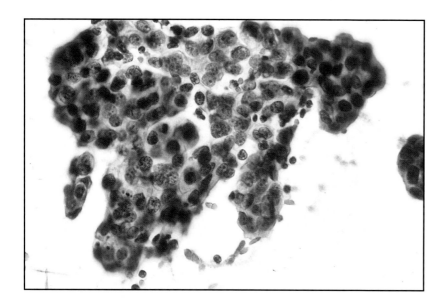

Image 12.41
Aspirate of a scalp lesion in a woman with a history of breast carcinoma shows clusters of neoplastic epithelial cells of uncertain origin (Papanicolaou, 200X).

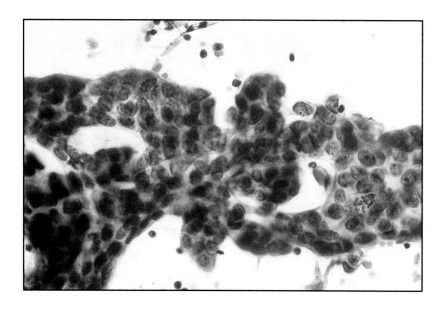

Image 12.42
Another view of the same case shows crowded clusters of tumor cells, suggesting a gland-like formation (Papanicolaou, 200X).

Image 12.43
Cell block preparation of the same case reveals no differentiating feature that indicates the site of the primary tumor (H&E, 200X).

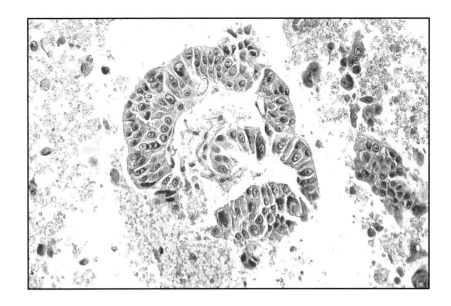

Image 12.44
Estrogen–receptor expression as evidenced by nuclear staining suggests that breast is the most likely site of the primary tumor (Immunoperoxidase, 400X).

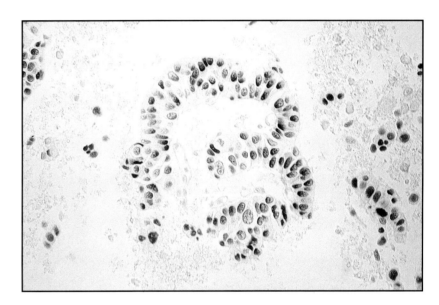

Image 12.45
Aspirate of the lung lesion shown in Figure 12.7 reveals clusters of neoplastic cells with no differentiating feature to indicate whether the lesion is a primary or a metastasis from breast (Papanicolaou, 200X). Reproduced with permission from: Masood S: Prognostic and diagnostic implications of estrogen and progesterone receptor assays in cytology. *Diagn Cytopathol* 10:263–267, 1994.

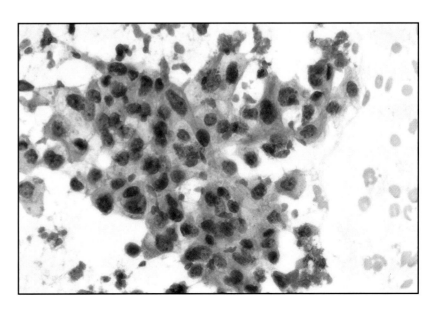

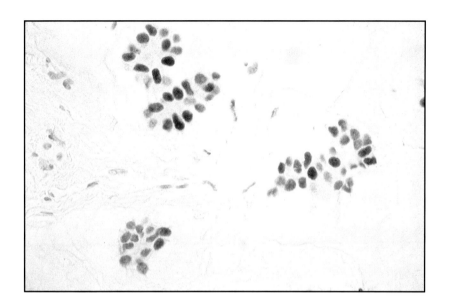

Image 12.46
Cell block preparation of the same case is positive for estrogen receptor, which suggests that the tumor originated in breast. The patient underwent tamoxifen therapy, and the lung lesion disappeared (Immunoperoxidase, 200X). Reproduced with permission from: Masood S: Prognostic and diagnostic implications of estrogen and progesterone receptor assays in cytology. *Diagn Cytopathol* 10:263–267, 1994.

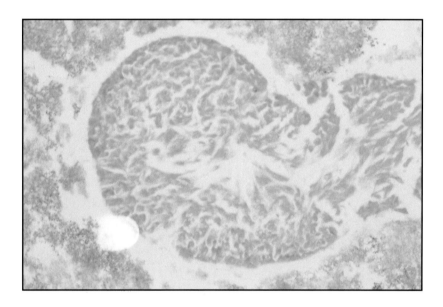

Image 12.47
Negative estrogen receptor immunocytochemical assay on cell block preparation from a bone aspirate of an 82-year-old woman with a lytic bone lesion and no obvious primary tumor (Immunoperoxidase, 200X). Reproduced with permission from: Masood S: Prognostic and diagnostic implications of estrogen and progesterone receptor assays in cytology. *Diagn Cytopathol* 10:263–267, 1994.

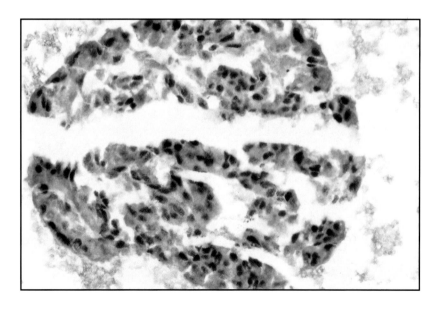

Image 12.48
Expression of progesterone receptor in the same tissue section suggests breast as the possible site of the primary (Immunoperoxidase, 200X). This was confirmed with a positive mammogram (Figure 12.8) and an excisional biopsy (Image 12.49). Reproduced with permission from: Masood S: Prognostic and diagnostic implications of estrogen and progesterone receptor assays in cytology. *Diagn Cytopathol* 10:263–267, 1994.

Image 12.49
Tissue section of needle-localizing excisional biopsy specimen from the same case shown in Figure 12.8 and Images 12.47 and 12.48 reveals an infiltrating duct cell carcinoma (H&E, 200X). Reproduced with permission from: Masood S: Prognostic and diagnostic implications of estrogen and progesterone receptor assays in cytology. *Diagn Cytopathol* 10:263–267, 1994.

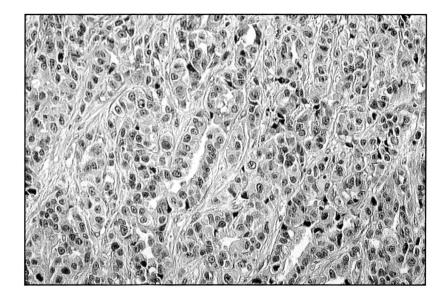

References

1. Hajdu S, Urban JA: Cancers metastatic to the breast. *Cancer* 20: 1691–1696, 1972.

2. Bohman LG, Bassett LW, Gold RH, et al: Breast metastases from extramammary malignancies. *Radiology* 144:309–312, 1982.

3. D'Orsi CJ, Feldhaus L, Sonnenfeld M: Unusual lesions of the breast. *Radiol Clin North Am* 21:7–80, 1983.

4. McIntosh IH, Hooper AA, Millis RR, et al: Metastatic carcinoma within the breast. *Clin Oncol* 2:393–401, 1976.

5. Silverman EM, Oberman HA: Metastatic neoplasm in the breast. *Surg Gynecol Obstet* 138:26–28, 1974.

6. Paulus DD, Libshitz I: Metastasis to the breast. *Radiol Clin North Am* 20:561–568, 1982.

7. Choudhury M, DeRosas J, Paosidero L, et al: Metastatic prostatic carcinoma to breast or primary breast carcinoma? *Urology* 3:297–299, 1982.

8. Drelichman A, Amer M, Pontes E, et al: Carcinoma of prostate metastatic to breast. *Urology* 16:250–255, 1980.

9. Naritoku WY, Taylor CR: Immunohistologic diagnosis of 2 cases of metastatic prostate cancer to the breast. *J Urol* 130:365–367, 1983.

10. Ordonez NG, Manning JT, Raymond AK: Argentaffin endocrine carcinoma (carcinoid) of the pancreas with concomitant breast metastasis: an immunohistochemical and electron microscopic study. *Hum Pathol* 16:746–751, 1985.

11. Charache H: Metastatic tumors in the breast with a report of 10 cases. *Surgery* 33:385–390, 1953.

12. Dardick L, Comer TP, O'Neill EJ, et al: Metastatic neoplasm presenting as primary cancer of the breast: case reports. *Milit Med* 149: 411–414, 1984.

13. McCrea ES, Johnston C, Haney PJ: Metastasis to the breast. *Am J Roentgenol* 141:685-690, 1983.

14. Schurch W, Lamauraux E, Lefevre R, et al: Solitary breast metastasis: first manifestation of an occult carcinoid of the ileum. *Virchows Arch [A]* 386:117–124, 1980.

15. Palgon NM, Novetsky AD, Fogler RJ, et al: Lung carcinoma presenting as a breast tumor. *NY State J Med* 83:1188-1189, 1983.

16. Schmitt FC, Tani E, Skoog L: Cytology and immunocytochemistry of bilateral breast metastasis from prostate cancer. Report of a case. *Acta Cytol* 33:899–902, 1989.

17. Deeley TJ: Secondary deposits in the breast. *Br J Cancer* 19:738–743, 1965.

18. Nielsen M, Andersen JA, Henriksen FW, et al: Metastases to the breast from extramammary carcinomas. *Acta Pathol Microbiol Scand (A)* 89:251–256, 1981.

19. Sandison AT: Metastatic tumors in the breast. *Br J Surg* 47:54–58, 1959.

20. Silverman JF, Feldman PS, Corell JL, Frable WJ: Fine needle aspiration cytology of neoplasms metastatic to the breast. *Acta Cytol* 31:291–300, 1987.

21. Gorczyca W, Olszewski W, Tuziak T, et al: Fine needle aspiration biopsy of rare malignant tumors of the breast. *Acta Cytol* 36: 918–926, 1992.

22. Cornillot M, Granier AM, Verhaeghe M: Aspect cytologie des metastases intramammaries. *Arch Anat Cytol Pathol* 27:234–238, 1979.

23. Yzadi HM: Cytopathology of endometrial adenocarcinoma metastases to the breast examined by fine needle aspiration. *Am J Clin Pathol* 38:559–563, 1982.

24. Leiman G: Squamous carcinoma of the breast: diagnosis by aspiration cytology. *Acta Cytol* 26:201–209, 1982.

25. Eisenberg AJ, Hajdu SI, Wilhelmus J, et al: Preoperative aspiration cytology of breast tumors. *Acta Cytol* 30:135–146, 1986.

26. Hoeven KV, Hibbard C, Jones J, et al: Fine needle aspiration diagnosis of tumors metastatic to the breast. *Acta Cytol* 35:613, 1991.

27. Sneige N, Zachariah S, Fanning T, et al: Fine needle aspiration cytology of metastatic neoplasms in the breast. *Am J Clin Pathol* 92: 27–35, 1989.

28. Kumar P, Esfahani F, Salimi A: Choriocarcinoma metastatic to the breast diagnosed by fine needle aspiration. *Acta Cytol* 35:239–242, 1991.

29. Koss LG, Woyke S, Olszewski W: *Aspiration Biopsy: Cytologic Interpretation and Histologic Bases.* New York, NY, Igaku-Shoin, 1984, pp. 53-104.

30. Krisnnan EU, Phillips AK, Randell A, et al: Bilateral metastatic inflammatory carcinoma in the breast from primary ovarian cancer. *Obstet Gynecol* 55(suppl):948–965, 1980.

31. Miura H, Konaka C, Kamate N, et al: Fine needle aspiration cytology of metastatic breast tumor originating from leukemia. *Diagn Cytopathol* 8:605–608, 1992.

32. London G, Sneige N, Ordonez NG, et al: Carcinoid metastatic to breast diagnosed by fine needle aspiration biopsy. *Diagn Cytopathol* 3:230–233, 1987.

33. Masood S: Prognostic and diagnostic implications of estrogen and progesterone receptor assays in cytology. *Diagn Cytopathol* 10:263–267, 1994.

34. Masood S: Estrogen and progesterone receptors in cytology. *Diagn Cytopathol* 8:475–491, 1992.

35. Masood S: Sex steroid hormone receptors in cytologic material. In: Schmidt WA, ed. *Cytopathology Annual 1992.* Baltimore, Md, Williams & Wilkins, 1992, pp. 77–102.

36. Kline TS, Joshi LP, Hunter SN: Fine needle aspiration of the breast: diagnosis and pitfalls: a review of 3,545 cases. *Cancer* 49:1458–1464, 1979.

37. Gritsman AY, Popok SM, Ro JY, et al: Renal cell carcinoma with intranuclear inclusions metastatic to thyroid: a diagnostic problem in aspiration cytology. *Diagn Cytopathol* 4:125–129, 1988.
38. Naritoku WY, Taylor CR: Immunohistologic diagnosis of 2 cases of metastatic prostate cancer to breast. *J Urol* 130:365–367, 1983.

CHAPTER THIRTEEN

Miscellaneous

Male Breast

Gynecomastia and carcinoma are the two most common lesions of the male breast. As with breast lesions in women, fine needle aspiration biopsy (FNAB) can be applied to the study of breast lesions in men. However, male breast lesions represent less than 1% of cases in breast fine needle aspirate studies.[1,2] Gynecomastia accounts for the majority of breast lesions in men, followed by malignant tumors, with a relatively equal frequency of primary and metastatic lesions.[3]

Gynecomastia

Gynecomastia, a potentially reversible enlargement of the male breast, is characterized by proliferation of ducts and stroma. It is the most common benign breast lesion in men and presents as either a unilateral or bilateral palpable mass.[4,5] Although the etiology is often unknown, in some cases there is a history of hormonal alteration, drug intake, or metabolic or endocrine disorders.[6-8] Gynecomastia has also been observed following chronic illness, starvation, malnutrition, weight loss, or hemodialysis and in patients with hepatic disorders or hyperparathyroidism.[9,10] A variety of benign or malignant neoplasms that produce estrogen, estrogen precursors, or human chorionic gonadotropin may also induce gynecomastia.[11]

Gynecomastia is most commonly seen during puberty and old age as a response to physiologic hormonal alteration. Morphologically, gynecomastia is divided into three categories based on the degree of proliferation.[12] The florid type is characterized by conspicuous proliferation of ductal epithelium and fibroblastic stroma. The fibrous type has inconspicuous epithelial proliferation; a cellular, fibrous stroma; and many dilated ducts. The intermediate type is a bridge between the florid and fibrous types.

In the majority of cases, aspirates of gynecomastia are modest in cellularity. The smears show monolayered, well-organized sheets of small uniform cells, tall columnar cells, and bare nuclei (Images 13.1 through 13.3). Apocrine metaplasia, histiocytes, tissue fragments with cribriform or micropapillary arrangements, and cystic changes have also been described in association with gynecomastia.[3,13,14] Abundant adipose tissue, occasionally seen in gynecomastia and pseudogynecomastia, may cause a misdiagnosis.[15] Pseudogynecomastia involves both breasts and occurs in obese men, without the evidence of ductal proliferation or fibrous tissue seen in gynecomastia.

Occasionally, the pattern of cells seen in gynecomastia resembles that of cells in fibroadenoma, with fronding and multilayering. More commonly, the cells appear in small groups. Isolated cells or a few cells in loosely cohesive aggregates are not unusual. When associated with this pattern of cellularity, the presence of small groups and scattered single epithelial cells with nuclear atypia may cause diagnostic difficulty. The presence of tall columnar cells may contribute to misinterpretation of the lesion as papillary carcinoma. In a series of 43 cases of gynecomastia, Rone et al[16] reported cases that were misinterpreted as suspicious for carcinoma. Gynecomastia may also be associated with atypical ductal hyperplasia, closely resembling noncomedo-type intraductal carcinoma (Images 13.4 through 13.6). Thus, a diagnosis of malignancy should be considered only if the aspirate shows obvious cytologic features of malignancy.

Cytomorphology of Gynecomastia
Moderate cellularity
Small groups of uniform epithelial cells
Tall columnar cells
Naked nuclei

Carcinoma

Primary breast cancers in men are similar to those in women but occur at an older age (mean, 60 years).[17] Typically, male breast cancer presents as a subareolar mass, since practically all cases arise from the major ducts. Except for lobular carcinoma, every variety of in situ and invasive carcinoma of the breast can occur in men.

Interestingly, intracystic papillary carcinoma accounts for 5% of breast carcinomas in men but less than 1% of all breast malignancies in women.[18] The cytologic features of male breast carcinoma are quite similar to those of female breast carcinoma (Images 13.7 through 13.10). However, FNAB smears of male breast carcinoma may present unique problems, including the relatively equal frequency of primary and metastatic lesions in the male breast and chest wall lesions masquerading as primary breast lesions.[3] The incidence of metastatic lesions in the female breast ranges from 0.5% to 5.1% of all breast cancers,[19,20] while up to 58% of male breast cancers represent metastases.[3] Lung cancer, prostate cancer, malignant lymphoma, and mesothelioma are the most frequently reported metastases to the male breast.[3,21]

Overall, FNAB is a reliable tool in the evaluation of male breast lesions. If the clinical setting is appropriate and the FNAB sample is adequate, cytology can offer a basis for correct diagnosis. It is also possible to separate primary male breast carcinoma from metastatic lesions by FNAB. An incorrect diagnosis of metastasis in a patient with primary breast cancer may have disastrous consequences. Nonepithelial tumors such as myofibroblastoma, hemangiopericytoma, and neurilemoma can also occur in male breast.[22–24]

Skin Tumors Over the Breast

Skin lesions occurring as breast nodules may simulate a breast neoplasm. Among the 20 cases studied by Ilie,[25] an eccrine spiradenoma and a leiomyoma were clinically misdiagnosed as primary breast carcinoma. Fine needle aspiration biopsy has been used in diagnosis of skin lesions of the breast.[26,27] In a case of eccrine spiradenoma of the breast reported by Bosch and Boon,[27] the smears displayed a bland group of cuboidal cells of uniform size, with scant cytoplasm and round to ovoid nuclei. Nucleoli were inconspicuous. The background was bloody, and the nuclei displayed a rosette-like arrangement. There were no foam cells, no naked nuclei, and no myoepithelial cells. The cytomorphology of this lesion did not resemble the pattern of any usual breast lesion. The lesion's well-defined bluish color and the absence of the characteristic features commonly seen in breast lesions suggested a diagnosis of skin lesion, which was confirmed by biopsy. Precise attention to cytomorphology may assist in arriving at a correct diagnosis.

Supernumerary Breast Lesions

Supernumerary mammary glands are uncommon and present on the front of the chest, mostly below and slightly medial to the normal site. Ectopic breast tissue has also been found in the axilla, the medial side of the thigh, and the vulva. Aberrant mammary gland tissue may not become apparent until pregnancy or lactation causes it to swell. Ectopic breast tissue undergoes changes during different phases of life and can become neoplastic.[28] Clinically, it is often mistaken for a lipoma or a large lymph node. Ectopic mammary tissue is often removed for cosmetic reasons[29] and has a number of different cytologic patterns.[30,31] In pregnancy and lactation, the smears show clusters of acinic cells, occasionally in a rosette-like pattern; apocrine cells; and naked nuclei in a secretory background (Images 13.11 and 13.12).

Nipple Secretion

A relatively common finding in women, nipple discharge may occur in a variety of physiologic and pathological disorders. Physiologic nipple discharge is most frequently due to hormonal influences. Pathologic conditions may lead to nipple discharge in the absence of pregnancy and lactation.[32-37] Puberty, galactorrhea-inducing drugs, breast nipple stimulation, and elevated levels of prolactin are the causes of abnormal physiologic nipple discharge. Oral contraceptives, phenothiazines, and major tranquilizers are also associated with nipple discharge.[33,35,36] Pathologic nipple discharge is frequently associated with papilloma. Carcinoma rarely causes nipple discharge,[32,38,39] but the incidence of carcinoma is higher in males with nipple discharge than in females.[40,41]

The majority of patients with nipple discharge are asymptomatic. However, patients with mastitis suffer from pain, and most patients with carcinoma have palpable lesions.[42] Breast cancer patients usually have abnormal mammograms; however, patients with fibrocystic change and papilloma may also have abnormal mammograms.

There are few reports on the cytology of nipple discharge.[40-47] The cytologic presentation of nipple discharge varies depending on the underlying cause. In a comprehensive study of 225 cases of nipple discharge, Johnson and Kini[42] reported that nipple cytology had a high specificity. They reported that finding malignant cells was the most specific means of detecting carcinoma. However, in contrast to its high specificity; nipple cytology had a low sensitivity. Three of the five cases of breast cancer in the study were not detectable in cytologic samples. Old age, male sex, unilaterality, bloody discharge, and abnormal mammograms are the clinical features that suggest malignancy.

The most frequent cause of nipple discharge is fibrocystic change.[42] Smears contain numerous foam cells, a proteinaceous background, and a small numbers of ductal epithelial cells (Image 13.13). Similar findings are reported in mammary duct ectasia.[46] Nipple discharge associated with mastitis has a significant number of neutrophils (Image 13.14). Papillomas present tight papillary clusters of slightly atypical ductal cells. Overall, however, nipple discharge due to benign conditions such as fibrocystic change, papilloma, or a physiologic mechanism cannot be distinguished cytologically.

The low sensitivity of nipple discharge cytology is a limiting factor. To identify patients with breast cancer and distinguish the various benign causes of abnormal nipple discharge, one should combine the cytologic features of nipple discharge with clinical findings. Nipple aspirate fluid cytology may offer a new way to study the spectrum of premalignant breast lesions and to identify women at risk for breast cancer.[47,48]

Image 13.1
Air-dried smear of gynecomastia reveals moderate cellularity; a cohesive cluster of uniform, small epithelial cells; and occasional isolated cells (Diff-Quik®, 200X).

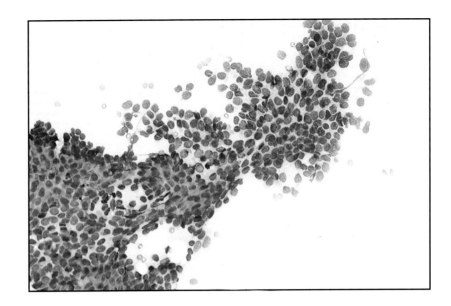

Image 13.2
Papanicolaou-stained smear of the same case shows almost monolayered, cohesive, organized sheets of epithelial cells (400X).

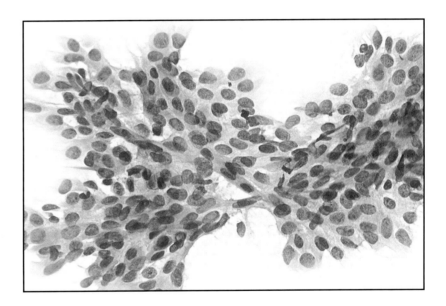

Image 13.3
Typical histologic appearance of gynecomastia: ductal proliferation surrounded by myxoid, loose stroma (H&E, 200X).

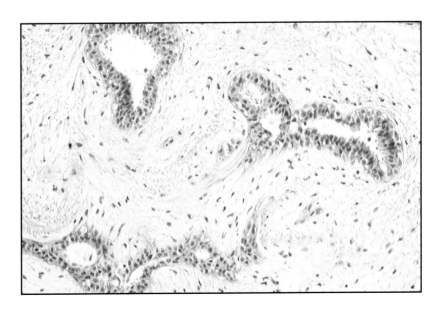

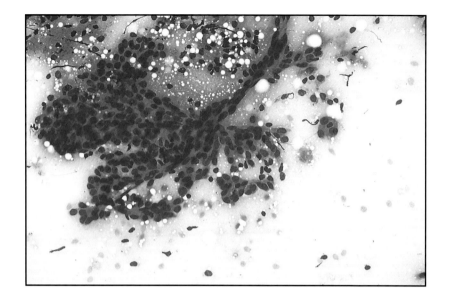

Image 13.4
The cytologic appearance of gynecomastia may sometimes simulate that of fibroadenoma, especially when there are fronds, cellular crowding, and naked nuclei in the background, as in this smear (Diff-Quik, 200X).

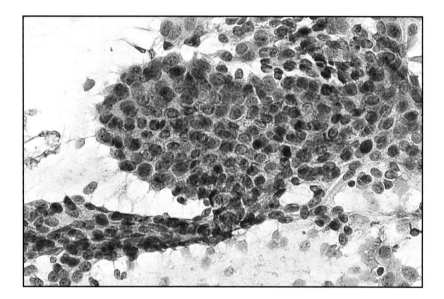

Image 13.5
Atypical cytologic features of gynecomastia: slight anisonucleosis, mild hyperchromasia, and overlapping of nuclei (Papanicolaou, 400X).

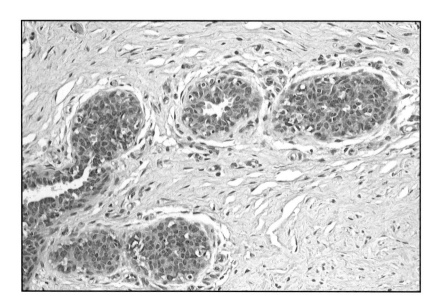

Image 13.6
Corresponding tissue section shows areas of ductal hyperplasia forming almost solid nests of cells (H&E, 200X).

Image 13.7
Aspirate of carcinoma in male breast reveals discohesive clusters of neoplastic cells with anisonucleosis and hyperchromasia (Diff-Quik, 1000X).

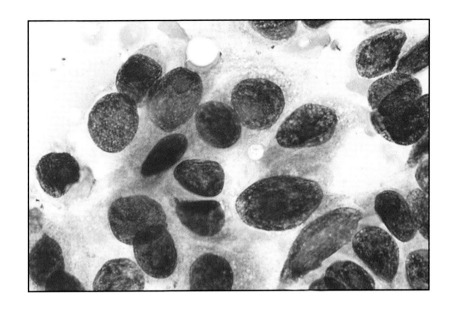

Image 13.8
Papanicolaou-stained smear of same case with occasional tumor giant cell formation (400X).

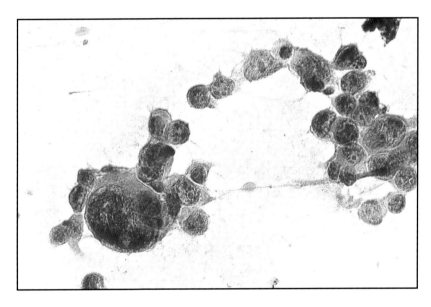

Image 13.9
Cell block preparation demonstrates the distinct cytologic features of malignancy in a male breast (H&E, 400X).

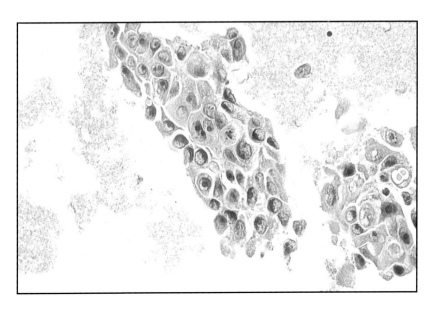

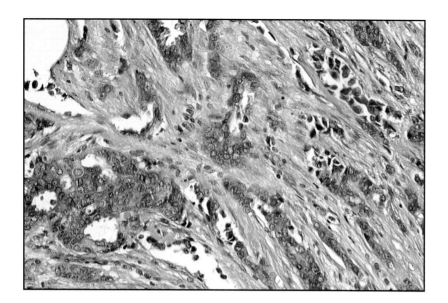

Image 13.10
Microscopic features of infiltrating duct cell carcinoma correlate with previous FNAB diagnosis of the same case (H&E, 200X).

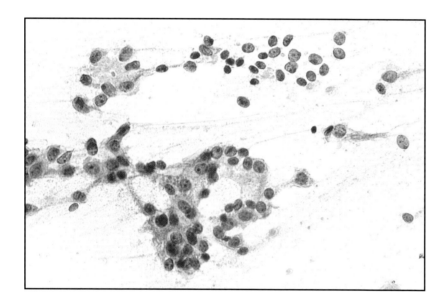

Image 13.11
An example of gestational changes diagnosed cytologically from aberrant mammary tissue needled after it had become prominent (Papanicolaou, 200X).

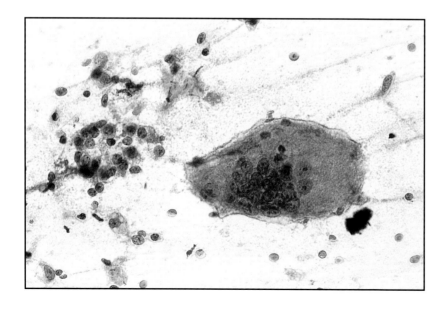

Image 13.12
Additional smear from the same case shows a multinucleated giant cell and proteinaceous background (Papanicolaou, 400X).

Image 13.13
Papanicolaou-stained smear of nipple discharge shows a few clusters of benign-looking epithelial cells in a proteinaceous background (200X).

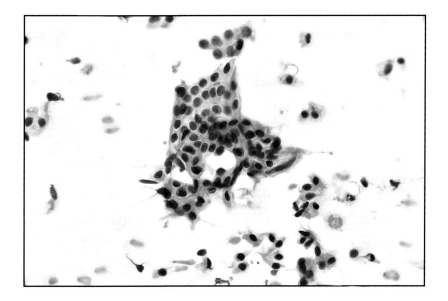

Image 13.14
Neutrophilic infiltrates associated with mastitis in a nipple discharge specimen (Papanicolaou, 1000X).

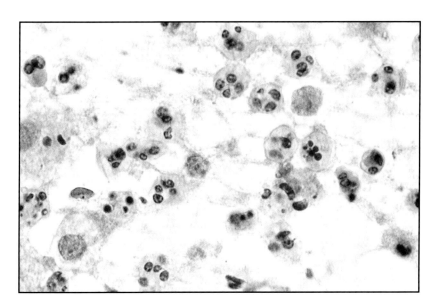

References

1. Gupta RK, Naran S, Dowle CS, et al: The diagnostic impact of needle aspiration cytology of the breast on clinical decision making with an emphasis on the aspiration cytodiagnosis of male breast masses. *Diagn Cytopathol* 7:637–639, 1991.

2. Eisenberg AJ, Hajdu SI, Wilhelmus J, et al: Preoperative aspiration cytology of breast tumors. *Acta Cytol* 30:135–146, 1986.

3. Sneige N, Holder PD, Katz R, et al: Fine needle aspiration cytology of the male breast in a cancer center. *Diagn Cytopathol* 9:691–697, 1993.

4. Carlson HE: Gynecomastia. *N Engl J Med* 303:795–799, 1980.

5. Sirtori C, Veronesi U: Gynecomastia, a review of 218 cases. *Cancer* 10:645–654, 1957.

6. Paulsen HS: Demonstration of hormonal sensitivity in gynecomastic tissue by thymidine incorporation in vitro. *Acta Pathol Microbiol Scand (A)* 85:19–24, 1977.

7. Menville IG: Gynecomastia. *Arch Surg* 26:1054–1083, 1933.

8. Glass AR, Berenberg J: Gynecomastia after chemotherapy for lymphoma. *Arch Intern Med* 139:1048–1049, 1979.

9. Schmitt GW, Shehadeh I, Sawin CT: Transient gynecomastia in chronic renal failure during chronic intermittent hemodialysis. *Ann Intern Med* 69:73–79, 1968.

10. Chopra JJ, Tulchinsky D: Status of estrogen-androgen balance in hyperthyroid men with Graves' disease. *J Clin Endocrinol Metab* 38:269–277, 1974.

11. Stepanas AV, Samaan NA, Schultz PN, et al: Endocrine studies in testicular tumor patients with and without gynecomastia: a report of 45 cases. *Cancer* 41:112–118, 1978.

12. Bannayan GA, Hajdu SI: Gynecomastia: clinicopathologic study of 351 cases. *Am J Clin Pathol* 57:431–437, 1972.

13. Russin VL, Lachowicz C, Kline TS: Male breast lesions: gynecomastia and its distinction from carcinoma by aspiration cytology (ABC). *Diagn Cytopathol* In press.

14. Gupta RR, Naron S, Simpson J: The role of fine needle aspiration cytology (FNAC) in the diagnosis of breast masses in males. *Eur J Surg Oncol* 14:317–320, 1988.

15. Johnson RL: The male breast and gynecomastia. In: Page DL, Anderson TJ, eds. *Diagnostic Histopathology of the Breast*. London, England, Churchill Livingstone, 1987, pp. 30–42.

16. Rone R, Ramzy I, Northcutt A: Gynecomastia: cytologic features and diagnostic pitfalls in aspiration biopsy. *Acta Cytol* 30:589, 1986.

17. Donegan WL: Cancer of the male breast. In: Donegan WL, Spratt JS, eds. *Cancer of the Breast,* 3rd ed. Philadelphia, Pa, WB Saunders Co, 1988, pp. 716–727.

18. Heller KS, Rosen PP, Schollenfeld D, et al: Male breast cancer. A clinicopathologic study of 97 cases. *Ann Surg* 188:60–65, 1978.

19. Sneige S, Zachariah S, Fanning TV, et al: Fine needle aspiration cytology of metastatic neoplasms in the breast. *Am J Clin Pathol* 92:27–35, 1989.

20. Silverman JF, Feldman PS, Cavell JL, et al: Fine needle aspiration cytology of neoplasms metastatic to the breast. *Acta Cytol* 31: 291–300, 1987.

21. Salyer WR, Salyer DC: Metastasis of prostatic carcinoma to the breast. *J Urol* 109:671–675, 1973.

22. Amin MD, Gottlieb CA, Fitzmaurice M, et al: Fine needle aspiration cytologic study of myofibroblastoma of the breast. Immunohistochemical and ultrastructural findings. *Am J Clin Pathol* 99:593–597, 1993.

23. Jimenez-Ayal M, Diez-Nau M, Larrad A, et al: Hemangiopericytoma in a male breast. Report of a case with cytologic, histologic and immunochemical studies. *Acta Cytol* 35:234–238, 1991.

24. Martinez-Onsurbe P, Fuentes-Vaamonde E, Gonzalez-Estecha A, et al: Neurilemoma of the breast in a man, a case report. *Acta Cytol* 36:511–513, 1992.

25. Ilie B: Neoplasms in skin and subcutaneous tissue over the breast: case reports and review of the literature. *J Surg Oncol* 31:191–198, 1986.

26. Bhalotra R, Jayaram G: Fine needle aspiration cytology of pilomatrixoma: a case report. *Diagn Cytopathol* 6:280–283, 1990.

27. Bosch MMC, Boon ME: Fine needle cytology of an eccrine spiradenoma of the breast: diagnosis made by a holistic approach. *Diagn Cytopathol* 8:366–368, 1992.

28. Kuzma JF: Breast. In: Anderson WAD, Kissan JM, eds. *Pathology.* St Louis, Mo, CV Mosby Co, 1977, pp. 1776–1801.

29. Zajicek J: Aspiration biopsy cytology, I. Cytology of supradiaphragmatic organs. In: Wied GL, ed. *Monographs in Clinical Cytology,* vol 4. Basel, Switzerland, S. Karger, 1974, pp. 1–5, 140.

30. Bhambhani S, Rajwanshi A, Pant L, et al: Fine needle aspiration cytology of supernumerary breasts. Report of three cases. *Acta Cytol* 31:311–312, 1986.

31. Dey P, Karmakar T: Fine needle aspiration cytology of accessory axillary breasts and their lesions. *Acta Cytol* 38:915–916, 1994.

32. Devitt JE: Management of nipple discharge by clinical findings. *Am J Surg* 149:789–792, 1985.

33. Leis HP Jr, Cammarata A, LaRaja RD: Nipple discharge: significance and treatment. *Breast* 11:6–12, 1985.

34. Murad TM, Contesso G, Mouriesse H: Nipple discharge from the breast. *Ann Surg* 195:259–264, 1982.

35. Newman HF, Klein M, Northrup JD, et al: Nipple discharge frequency and pathogenesis in ambulatory population. *NY State J Med* 83:928–933, 1983.

36. Urban TA, Egeli RA: Nonlactational nipple discharge. *CA Cancer J Clin* 28:130–140, 1978.

37. Rimsten A, Skoog V, Stenkvist B: On the significance of nipple discharge in the diagnosis of breast disease. *Acta Chir Scand* 142: 513–518, 1976.

38. DiPietro S, DeYoldi GC, Berganzi S, et al: Nipple discharge as a sign of preneoplastic lesion and occult carcinoma of the breast. Clinical and galactographic study in 103 consecutive patients. *Tumori* 65:317–324, 1979.

39. Ciatto S, Bravetti P, Cariaggi P: Significance of nipple discharge clinical patterns in the selection of cases for cytologic examination. *Acta Cytol* 30:17–20, 1986.

40. Fujii, Ishii Y, Wakabayashi T, et al: Cytologic diagnosis of male breast cancer with nipple discharge. A case report. *Acta Cytol* 30:21–24, 1986.

41. Johnson TL, Kini SR: Significance of bloody breast nipple discharge in men. *ASCP Cytopathology Check Sample* C87-15 (C-173). Chicago, Ill, American Society of Clinical Pathologists, 1987.

42. Johnson TL, Kini SR: Cytologic and clinicopathologic features of abnormal nipple secretions: 225 cases. *Diagn Cytopathol* 7:17–22, 1991.

43. Knight DC, Lowell DM, Heimann A, et al: Aspiration of the breast and nipple discharge cytology. *Surg Gynecol Obstet* 163:15–20, 1986.

44. Takeda T, Suzuki M, Sato Y, et al: Cytologic studies of nipple discharges. *Acta Cytol* 26:35–36, 1982.

45. Vei Y, Watanake Y, Hirota Y, et al: Cytologic diagnosis of breast carcinoma with nipple discharge. Special significance of the spherical cell cluster. *Acta Cytol* 24:522–528, 1980.

46. Insabato L: Nipple secretions in breast diseases. *Diagn Cytopathol* 8:200–202, 1992.

47. Takeda T, Matsui A, Irumagama H, et al: Nipple discharge cytology in mass screening for breast cancer. *Acta Cytol* 34:161–164, 1990.

48. King EB, Chew KL, Petrakis NL, et al: Nipple aspirate cytology for the study of breast cancer precursors. *J Natl Cancer Inst* 71:1115–1121, 1983.

CHAPTER FOURTEEN

Prognostic Factors in Breast Cancer

Rationale Behind the Use of Prognostic Factors

During the past few years, there have been significant changes in the medical approach to and management of breast cancer patients. Advances in radiologic imaging, increased experience in fine needle aspiration biopsy and other sampling techniques, conservation in breast surgery, and the availability of new chemotherapeutic and radiotherapeutic options as well as bone marrow transplants have revolutionized the primary treatment of this devastating disease. The heterogeneous nature of breast cancer has also resulted in an overwhelming interest in prognostic markers that can identify patients who might benefit most from available therapeutic modalities.

During the past few years, systemic adjuvant chemotherapy has played a major role in improving the prognosis of patients with breast cancer.[1-5] Table 14.1 summarizes the 5-year disease-free survival rates associated with modern chemotherapy regimens. As can be seen, chemotherapy is associated with a considerably better prognosis than local treatment alone.[6,7] The potential value of adjuvant systemic therapy for node-negative breast cancer patients is confirmed in the updated overview analysis recently published by the Early Breast Cancer Trialists' Collaborative Group.[1] Recurrence-free survival and overall survival were significantly improved in the women treated with chemotherapy and tamoxifen.

However, recommending adjuvant chemotherapy for node-negative breast cancer patients is controversial for three reasons. First, 70% of node-negative breast cancer patients are cured without any adjuvant therapy.

371

Table 14.1
The Effect of Adjuvant Chemotherapy on Breast Cancer Patient Outcome★

No. of Nodes	5-Year Disease-Free Survival	
	After Surgery +/− Radiotherapy (%)	Chemotherapy After Surgery +/− Radiotherapy (%)
0	55–65	80–90
1–3	35–40	70–75
4–10	25–35	65–67
>10	10–15	45–50

★Modified from: Bonadonna G: Karnofsky memorial lecture. Conceptual and practical advances in the management of breast cancer. *J Clin Oncol* 7:1380–1397, 1989. Salmon SE: *Adjuvant Therapy of Cancer,* vol 6. Philadelphia, Pa, WB Saunders Co, 1990.

Thus, many women who would be cured anyway would be subject to the toxic effect of chemotherapy, and a few might die of it. Second, some patients do not benefit from chemotherapy; they relapse. Third, the cost of treatment for women who do not benefit could amount to over $500 million each year in the United States alone. These factors underscore the need to identify prognostic factors that can separate patients into low-risk and high-risk groups in terms of the probability of recurrence. Adjuvant chemotherapy should be offered to patients at high risk. Attempts should also be made to identify parameters that predict a patient's response to therapy, since even high-risk patients should be spared treatment if it can be reliably determined that they will not benefit from it. In locally advanced and systemic breast disease, prognostic factors could be used to determine which patients should receive hormonal therapy or chemotherapy.

Prognostic testing is commonly performed on surgically excised lesions. However, there are clinical conditions in which a surgical specimen may not be suitable or available for such analysis. In these circumstances, fine needle aspiration biopsy and imprint preparation provide attractive samples for prognostic testing.

Prognostic Factors

The National Institute of Health's 1990 Consensus Conference on Early-Stage Breast Cancer recognized six prognostic markers[8]: (1) the presence or absence of lymph node metastases, (2) tumor size, (3) nuclear grade, (4) steroid receptor content, (5) histologic tumor type, and (6) cellular proliferation rate. In small samples, particularly in cytologic preparations, the cytologic and/or histologic diagnosis should not be compromised for measurement of a prognostic factor.[9] If the samples are highly cellular, cytologic preparations of breast fine needle aspirates can provide prognostic information, which is particularly important in patients selected for preoperative chemotherapy or radiotherapy.

Lymph Node Status

The single most important prognostic factor in breast cancer is axillary lymph node involvement. Table 14.2 presents the 10-year relapse-free sur-

Table 14.2
The Effect of Lymph Node Status on Breast Cancer Patient Outcome★

Number of Involved Nodes	10-Year Disease-Free Survival (%)
0	75–80
1–3	35–40
4–10	25–35
>10	10–15

★Modified from: Bonadonna G: Karnofsky memorial lecture. Conceptual and practical advances in the management of breast cancer. *J Clin Oncol* 7:1380–1397, 1989.

vival rate relative to the number of axillary lymph nodes detected by microscopic examination.[6] Reports in the literature indicate that survival, recurrence, metastasis, and treatment failure correlate with the number of positive axillary nodes.[6,10,11]

Gross identification of lymph node involvement and the presence of fixed axillary nodes are also associated with poor prognosis.[12,13] Some studies suggest that the presence of micrometastasis detected by serial sectioning of the lymph nodes and immunostaining the sections for epithelial markers is associated with higher recurrence and poorer survival rates than in lymph node–negative breast cancer patients.[14–17] The involvement of Rotter's node by metastatic carcinoma does not influence the prognosis regardless of the axillary lymph node status.[18] In contrast, the presence of metastatic tumor in the internal mammary nodes with or without axillary node involvement is associated with unfavorable prognosis.[19,20] Other features associated with poor prognosis are supraclavicular lymph node involvement,[21,22] spilling of the tumor to the extranodal tissue in patients with three or fewer involved nodes,[23] and presence of metastasis in the apical lymph nodes.[24]

As mentioned earlier, although lymph node status is a powerful prognostic indicator, there are subsets of axillary lymph node–negative breast cancer patients whose risk of relapse is similar to that of patients with node-positive disease. These patients should receive further therapy. Thus, one of the most important practical applications of prognostic factors is determining which node-negative breast cancer patients should receive adjuvant treatment.

Tumor Size

It has been known for many years that tumor size is a good predictor of outcome in patients with breast cancer.[25–27] In a retrospective study of more than 2,600 patients with 20 years' follow-up, only 25% of patients with tumors that had a diameter less than 2.5 cm developed metastases. In contrast, the metastatic rate increased to 40% in patients with tumor diameters between 2.5 and 3.5 cm. Among lymph node–negative breast cancer patients, less than 20% of patients with tumors less than 2 cm in diameter developed metastasis. Only 15% of patients with histologically well differentiated tumors suffered from metastases.[28]

The prognostic significance of tumor size has been confirmed by other large studies with long follow-up.[29,30] The relationship between tumor size and lymph node status was also the subject of the Surveillance Epidemiology and End Results program at the National Cancer Institute.[25] Tumors measuring fewer than 2 cm in lymph node–negative breast cancer patients were associated with a 96.3% 5-year survival rate. Similarly, fewer than 2% of patients with tumors fewer than 1.0 cm died of breast cancer within 5 years. In another study, when compared with other prognostic factors such as the number of nodes, hormone receptor status, patient age, and adjuvant chemotherapy or endocrine therapy, tumor size remained an independent prognostic indicator.[26] These data indicate that tumor size is an extremely important prognostic factor and may play a role in decisions about therapy.

Tumor Type

According to the 1990 National Institute of Health Consensus Conference,[1] tubular, colloid and papillary carcinomas are associated with a favorable prognosis and should be recognizable in cytologic preparations. The cytologic features of these tumors are well described. Tubular carcinomas are relatively rare tumors with a well-differentiated pattern that can be mistaken for that of a benign proliferative breast lesion. The recognition of tubular carcinoma has therapeutic implications, since it may not require mastectomy or axillary dissection.[31,32] It is also important to differentiate between lobular and ductal carcinoma, because invasive lobular carcinomas have a different pattern of metastatic spread.[32] In addition, poorly differentiated tumors and signet ring and inflammatory carcinomas behave aggressively. Despite the use of chemotherapy, which has improved survival rates, inflammatory carcinoma is still considered the most aggressive breast carcinoma, with a 5-year survival rate of only 11%.[29,30]

Nuclear Grade

Nuclear grade can be assessed in breast fine needle aspirates.[33–48] Some investigators have proposed the development of cytologic scoring systems for breast fine needle aspirates that would incorporate variables such as cell dissociation, cell size, cell uniformity, nucleoli, nuclear margin, chromatin pattern, and the presence of necrosis and inflammatory cells.[44,45] The Scarff-Bloom Richardson tumor grading system has been applied to breast fine needle aspirates to assess the reproducibility of nuclear grade, tubule formation, and mitosis.[42,45,46] In the majority of studies, characteristics of the nucleus or nuclear grade have been shown to be superior to tubule formation and mitosis. When compared with corresponding tissue specimens, nuclear grade is the parameter with the highest degree of reproducibility (up to 95%).[43,46] The relative lack of mitoses may be attributable to the fact that tumor cells are fragile and less likely to survive smear preparation or because fewer cells are examined in smears than in surgical biopsy material, so mitoses are less likely to be detected. Tubular structures are also difficult to identify in cytologic preparations.[43,46] Robinson et al[45] however, advocate the use of a cytologic grading system for ductal carcinoma not otherwise specified (NOS), using wet-fixed, Papanicolaou-stained breast aspirates. Examining smears for the extent of cell dissociation, cell size, and uniformity, as well as the appearance of nucleoli, the nuclear margin, and the chromatin pattern, Elston and Ellis[49] found a good correlation between nuclear grade and established histologic grades (Elston's modified Bloom and Richardson method).

Using preparations stained with Papanicolaou and hematoxylin and eosin stains, New and Howart[47] introduced another system for assessing nuclear grade in breast cytologic specimens. Excluding the presence of nucleoli, the authors compared nuclear size and the degree of nuclear pleomorphism with the corresponding histologic criteria of tubule fraction, nuclear pleomorphism, and number of mitoses. The authors found 100% agreement between cytologic and histologic diagnosis of grade I carcinoma. Seventy-seven percent of carcinomas assessed as grade II histologically were assessed as low grade cytologically, while 72% of carcinomas assessed as grade III histologically were considered high grade cytologically.

The most commonly used nuclear grading system is Fisher's modification of Black's nuclear grading scheme.[50] Black's nuclear grading system includes four grades, with grade I equal to anaplasia and grade IV as the best-differentiated grade. Fisher's scheme employs a three-tier nuclear grading system, with grade I representing the highest level of differentiation and grade III equivalent to anaplasia. In nuclear grade I, the nucleus is similar to but usually slightly larger than nuclei in normal duct epithelium. The nucleus is round or ovoid with no nuclear membrane abnormality and no nucleoli (Images 14.1 and 14.2). Grade II nuclei may be twice the size of grade I nuclei and may show small nucleoli. The nuclear membrane is smooth, and mild anisonucleosis may be seen (Images 14.3 and 14.4). The features that distinguish grade III nuclei from nuclei in grades I and II are anisonucleosis, hyperchromasia, and macronucleoli. Grade III nuclei have irregular membranes and coarse chromatin. Mitoses may be frequent (Images 14.5 and 14.6).

A review of the literature yields sufficient evidence to support the reliability of nuclear grading in cytologic specimens when the results are compared with those in corresponding surgical specimens.[34–36,40–42] The prognostic significance of nuclear grade is still under investigation, however. While there are studies that demonstrate a difference in patient outcome based on the results of nuclear grading in cytologic specimens,[9,34] Ciatto et al[37] believe that cytologic grading does not improve prognostic judgment of breast cancer patients. These authors reviewed 213 consecutive breast cancer patients with fine needle aspirates positive for malignancy. When compared with other prognostic factors such as size and clinical stage, the prognostic significance of nuclear grading was negligible. In a retrospective study, we reviewed 110 node-negative breast cancer patients with histologic and clinical follow-ups. We found a difference in 5-year survival between patients with nuclear grades I and II (94%) and those with nuclear grade III (83%) (Tables 14.3 and 14.4). Since grades I and II are prognostically similar, perhaps these two grades should be lumped together and breast fine needle aspirates classified as either low or high nuclear grade.[42]

Obtaining information on nuclear grade is particularly important for patients who are treated with chemotherapy prior to definitive surgery.[51,52] It has already been suggested that high-grade, fast-growing tumors are more likely to respond to chemotherapy than low-grade, slow-growing tumors, which may be better suited to pretreatment with tamoxifen. Cytologic nuclear grading may provide information about a tumor's biologic aggressiveness and likely response to therapy.

Table 14.3

Comparison of Nuclear Grading in Cytologic and Histologic Specimens from 100 Node-Negative Breast Cancer Patients

Nuclear Grading	Cytology	Histology
I	20	19
II	25	23
III	65	68

Concordance, 105/110 = 95%.

Estrogen and Progesterone Receptors

The first published report on hormonal therapy for breast carcinoma appeared in 1896, when Beatson[53] reported remission of metastatic breast cancer following oophorectomy. In the 1940s, orchiectomy was introduced for the treatment of prostate cancer.[54] Huggins and Bergenstal[55] in 1952 and Luft et al[56] in 1958 reported on the efficacy of adrenalectomy and hypohysectomy in the management of metastatic breast disease.

By the early 1960s, endocrine ablation became the preferred treatment for advanced breast cancer. However, clinical experience indicated that only 20% to 30% of patients responded favorably to such treatment.[57] This led to various investigations to distinguish between responsive and nonresponsive tumors. The work of Folca et al[58] in 1961 demonstrated binding of radioactive estrogen in patients who benefited from ablative surgery, suggesting a practical method for predicting a patient's response to therapy. Following Toft and Gorski's[59] description of estrogen receptor (ER) protein in the rat uterus, Jensen[60] reported detection of ER in human breast tumors. Since then the correlation between the ER content of breast carcinomas and clinical responsiveness to endocrine therapy has been well established by many investigators.[61–64]

Soon it was also recognized that progesterone receptor (PgR) synthesis is an estrogen-dependent process and that the presence of PgR is an expression of a fully functional ER mechanism.[65] Thus, it seemed reasonable to assume that assessment of PgR could improve the predictive value of hormone receptor determination. Indeed, it has been shown clinically that PgR is a more important prognostic indicator than ER.[66]

Like other steroid hormones, estrogens regulate gene expression in target cells through their interaction with specific macromolecular binding proteins called receptors. Receptors are normally found in target tissue such as breast and female reproductive organs. Because receptors appear in

Table 14.4

Survival in Relation to Nuclear Grade in Breast Cytology

Nuclear Grade	No. of Cases	5-Year Survival Rate
I and II	45	94%
III	65	83%

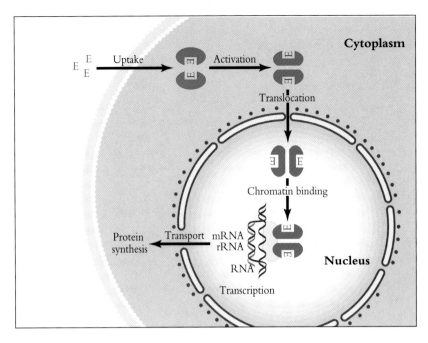

Figure 14.1
Old model for the sequence of events in steroid hormone action on a target. E = estrogen. Reproduced with permission from: Masood S: Sex-associated hormones. In: Stewart Sell, ed. *Serological Cancer Markers.* Totowa, NJ, Humana Press, 1992, pp. 155–192.

the supernatant or cytosol fraction of tissue homogenates, it was originally thought that estrogen binds to its receptor in the cytoplasm of target cells and then enters the nucleus by a process termed translocation (Figure 14.1).[59] Recent studies have suggested that the estrogen receptor is localized predominantly in the nucleus, where it is loosely bound until its association with estradiol converts the receptor to an active form with the ability to bind tightly in the genome.[65,67] Initially, the estrogen receptor associates with low-affinity type II receptors in the cytoplasm and then enters the nucleus by means of high-affinity receptors in the nucleus. The activated ER complex is believed to bind with chromatin, resulting in specific changes in gene expression and leading to synthesis of new messenger RNA (mRNA), such as progesterone receptor mRNA. Binding of PgR with progesterone induces synthesis of up to 100 proteins, including growth and mitogenic factors (Figure 14.2).[65,67]

There are at least two ERs, each with different affinities for estrogen.[68,69] Type I, the "true" receptor, is routinely measured in specimens (cytosolic ER) and has the greatest affinity for estrogen. Type II, the low-affinity receptor, is present in the cytoplasm and nucleus and represents a different group of proteins that were first reported in the cytosol of rat uterus in 1966.[59] The functional significance of type II ER is not yet clear. At present, it is also not clear why some hormone-dependent tumors fail to express ER. Gene mutation, heterogeneity of receptors in tumors, and effects secondary to transfection with the *ras* oncogene are suggested hypotheses.[71–73]

In the past few years, hormone receptors have been well described. Monoclonal antibodies specific to both estrogen and progesterone have been developed.[67,68] Human genes for the receptors have been cloned.[69,70] The ER gene on chromosome 6 produces two 65-kd subunits. The PgR

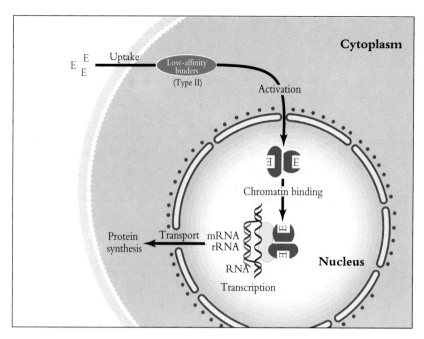

Figure 14.2
New model for the sequence of events in the interaction of steroid hormone with a target cell. E = estrogen. Reproduced with permission from: Masood S: Sex-associated hormones. In: Stewart Sell, ed. *Serological Cancer Markers.* Totowa, NJ, Humana Press, 1992, pp. 155–192.

gene on chromosome 11 transcribes two dissimilar subunits of 95 and 120 kd. Each cell contains about 10,000 ERs and 50,000 to 100,000 PgRs. With this new information, we can more precisely study the expression of sex steroid hormone receptors in hormone-dependent tumors.

The most commonly used biochemical assay is dextran-coated charcoal (DCC) assay, which requires 0.5 to 1 g of tissue. This technique is not suitable for hormone receptor analysis of small tumors or the small quantity of material obtained by fine needle aspiration biopsy (FNAB). Biochemical assays are also time consuming and expensive and cannot provide information regarding tumor hormone receptor heterogeneity. The results obtained by biochemical assay may not reflect the actual values of the tumor's hormone receptor proteins. Many variables influence these results, including the presence of endogenous estrogen, tumor necrosis and fibrosis, and contamination with the hormone receptors commonly found in benign epithelial components surrounding the tumor.[71] The predictive value of the biochemical assay is somewhat limited, since only 55% to 60% of patients with biochemical-positive tumors respond to endocrine therapy, while 10% of patients with receptor-negative tumors respond to hormonal manipulation.[72] Thus, the need for practical tests that are simpler, less expensive, and less sensitive to variation than the commonly used biochemical assay has been well recognized. This has resulted in the development of new immunocytochemical producers.

Immunocytochemical assays may be performed with either the immunoperoxidase or the immunofluorescence technique. In these methods, tissue sections or cells are incubated with estradiol, and antiestradiol antibody is added. Hormone receptors are detected when either a fluorescein-labeled anti-IgG or an unlabeled antibody binds to a peroxidase-antiperoxidase complex.

The fluorescent technique introduced by Lee[74] in 1978 links estradiol to bovine serum albumin (BSA) coupled with fluorescein isothiocyanate (FITC). Progesterone is linked to BSA and coupled with tetramethylrhodamine isothiocyanate (TMRITC). The expression of hormone receptors is shown by the presence of cytoplasmic fluorescent staining (Images 14.7 and 14.8). This procedure is now patented as FluoroCep® (Zeus Technologies Inc, Raritan, NJ). In a number of studies, the fluorescent technique has shown good correlation with the biochemical assay.[75–77] Indeed, reported sensitivity, specificity, and positive and negative predictive values for the clinical response rate are almost comparable to those reported for the biochemical assay.[78–81] The fluorescent technique may identify the low-affinity, type II cytoplasmic estrogen binding proteins rather than the high-affinity, type I nuclear ER measured biochemically. This has been raised as an argument against the fluorescent technique. However, the good results of the fluorescent assay as reported in the literature may be explained by the frequent coexistence of cytoplasmic and nuclear ERs, as demonstrated by Lee[82] in 1989.

The recent production of specific monoclonal antibodies against ER and PgR has provided another approach to the study of hormone receptor proteins. This technique, which utilizes a monoclonal antibody to nuclear ER or PgR and peroxidase-antiperoxidase for visualization, can be applied to paraffin-embedded or frozen tissue sections and to cytologic preparations. Estrogen receptor monoclonal antibodies are produced by hybridomas in rats immunized with purified receptor from an MCF 7–type human breast cancer cell. Typically, a rat monoclonal antibody binds to human estrophilin in tissue or cells on a microscope slide. A goat antibody forms a bridge between the antiestrophilin monoclonal antibody and a rat antibody bound to horseradish peroxidase. After washing, the bound, enzyme-bearing complex reacts with a chromogenic substance to form a colored substance at the receptor site, causing brown nuclear staining (Figure 14.3).[73]

The immunoperoxidase technique is attractive not only for its binding to the nuclear ERs or PgRs but also because it can be applied to fresh frozen or formalin-fixed, paraffin-embedded specimens. Imprint preparations have also been utilized for hormone receptor analysis and are recommended for tumors that are too small or ill defined to permit conventional sampling. This is particularly important for nonpalpable breast lesions discovered by mammography and sampled via radiologic imaging devices. It has also been possible to show expression of hormone receptors in cytologic specimens from malignant effusions (Images 14.9 through 14.11).[83–90]

Unlike biochemical assays, immunocytochemical assays provide information about hormone receptor heterogeneity, which is important not only in understanding the biology of tumors but also in explaining the different responses to endocrine therapy that are commonly observed in clinical practice (Image 14.12). Reports in the literature have confirmed an acceptable correlation between immunocytochemical hormone receptor assay and biochemically determined analysis, with an average of 84% and a range of 66% to 98%.[86–90] Cellular paucity due to presence of fibrosis and necrosis in the tissue sample and the prevalence of mixed benign epithelial and stromal elements are the most important reasons for the discrepancy

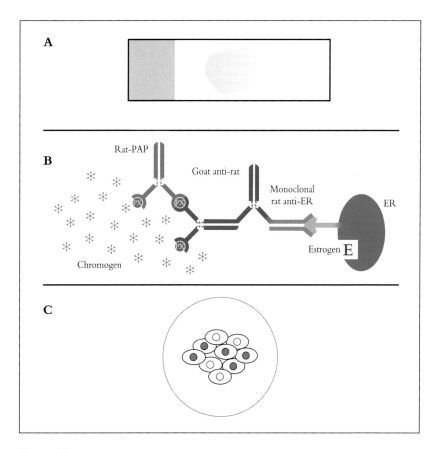

Figure 14.3
Schematic illustration of immunocytochemical hormone receptor assay. A, Estrogen receptor (ER) immunocytochemical assay can be applied to frozen sections, fine needle aspirates, imprint preparations, permanent sections, and cytospin preparations. B, Schematic presentation of peroxidase-antiperoxidase (PAP) technique utilizing monoclonal antibody directed against estrogen. C, Estrogen receptor expression is seen exclusively as brown nuclear staining. Reproduced with permission from: Masood S: Sex steroid hormone receptors in cytologic material. In: Schmidt WA, ed. *Cytopathology Annual 1992.* Baltimore, Md, Williams & Wilkins, 1992, pp. 77–102.

between biochemical and immunocytochemical assays. We have frequently demonstrated nuclear staining in benign epithelial cells adjacent to a non-expressive malignant component in cases reported positive by biochemical assay (Image 14.13).

The prognostic significance of immunocytochemically assessed hormone receptors in early-stage breast cancer patients has been well-demonstrated by Pertschuk et al,[90] who showed that PgR immunocytochemical assay is an even better predictor of survival than ER immunocytochemical assay and biochemical hormone receptor assay. More important, they documented that immunocytochemically determined hormone receptors are better predictors of response to endocrine therapy than hormone receptors that are measured biochemically.

On the other hand, the lack of adequate standardization and quantitation remain limiting factors in the use of immunocytochemical hormone receptor assays. In a well-designed study, Elias et al[91] demonstrated significant intralaboratory variation in the results of ER immunocytochemical assays. Positive results were only 55% reproducible among the laboratories in the study, highlighting the need for standardization of this technology.[92] Because of this variation, many national cancer therapy protocol studies still require biochemical assays for determination of hormone receptor proteins. Recently, however, immunocytochemical hormone receptor assays for ER and PgR were incorporated into the National Surgical Adjuvant Breast Project. In addition, reports in the literature suggest that it may be possible to use computerized image analysis systems in quantitation of cytochemical hormone receptor assays.[93,94] Thus, it seems reasonable to assume that immunocytochemical hormone receptor assays will continue to evolve and may eventually replace biochemical assays.

Direct smears and cytospin preparations are suitable for hormone receptor analysis using the immunoperoxidase technique (Images 14.14 and 14.15). The adaptability of immunocytochemical hormone receptor assays to formalin-fixed, paraffin-embedded tissue has provided an effective means of using cell block preparations for such analysis (Images 14.16 and 14.17).[85,95] Hormone receptor–positive tumors are often well differentiated and diploid, with low proliferative indices such as S-phase fraction. They also have a low propensity for visceral recurrence, especially in liver and brain, and frequently respond to endocrine therapy.[96–98] In contrast, hormone receptor–negative tumors are often poorly differentiated histologically and aneuploid, with high proliferative indices. They tend to recur in visceral sites and are often unresponsive to hormonal manipulation. Regardless of nodal status, cumulative data from several clinical trials indicate that hormone receptor–positive tumors have a more indolent natural course, and patients with such tumors are disease free longer and have higher overall survival rates.[99]

The prognostic significance of hormone receptors in early-stage breast cancer has been well studied.[26,100,101] It has been suggested that combining hormone receptor status with other prognostic factors may identify subgroups of breast cancer patients who may be at higher risk for recurrence and metastasis and may benefit from adjuvant chemotherapy. For example, in an updated, multivariate analysis of a clinical trial with 10-year follow-up, it was found that PgR and the number of positive nodes were the only significant prognostic factors.[102]

Several investigators have studied whether hormone receptors can predict response to endocrine therapy in patients with advanced breast cancer.[103–108] In 1991, Bezwada et al[106] reported their experience with 415 women with recurrent or metastatic breast cancer and known hormone receptor levels. They found that quantitation of ER is the most important predictor of response to hormone therapy, with response rate increasing from approximately 20% in patients with ER values of 3 to 10 fmol/mg of protein to approximately 75% in patients with ER levels greater than 30 fmol/mg of protein. Breast cancer patients with PgR levels greater than 10 fmol/mg of protein showed a significantly higher response rate than those with a lesser value. However, in a multivariate analysis that included age, site, and number of metastases, only the ER level was significant in predicting patient response to treatment with tamoxifen. It was postulated that the 25% of patients with ER-rich tumors that remained refractory to treatment may possess a defective receptor. Production of hormone receptors by these tumor cells may also be an epiphenomenon not related to tumor cell growth requirements. The median duration of response for all levels of hormone receptors was approximately 14 months. The limited duration of hormone responsiveness is a major obstacle to managing breast cancer patients with hormone therapy. This limitation may be due to tumor hormone receptor heterogeneity, demonstrating coexistence of ER-positive and ER-negative tumor cells. Unaffected by therapy, ER-negative clones of tumor cells emerge and continue to grow.[109,110]

The availability of immunocytochemical hormone receptor assays and techniques for assessing the pattern of expression and degree of heterogeneity of hormone receptors make it possible to initiate new studies to enhance our understanding of the role that hormone receptors can play in the management of breast cancer patients.

DNA Ploidy and Proliferation Rate

Tumor cell proliferative activity and ploidy have an inverse relationship with survival in patients with breast cancer. The methods used to assess these factors include mitotic figure counts, thymidine-labeling index (TLI), DNA flow cytometric analysis, and immunocytochemical detection of proliferation-associated nuclear proteins.

Counting the number of mitoses in a well-fixed, hematoxylin and eosin–stained slide remains the most inexpensive method of assessing tumor cell proliferation. However, the variability of the results obtained with this method is a limiting factor. Variability can be effectively reduced by employing a carefully standardized quantitative measure, such as the mitotic figure index (number of mitoses per 1000 cells), instead of simply counting the mitotic figures in high-power fields.[111–113] The TLI measures the fraction of cells actively engaged in DNA synthesis and correlates the result with the S-phase fraction as measured by flow cytometry. Thymidine labeling index is recognized as a strong independent prognostic indicator in patients with any stage breast cancer.[114] Several studies have clearly demonstrated that as a method of predicting relapse and survival, TLI is superior to other prognostic indicators, including tumor size and hormone receptors in both early stage and advanced breast cancer.[114–116] However, TLI is technically cumbersome and difficult to apply in routine analyses of tumor specimens.

A more recent technique, flow cytometry, determines proliferative rate by assessing the percentage of cells in the DNA synthesis phase (S-phase) of the cell cycle and the status of the tumor cells' DNA. Flow cytometry measures DNA within a nucleus by using fluorescent dyes that bind with the DNA. The intensity of each cell's fluorescence is proportional to its DNA content. By compiling the DNA content in several thousand nuclei, a histogram can be generated. Tumor cells with normal DNA content are called diploid, while tumor cells with abnormal DNA content are called aneuploid. DNA content abnormality, or aneuploidy, is usually expressed in terms of the DNA index, ie, the ratio of the DNA content of G_0/G_1 cells in the abnormal population to G_0/G_1 cells in a normal diploid population.

As shown in Figure 14.4, after a cell has completed mitosis, it enters the presynthetic, or G_1, phase of cell growth, in which the nucleus is diploid—ie, it has twice the normal amount of DNA (23 chromosome pairs). These cells are cycling. Cells in G_0 are in a resting state and have a normal amount of DNA. At some point, the cells begin to duplicate their DNA. This is the synthesis phase, or S-phase, in which the cells have an intermediate amount of DNA, between two times and four times the normal amount. After DNA replication is complete, the cells enter the post-

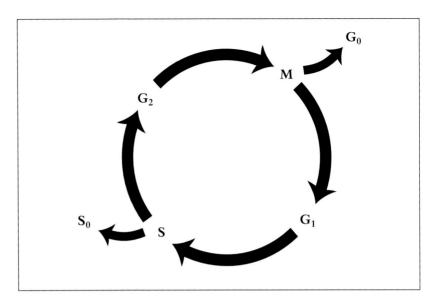

Figure 14.4
Schematic representation of a cell cycle. Reproduced with permission from: Bedrossian CWM, Masood S: Immunocytochemistry applied to cytological specimens. In: Leong AS-Y, ed. *Applied Immunocytochemistry for the Surgical Pathologist*. London, England, Edward Arnold, 1992, pp. 342–372.

synthetic, or G_2, growth phase, in which they have four times the normal amount of DNA. In flow cytometry, there is no distinction between G_2 nuclei and M nuclei, since they both have four times the normal amount of DNA. This phase is described as $G_2 + M$.

Figure 14.5 shows a histogram of a diploid tumor. To the left is a small peak created by chicken erythrocyte nuclei (CEN), which are added to the sample as the fluorescence standard. The majority of cells are diploid and in the G_0/G_1 phase (91.2%). A small percentage (3.2%) of tumor cells contain exactly twice the amount of DNA in diploid cells. These cells are in the G_2 phase, undergoing mitosis. Cells with intermediate DNA content are in the S-phase (5.7%). The DNA index in these cells is 1.0, which represents normal DNA content. Hyperdiploid tumors have a DNA index greater than 1.00, hypodiploid tumors have a DNA index less than 1.00, and tetraploid tumors have a DNA index of 2.00.

Figure 14.6 is a histogram of an aneuploid tumor. On the left a normal diploid G_0/G_1 peak is seen. The aneuploid G_0/G_1 population of the tumor cells is displaced to the right of the diploid, G_0/G_1 population, reflecting a higher amount of DNA per nucleus. Aneuploid tumor cells constitute 64.8% of cells examined. The percentage of cells in S-phase is 18.4%, and the percentage of cells in G_2M phase is 16.8%. Cell cycle distribution within clonal populations can be calculated by a variety of computer programs, and models have been suggested for estimating the distribution of cells in the different cell cycles based on flow cytometry–generated DNA histograms.

It is generally believed that tumors with grossly abnormal DNA content, or aneuploidy, are biologically more aggressive than tumors with normal DNA content, or diploidy. Thus, assessing ploidy status in patients with breast cancer is a common practice and has been the subject of extensive

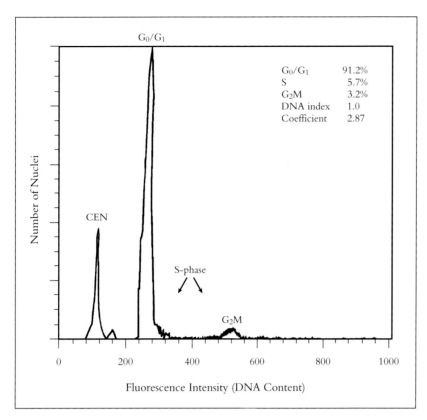

G₀/G₁ values shown in figure:

G_0/G_1	91.2%
S	5.7%
G_2M	3.2%
DNA index	1.0
Coefficient	2.87

Figure 14.5
Histogram of a diploid DNA pattern. Reproduced with permission from: Bedrossian CWM, Masood S: Immunocytochemistry applied to cytological specimens. In: Leong AS-Y, ed. *Applied Immunocytochemistry for the Surgical Pathologist.* London, England, Edward Arnold, 1992, pp. 342–372.

investigation. However, despite numerous reports in the literature, the value of DNA ploidy analysis remains controversial.[117–125]

In 1992, the DNA Cytometry Consensus Conference met to define the role of DNA cytometry in predicting outcome in breast cancer patients.[126] Based on the recommendations of this conference, DNA ploidy status alone is not considered a strong independent prognostic indicator in patients with breast cancer. In contrast, there is a clear association between high S-phase fractions and an increased risk of recurrence and mortality for both axillary node–negative and node–positive breast cancer patients.[126–133]

The prognostic significance of DNA ploidy and proliferation rate in advanced and metastatic breast disease is also controversial. There are studies suggesting that DNA ploidy and proliferation index are helpful in predicting response to chemotherapy.[108,134–136] It has also been shown that diploid and tetraploid tumors have a higher remission rate following endocrine therapy than do aneuploid tumors.[137] However, several studies have failed to confirm the influence of DNA ploidy on survival of patients with metastatic disease.[138–141] In a review of 55 patients with metastatic breast disease, DeLena et al[142] showed that DNA ploidy of a primary tumor did not predict the metastatic pattern and had no influence on response to treatment, duration of response, time to progression of disease, or overall survival. However, in the group of patients with

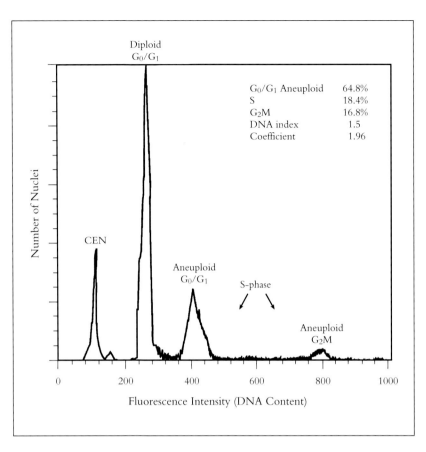

G0/G1 Aneuploid   64.8%
S   18.4%
G2M   16.8%
DNA index   1.5
Coefficient   1.96

Figure 14.6

Histogram of an aneuploid DNA pattern. Reproduced with permission from: Bedrossian CWM, Masood S: Immunocytochemistry applied to cytological specimens. In: Leong AS-Y, ed. *Applied Immunocytochemistry for the Surgical Pathologist.* London, England, Edward Arnold, 1992, pp. 342–372.

extraosseous metastasis, statistics showed that patients with diploid DNA content had better survival rates.

Overall, studies on the value of ploidy status in locally advanced and metastatic breast cancer are somewhat limited, warranting further investigation. Existing studies are based on the results of ploidy study in primary tumors, but attempts should also be made to assess the DNA content of metastatic tumor cells, since the discrepancy between ploidy of primary tumors and their metastases has been reported to be as high as 44%.[143]

Another way to measure proliferative activity in breast cancer is to use antibodies directed against nuclear antigens newly expressed during each phase of the cell cycle.[144] Several such antibodies (eg, Ki-67) are commercially available and may be applied via immunocytochemical assay. Originally prepared by immunizing mice with a Hodgkin's disease cell line, Ki-67 recognizes a nuclear antigen expressed in cycling cells but not in resting cells. Recent studies have shown excellent correlation between Ki-67 staining, mitoses counts, and TLIs. It seems that Ki-67 or similar antibodies to proliferation-associated markers such as p120 may be important in determining the prognostic significance of cell cycle activity in breast cancer.[145–147]

To determine the optimal technique for measuring tumor cell proliferation rate, multiparametric analysis must be performed, comparing various measures with survival outcome. Each laboratory must establish its own distribution of S-phase values for diploid and aneuploid tumors, and the cutoff levels must be carefully selected. In a study of breast cancer patients conducted by myself and my colleauges, 10% was the cutoff value.[125] Of the various modalities available to assess the proliferation rate in cytologic preparations, flow cytometry for assessing the percentage of cells in S-phase and immunocytochemistry for detecting proliferation-associated antigens are most useful.[148] Flow cytometry can be applied to cytologic or cell block preparations, producing a histogram with information regarding the S-phase fraction of tumor cells.[149] The technique is rapid, and the results are based on the study of large numbers of nuclei. One limitation of flow cytometry, however, is that it cannot be used to distinguish nontumor cells from tumor cells. In addition, the presence of an aneuploid peak in a histogram may complicate the established mathematical analysis and result in an inaccurate assessment.

To overcome this shortcoming, S-phase fraction determination is now complemented by flow cytometric determination of tumor cell Ki-67 positivity.[150,151] Immunostaining with Ki-67 has been performed on routinely prepared, air-dried, breast fine needle aspirate smears.[152,153] If necessary, the smears can be stored at −70°C and immunostaining can be performed later. A commercially available mouse antihuman monoclonal antibody can be coupled with standard development procedures. Smears prepared from fresh surgical tonsillectomy specimens are an effective positive control. The expression of Ki-67 is indicated by strong nuclear staining (Images 14.18 and 14.19). Quantitation of Ki 67–positive cells can be performed by visually assessing the percentage of nuclear positivity or by cell image analysis. A good correlation between Ki-67 immunostaining of cytologic preparations and tissue sections of breast carcinoma has been reported.[154,155] Ki-67 immunostaining can also be applied to imprint preparations of small tumors and provide prognostic information.[154]

The difficulties inherent in the use of immunocytochemical techniques and in the subsequent interpretation of results are limiting factors. In addition, since formaldehyde destroys Ki-67 antigen, solutions that contain this fixative, such as Bouin's, interfere with accurate measurements of Ki 67–positive cells. Fortunately, new monoclonal antibodies are now commercially available that can highlight the Ki-67 antigen in formalin-fixed, paraffin-embedded tissue.[152] Thus, in addition to direct smears, cell block preparations obtained from breast fine needle aspirates can also be subjected to Ki-67 immunostaining.

Newly Recognized Prognostic Factors

In addition to the established prognostic factors are new biologic markers that can also be detected in samples obtained from breast fine needle aspirates. As previously mentioned, standard immunocytochemistry applied to direct smears, cytospins, or cell block preparations is the technique used most frequently to obtain prognostic information from cytologic specimens. We prefer the use of cell block preparations, since they allow for multiple immunostaining and appropriate tissue controls.[156]

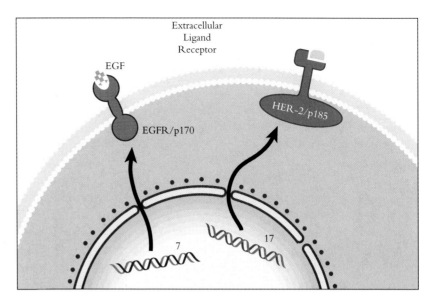

Figure 14.7

Schematic representation of the characteristics of HER/2-*neu* oncogene. EGF = epidermal growth factor; EGFR = epidermal growth factor receptor.

HER-2/*neu* (*c-erb*B-2) Oncogene

The activation of several proto-oncogenes has been shown to play a role in the pathogenesis of a variety of human malignancies, including breast cancer. These genetic alterations may also be important in assessing the biologic aggressiveness of the tumor and thus in predicting the patient's clinical outcome. HER-2/*neu* is a proto-oncogene homologous to the epidermal growth factor–receptor gene. It encodes a 185 kd transmembrane protein with an intracellular tyrosine kinase domain and an extracellular domain that may bind with a growth factor (Figure 14.7).[157]

Several studies have examined the role of HER-2/*neu* as a prognostic factor in breast cancer patients.[158–162] In 1987, Slamon et al[158] published a pilot study of 86 node-positive breast cancer patients and showed that amplification of HER-2/*neu* oncogene is associated with tumor recurrence and shortened survival. In a well-designed study by Tandon et al[159] involving 350 node-positive patients, a strong connection between HER-2/*neu* expression and both early recurrence and decreased survival was found. Subsequent attempts to confirm these data were successful, marginally successful, or completely unsuccessful.[160–162]

The role of HER-2/*neu* oncogene in predicting outcome in node-negative breast cancer patients remains controversial. Although the majority of reports are negative, Paik et al[160] found that HER-2/*neu* oncogene overexpression is associated with decreased survival among women with tumors of a low nuclear grade. Similarly, Allred et al[161] retrospectively evaluated a group of 325 node-negative patients assigned to the observation arm of a cooperative group clinical trial. These patients had tumors that were smaller than 3 cm and ER positive. HER-2/*neu* overexpression in purely invasive tumors in this otherwise low-risk group was associated with early recurrence. Thus, despite the controversy regarding the prognostic significance of HER-2/*neu* expression, this oncogene may identify a subset of node-negative patients with small, predominantly invasive tumors that are estrogen-receptor positive. Patients with such tumors may be more likely to develop early tumor recurrence.

The clinical significance of HER-2/*neu* oncogene expression must be further studied in locally advanced and metastatic breast disease. Strong correlation between HER-2/*neu* oncogene expression and the prognosis of patients with node-positive breast cancer suggests that HER-2/*neu* oncogene expression could be a means of selecting patients for aggressive treatment regimens, such as high-dose chemotherapy followed by bone marrow transplantation.

Several antibodies for detecting HER-2/*neu* oncogene are commercially available. Standard immunocytochemical stains can be performed on cytologic preparations, fresh frozen or formalin-fixed tissue. Although preliminary studies used cell block preparations, later investigators used destained, alcohol-fixed, Papanicolaou-stained direct smears for detecting HER-2/*neu* oncogene in breast lesions. These investigators found a good correlation between the expression of HER-2/*neu* oncogene in cytologic preparations and in corresponding tissue sections.[156–158]

As in tissue sections, the expression of HER-2/*neu* oncogene in cytologic preparations is evidenced by membrane staining (Images 14.20 and 14.21). Immunocytochemical localization of HER-2/*neu* oncogene in previously destained direct smears of breast carcinoma may be more sensitive than such localization in formalin-fixed, paraffin-embedded tissue.[157] In tumors with lower levels of amplification, the antigen may be better preserved with the alcohol-based fixatives used with cytologic preparations than with the routine formalin fixative used with tissue specimens. Length of fixation may also play a role: cytologic preparations are fixed for short periods of time (minutes), while tissue sections are kept in fixative for longer periods of time (hours). The possibility of intramural heterogeneity may also explain the differences between breast cytology smears and formalin-fixed tissue in HER-2/*neu* oncogene staining. However, several studies have found that there is not a significant degree of heterogeneity of HER-2/*neu* oncogene expression in breast carcinoma.[159–161] Cytologically, the pattern of HER-2/*neu* oncogene expression also appears to be relatively uniform. Assessing the status of HER-2/*neu* oncogene expression in breast cytologic preparations may be of some value in predicting response to therapy, since there is some evidence that HER-2/*neu* oncogene-positive tumors may be drug resistant.[163] However, this awaits further investigation.

p53

Scientific evidence suggests that the growth of normal cells is regulated by a precise balance of proto-oncogenes, which promote cell growth, and tumor suppressor genes, which constrain cell proliferation. Alterations of proto-oncogenes that enhance growth potential create oncogenes that force the growth of tumor cells. Inactivation or loss of tumor suppressor genes, on the other hand, results in uncontrolled growth of tumor cells (Figures 14.8 and 14.9).

The p53 protein, a tumor-suppressor gene product, is found predominantly in the nuclei of different tumors. Due to its increased half-life and altered conformational structure, the mutant form of p53 protein accumulates in malignant cells and can be visualized using immunocytochemical techniques (Images 14.22 and 14.23). The normal allele of p53 encodes a

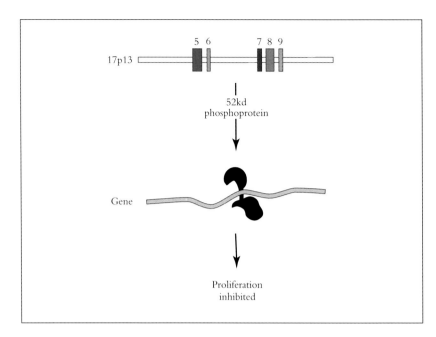

Figure 14.8
Schematic illustration of the function of p53.

53-kd nuclear phosphoprotein involved in the control of cell proliferation. The p53 gene is located on human chromosome 17p, and partial or complete loss of one allele on chromosome 17p is frequently seen in breast carcinoma. p53 is the most frequently mutated gene in human cancer.[164–166]

Recent studies suggest that p53 expression is associated with hormone receptor negativity, high nuclear grade, DNA aneuploidy, and high prolifer-

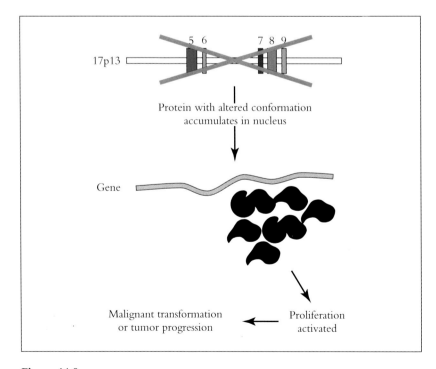

Figure 14.9
Schematic illustration of p53 mutation.

ative rate. p53 has also been reported as a strong predictor of early recurrence and reduced survival.[167–172] Several investigators have emphasized an association between p53 expression and late-stage metastatic disease in breast cancer,[172,173] which may imply that p53 metastasis is a late event in the nonfamilial form of breast cancer.[173] However, demonstration of p53 overexpression in the earliest recognizable phase of breast cancer and through progression to metastatic stage creates a paradox. The paradox could perhaps be resolved if p53 mutations were an early event in tumor progression that gives tumor cells a more aggressive phenotype. The tumor cells would then rapidly progress through early stages and would have a higher frequency of p53 expression.[172,174] In this scenario, alterations in p53 provide important prognostic information. In locally advanced breast cancer, p53 overexpression has been strongly associated with large tumor diameter ($p = 0.0002$) and the presence of distant metastasis ($p = 0.0015$). Less significantly, tumors with p53 mutations showed an association with negative hormone receptors and a lower rate of response to therapy.[173]

nm23

The suppressor gene nm23 was identified on the basis of its reduced, steady-state RNA levels in five highly metastatic melanoma cell lines, as compared with tumor-related, low metastatic potential melanoma cell lines.[175] Low nm23 RNA levels are associated with the presence of lymph node metastasis.[176,177] We have studied the pattern of nm23 expression in breast cancer via immunocytochemistry and have shown that low nm23 expression correlates with reduced patient survival (Images 14.24 and 14.25).[178] These studies suggest the potential value of nm23 in predicting prognosis in breast cancer; however, the results remain preliminary.

Epidermal Growth Factor Receptor

Epidermal growth factor receptor (EGFR) is a 170 kd transmembrane glycoprotein with an extracellular region that binds to EGF and an intracellular region that exhibits tyrosine kinase activity. Epidermal growth factor receptor, which can be detected by immunocytochemistry (Images 14.26 and 14.27), is frequently overproduced in breast tumors and is inversely related to ER status.[179,180] The presence of high levels of EGFR in ER-negative breast cancer patients has been associated with poor prognosis. Overall, studies on breast tumors have shown that overaccumulation of EGFR protein in a tumor indicates poor differentiation and increased tumor aggressiveness.[181] The prognostic value of EGFR in advanced breast cancer is not yet well established.

Cathepsin D

Cathepsin D is an estrogen-induced, lysosomal protease that is secreted as a 52 kd precursor. The cathepsin-D gene, which is located at the extremity of the short arm of chromosome 11 near the H-*ras* oncogene, may facilitate cancer cell migration and promote invasion by digesting the basement membrane, extracellular matrix, and connective tissue.[182] The presence of this protein can be detected by biochemical as well as immunocytochemical assays (Images 14.28 and 14.29).

In 1989, Thorpe et al[183] analyzed 396 breast tumors for cathepsin D using a two-site, solid-phase immunoenzymatic assay. They showed that patients with elevated cathepsin-D levels had shorter disease-free and overall survival rates. However, in an analysis of 94 breast cancer patients using immunocytochemical technique, Henry et al[184] reported in 1990 that positive cathepsin-D immunostaining was associated with a significantly better prognosis in patients with confirmed lymph node metastasis but not in node-negative patients.

Over the past few years, reports on the prognostic value of cathepsin D have been inconsistent. While there is convincing evidence suggesting a strong relation between increased cytosolic levels of cathepsin D and poor prognosis, most immunocytochemical studies have failed to confirm the results of cytosolic studies.[183–199] This discrepancy raises serious questions about the dependability of cathepsin D as a prognostic indicator, and the value of cathepsin D in breast cancer evaluation remains to be determined.

Angiogenesis

Experimental evidence suggests that tumor growth depends on the growth of new vessels, or neovascularization.[200] Tumor neovascularization is caused by the release of angiogenesis factor by the tumor cells and/or tumor-associated inflammatory cells.[201,202] Angiogenesis is also necessary for a tumor to metastasize.[203]

The intensity of angiogenesis can be quantitated by determining the number of capillaries and small venules (microvessels) per area of the tumor. The microvessels can be highlighted by staining the endothelial cells for factor VIII–related antigen using a standard immunoperoxidase technique (Images 14.30 and 14.31). Correlating the mean microvessel count of the tumor with the incidence of metastasis, Weidner et al[204] were the first to demonstrate the prognostic significance of angiogenesis in breast carcinoma. In a study that was subsequently confirmed by others,[205,206] Weidner showed microvessel density to be the best predictor of metastasis when compared with tumor grade and tumor size. Similar studies have shown a statistically significant association between microvessel density, overall survival, and relapse-free survival in breast cancer patients.[207,208] Based on these studies, angiogenesis is viewed as an independent, highly significant, and accurate predictor of metastasis as well as overall and disease-free survival in early-stage breast carcinoma. Further studies are required to assess the value of angiogenesis in late-stage breast carcinoma.

pS2

The small secreted protein pS2 is a 6.5 kd, estrogen-inducible, cytoplasmic polypeptide of unknown function. The expression of pS2 may be analogous to expression of PgR, as there is a significant correlation between the presence of pS2 mRNA and ER. The expression of pS2 may reflect a functional estrogen regulatory system and therefore define another subset of ER+/PgR+ patients who may show an even greater degree of hormone responsiveness.[209–211]

The functional significance of ER+/PgR+/pS– tumors is presently unknown. A recent report suggests that pS2 is already highly expressed in malignant cells before they have acquired a propensity for invasion that may be prognostically significant.[211] Using an immunocytochemical technique, Abbondanzo et al[210] studied 598 axillary node–negative breast cancers and found that high expression of pS2 in node-negative breast cancer is associated with significantly longer disease-free survival and several low-risk clinical pathologic features. Whether pS2-negative breast cancer patients benefit from aggressive adjuvant therapy with or without the addition of hormonal therapy awaits further study.

p-Glycoprotein

The need for a sensitive and rapid assay to assess the level of responsiveness to chemotherapy in patients with breast cancer is well recognized. With such an assay, individualized chemotherapy for breast cancer patients would be possible. The expression of the multidrug resistance (MDR) phenotype in human breast cancer is is one possiblity under intense investigation. Expression of the MDR gene (p-glycoprotein) is one of the mechanisms involved in the chemoresistance phenomenon. Two closely related MDR genes have been identified, although MDR1 is the only one linked to MDR phenotype.[212,213] The p-glycoprotein, a 170,000 daltons protein, consists of a hydrophobic region containing potential nucleotide binding sites.[214] It functions as an energy-dependent efflux pump that decreases intracellular drug accumulation,[215] overcoming resistance to antineoplastics, antimetabolites, and the synthetic dihydroxyanthracenedione-derivative mitoxantrone.[216]

Expression of MDR1 has been detected by a variety of techniques, such as polymerase chain reaction (PCR), Southern blot analysis, in situ hybridization, and immunocytochemistry.[216–218] Although PCR is the most promising detection technique, immunocytochemistry offers an advantage because it permits visualization of the protein on a per-cell basis. This allows the degree of heterogeneity of MDR1 expression to be assessed and discounts the contribution of stromal cells and nonneoplastic components. Immunostaining is apparent on the cell membrane and in the Golgi apparatus of the cytoplasm (Images 14.32 and 14.33).

The frequency of p-glycoprotein expression in breast cancer varies and is influenced by therapy.[216–218] Although patients who have received therapy show a greater degree of staining intensity, it has also been shown that in patients who have relapsed there is an increase in both the amount and intensity of staining, regardless of prior therapy.[216–218] This suggests the possibility of genomic instability induced by cancer progression as well as chemotherapy.[219] Determining the clinical value of MDR expression in breast cancer requires further study to correlate pretreatment MDR with subsequent chemotherapy response.[215,220]

bcl-2

The bcl-2 gene encodes a protein that suppresses programmed cell death, or apoptosis. Therefore, it may play a role in the modulation of hormonal/antihormonal responsiveness.[221] Studies utilizing immunocytochemistry to detect the presence of bcl-2 protein have shown a strong positive relationship between the expression of bcl-2 and estrogen and progesterone receptors.[221–224] Expression of bcl-2 in breast cancer has also been associated with reduced cell proliferation, lower-grade carcinomas, and tumors with low expression for p53 suppressor genes.[221–224]

Gee et al[221] demonstrated a highly signficant relationship between response to endocrine therapy and the presence of bcl-2 protein in breast cancer cells. Indeed, the expression of bcl-2 proved to be a more accurate predictor of response to endocrine therapy than estrogen receptor status. The prognostic significance of bcl-2 expression in node-negative breast cancer patients remains to be proven. However, in a study of 251 invasive breast cancers, Hellemans et al[225] showed that the absence of bcl-2 expression is an independent predictor of shortened disease-free survival ($p = 0.003$) and reduced overall survival ($p < 0.0001$) in axillary node–positive breast cancer patients. These studies suggest that bcl-2 may play an important role in modulating response to adjuvant therapy for breast cancer.

How to Use Prognostic Factors in Breast Cancer

A variety of tumor characteristics can provide prognostic information in patients with breast cancer. Although some characteristics are firmly established, others require large-scale, controlled studies before they can be appropriately utilized. No single marker is available to define which patients with primary breast cancer will relapse, and the prognostic value of the new markers remains controversial.

Recognition of high-risk breast cancer is particularly important in node-negative breast cancer patients. As we move from the age of clinical and morphologic indicators to the era of cell biology and molecular pathology, our understanding of the natural history of breast cancer is evolving. It is important to refine prognostic factors and reproducibility, to integrate new and old indicators, and to carefully evaluate prospective trials. We must be certain of the data on which patient stratification is based. For prognostic factors to become reproducible, it is necessary to standardize methods, scoring system, and data analysis. The relative importance of prognostic factors should also be based on large-scale prospective, multiparameter studies.

Since there is no single prognostic marker that can discriminate between low- and high-risk subgroups of patients with node-negative breast cancer, a major thrust in future research will be the development of panels of prognostic markers that will maximize the benefit of prognostic markers in clinical decision making. O'Reilly et al[226] already attempted this in a study that combined the results of DNA ploidy study with tumor size as a means of predicting outcome in 169 node-negative breast cancer patients who received local therapy alone. The 5-year recurrence-free survival rate was 95%, 78%, and 52%, respectively, for patients with tumors with a diameter of 1.0 cm or less, tumors with a diameter greater than 1.0 cm with S-phase fraction (SPF) of 10% or less, and tumors with a diameter greater than 1.0 cm with SPF over 10%. Similarly, Clark et al[119] reported that SPF can be used to identify higher- and lower-risk groups of women with ER-positive tumors measuring less than 3 cm. Paik et al[160] demonstrated the prognostic value of HER-2/*neu* oncogene expression in the subset of node-negative patients with low nuclear grade tumors.

Factors associated with a low risk include ductal carcinoma in situ; pure tubular, papillary, or typical medullary carcinoma; tumors measuring less than 1 cm in diameter; diploid tumors with a low S-phase fraction; tumors of nuclear grade I; and tumors of intermediate size without any high-risk features. Factors associated with a high risk include aneuploidy, a high S-phase fraction, a high cathepsin-D level, the absence of estrogen receptors, and tumors larger than 3 cm. Unfortunately, it is somewhat difficult to assess tumors with mixed characteristics.

In 1990, McGuire et al[227] proposed that the first step in arriving at a clinical treatment decision based on the merits of prognostic factors in breast cancer is determining the probability of tumor recurrence. The second step is to determine the anticipated benefit of adjuvant chemotherapy or endocrine therapy. The third step requires weighing the anticipated benefit of treatment against the risks and costs. The final decision on whether to initiate or withold therapy remains the responsibility of the well-informed breast cancer patient (Figures 14.10 through 14.12).

The probability of recurrence may be determined by using a rank-order bar chart of prognostic factors and a combination of factors that give the approximate risk of recurrence based on results from the literature. After estimating the likelihood of recurrence, the next step is to estimate the potential benefit from different types of treatment using data from published adjuvant trials in node-negative breast cancer patients. Overall, the anticipated benefit from adjuvant therapy is greatest when the probability of recurrence is high. For example, a patient with favorable prognosis and a recurrence probability of 5% has an anticipated benefit of less than 2% for adjuvant tamoxifen therapy or less than 3% for adjuvant chemotherapy. In

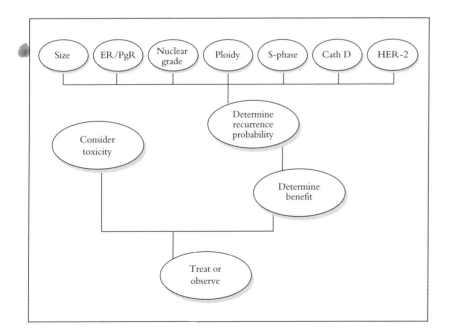

Figure 14.10
A diagram of the process involved in deciding on a therapy for node-negative breast cancer. Reproduced from: McGuire WH, Tandon AK, Allred DC, et al: How to use prognostic factors in axillary node negative breast cancer patients. *J Natl Cancer Inst* 82:1006, 1991.

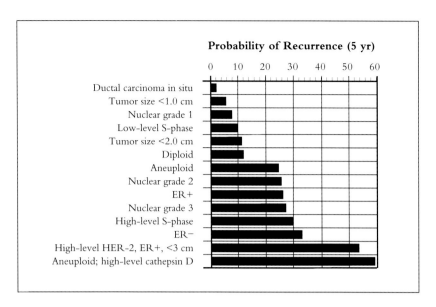

Figure 14.11
Schematic representation of recurrence probability in breast cancer patients. Reproduced from: McGuire WH, Tandon AK, Allred DC, et al: How to use prognostic factors in axillary node negative breast cancer patients. *J Natl Cancer Inst* 82:1006, 1991.

contrast, a patient with a risk probability of 60% has an anticipated benefit of 15% for adjuvant tamoxifen therapy and 30% for adjuvant chemotherapy.

The third step is to weigh the anticipated benefit of treatment against the risks and costs. Relatively few patients who receive chemotherapy or endocrine therapy will benefit, but all must bear its toxicity and cost. Toxicity-related deaths have been reported.

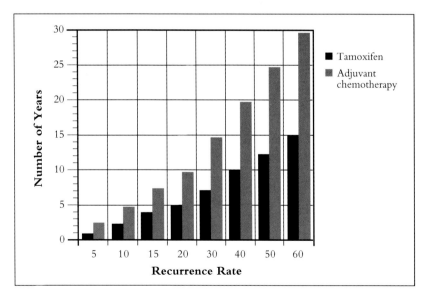

Figure 14.12
A diagram of the relationship between patient benefit and recurrence probability. Reproduced from: McGuire WH, Tandon AK, Allred DC, et al: How to use prognostic factors in axillary node negative breast cancer patients. *J Natl Cancer Inst* 82:1006, 1991.

The long-term consequences of cytotoxic therapy remain to be determined. Even tamoxifen, commonly regarded as a drug with little risk, is associated with a few side-effects. These include the striking increase in low-grade endometrial carcinoma in more than 1 of 100 tamoxifen-treated women; thrombophlebitis in 1 of 100 tamoxifen-treated women, with rare deaths from pulmonary embolism; the unknown long-term effects of tamoxifen administration on the liver and cardiovascular and skeletal systems; and the financial burden to the patient—more than \$5000 for a complete 5-year course of the drug alone.[227]

According to the recommendations of the NIH's 1991 Consensus Conference on Early Stage Breast Cancer,[8] patients with node-negative breast cancer should be aware of the risks and benefits of adjuvant systemic therapy. Patients who choose to undergo adjuvant systemic therapy should do so in the context of a clinical trial. The need to develop better methods of risk assessment for breast cancer patients was also emphasized. Although current clinical trials suggest that adjuvant therapy can change the natural history of node-negative breast cancer, the use of prognostic factors to define low- and high-risk subgroups is still problematic, and delineation of optimal treatment strategies is critical. Patients should be fully apprised of the risk of recurrence with local therapy alone and the anticipated benefits and potential toxicities of adjuvant therapy, so that they can actively participate in the decision-making process.

Future Considerations

A review of the literature on the clinical validity of different biologic markers reveals contradictory results (Tables 14.5 and 14.6). Among the various causes for these conflicting results, such as differences in study populations and data analysis, lack of uniform standardized procedures remains the most important factor. By creating a research consortium, a network of investigators interested in the study and management of breast cancer, the need for randomly oriented, well-controlled studies that incorporate sufficient numbers of breast cancer patients at different stages of the disease could be met. Technology and result interpretation could be standardized, and data could be analyzed with an emphasis on patient outcome.[228–230]

This is an exciting time for pathologists and cytopathologists. We can become more visible in our role as consultants to other physicians and more engaged in our role as researchers. Recent advances in computer science coupled with the availability of new biologic markers provide unique opportunities for us to expand our diagnostic abilities and predict the biologic behavior of a given tumor. Thus, we must become more familiar with emerging concepts and technologies in different disciplines.

Table 14.5
Results of Studies Measuring Cathespin D by Cytosolic Assay

Reference	Results
Thorpe et al (1989)[183]	Increased cathespin D, decreased survival
Spyratos et al (1989)[185]	Increased cathespin D, decreased metastasis-free survival
Duffy et al (1991)[186]	Increased cathespin D, decreased survival
Romain et al (1990)[187]	Increased cathespin D, decreased survival in lymph node–positive and estrogen receptor–negative tumors
Namer et al (1991)[188]	Increased cathespin D, decreased survival in lymph node–positive tumors
Pujol et al (1993)[189]	Increased cathespin D, decreased survival in lymph node–positive tumors
Tandon et al (1990)[199]	Increased cathespin D, decreased survival in lymph node–negative tumors
Granata et al (1991)[190]	Increased cathespin D, decreased survival in estrogen receptor–positive tumors

Table 14.6
Results of Studies Measuring Cathespin D by Immunocytochemistry

Reference	Results
Kandalaft et al (1992)[194]	No correlation with survival
Tetu et al (1992)[195]	Increased stromal cathespin D, decreased metastasis-free survival
Sahin et al (1992)[196]	No correlation with survival
Isola et al (1993)[197]	Increased cathespin D, decreased survival
Armas et al (1994)[198]	No correlation with survival
Henry et al (1990)[184]	Increased cathespin D, increased survival in lymph node–positive and estrogen receptor–positive tumors
Domagala et al (1992)[191]	No correlation with survival
Cowan et al (1991)[192]	Increased cathespin D in screen-positive, asymptomatic tumors
Martin et al (1992)[193]	Increased cathespin D, increased survival

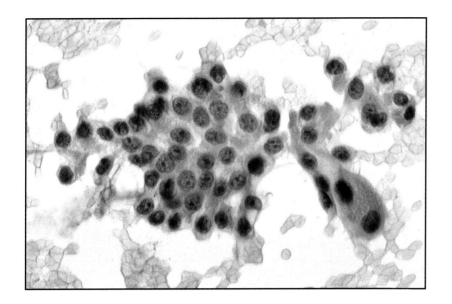

Image 14.1
Nuclear grade I (Papanicolaou, 200X).
Reproduced with permission from:
Masood S: Is nuclear grading worthwhile in breast cytology? *Adv Anat Pathol* 2:382–385, 1995.

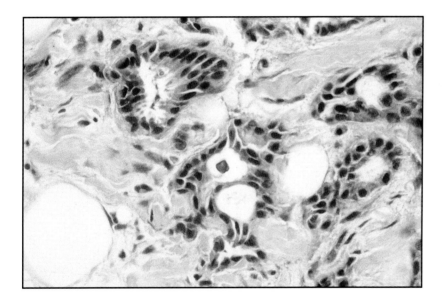

Image 14.2
Corresponding tissue section (H&E, 200X). Reproduced with permission from: Masood S: Is nuclear grading worthwhile in breast cytology? *Adv Anat Pathol* 2:382–385, 1995.

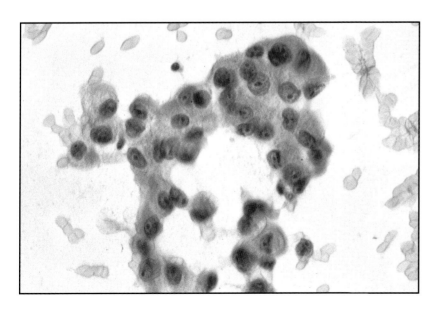

Image 14.3
Nuclear grade II (Papanicolaou, 200X). Reproduced with permission from: Masood S: Is nuclear grading worthwhile in breast cytology? *Adv Anat Pathol* 2:382–385, 1995.

Image 14.4
Corresponding tissue section (H&E, 400X). Reproduced with permission from: Masood S: Is nuclear grading worthwhile in breast cytology? *Adv Anat Pathol* 2:382–385, 1995.

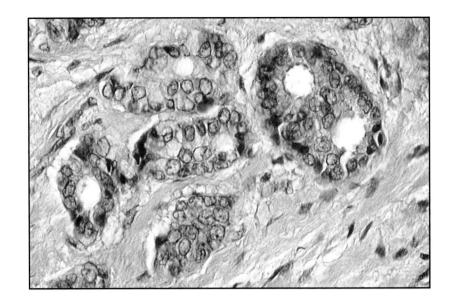

Image 14.5
Nuclear grade III (Papanicolaou, 400X). Reproduced with permission from: Masood S: Is nuclear grading worthwhile in breast cytology? *Adv Anat Pathol* 2:382–385, 1995.

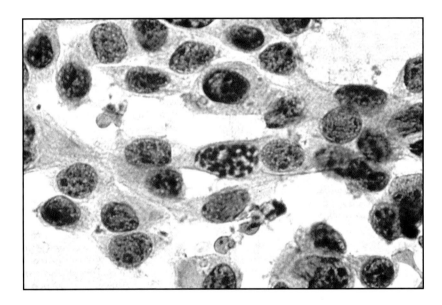

Image 14.6
Corresponding tissue section (Papanicolaou, 400X). Reproduced with permission from: Masood S: Is nuclear grading worthwhile in breast cytology? *Adv Anat Pathol* 2:382–385, 1995.

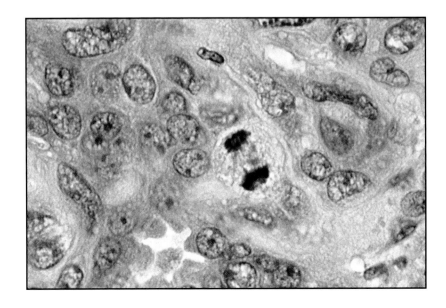

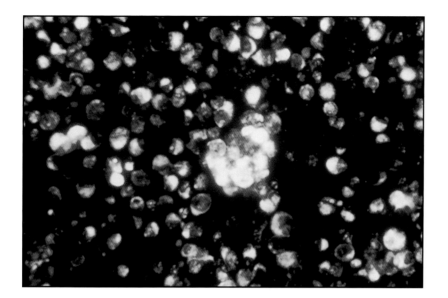

Image 14.7
Fluorescent cytochemical staining for demonstration of estrogen receptor protein in the cytoplasm of breast tumor cells (100X).

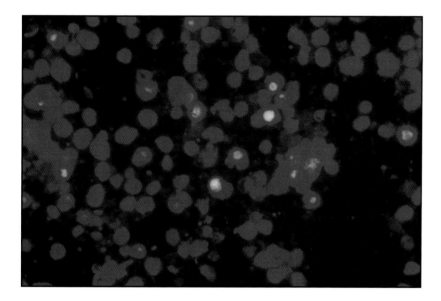

Image 14.8
An example of a progesterone receptor–positive breast tumor with bright red illumination in the cytoplasm (100X).

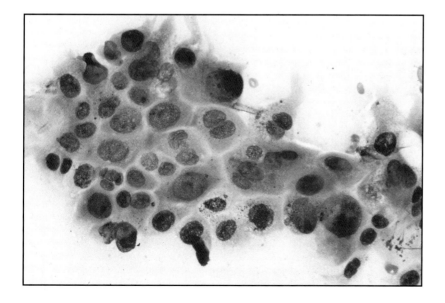

Image 14.9
Direct smear of breast FNAB shows clusters of neoplastic epithelial cells (Diff-Quik®, 400X). Reproduced with permission from: Masood S: Cytomorphology of fibrocystic change, high risk and premalignant breast lesions. *Breast J* 1:210–221, 1995.

Image 14.10
Direct smear of breast FNAB: expression of estrogen receptor evidenced by presence of nuclear staining (Immunoperoxidase, 400X). Reproduced with permission from: Masood S: Use of monoclonal antibody for assessment of estrogen receptor content in fine needle aspiration biopsy specimens from patients with breast cancer. *Arch Pathol Lab Med* 113:26–30, 1989.

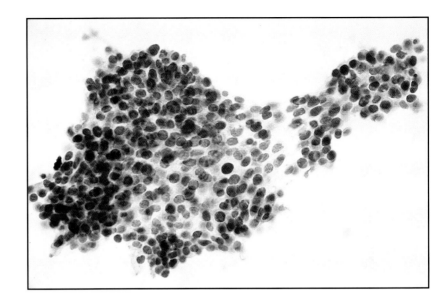

A   B

Image 14.11
Expression of hormone receptor in an unsuspected breast cancer. A. Infiltrating duct cell carcinoma (H&E, 400X). B. Nuclear staining in hormone receptor–positive tumor cells (Immunoperoxidase, 400X). Reproduced with permission from: Masood S: Prediction of recurrence for advanced breast cancer. In: Bland K, ed. *Surgical Oncology Clinics of North America*. Philadelphia, Pa, WB Saunders Co, 1995, pp. 601–632.

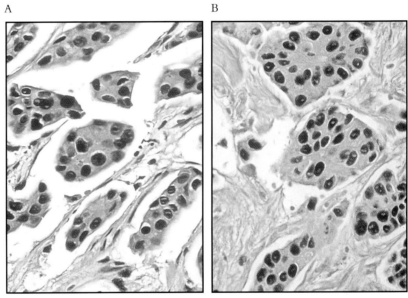

Image 14.12
Demonstration of the heterogeneity of hormone receptor expression in a patient who failed to respond to endocrine therapy (Immunoperoxidase, 400X). Reproduced with permission from: Masood S: Prognostic and diagnostic implications of estrogen and progesterone receptor assays in cytology. *Diagn Cytopathol* 10:263–267, 1994.

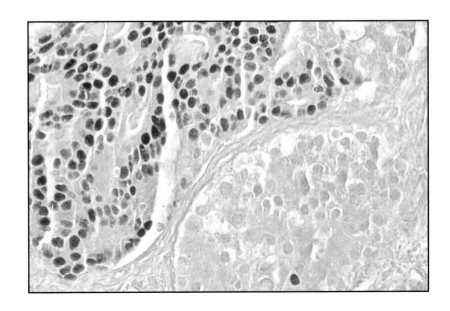

A   B

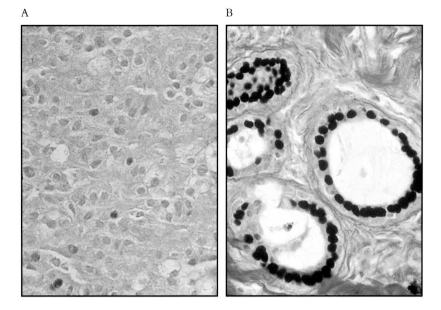

Image 14.13
An example of a biochemically hormone receptor–positive breast cancer patient who did not respond to endocrine therapy. A. Tumor cells with no or a small amount of estrogen receptor protein (Immunoperoxidase, 400X). B. Positive expression of hormone receptor in mixed benign epithelial elements of the same case, contributing to a false-positive biochemical assay (400X). Reproduced with permission from: Masood S: Prognostic and diagnostic implications of estrogen and progesterone receptor assays in cytology. *Diagn Cytopathol* 10:263–267, 1994.

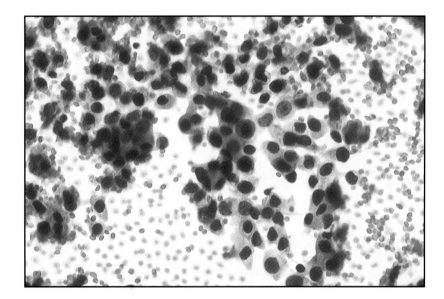

Image 14.14
Cytospin preparation of breast FNAB shows neoplastic epithelial cells isolated and in clusters (Diff-Quik, 200X).

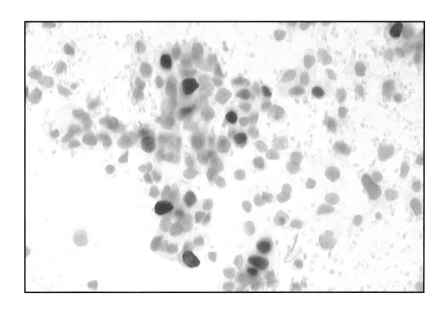

Image 14.15
Cytospin preparation for demonstration of estrogen receptor in the same tumor cells (Immunoperoxidase, 200X).

Image 14.16
Cell block preparation of a breast aspirate demonstrates the presence of tumor cells (H&E, 200X).

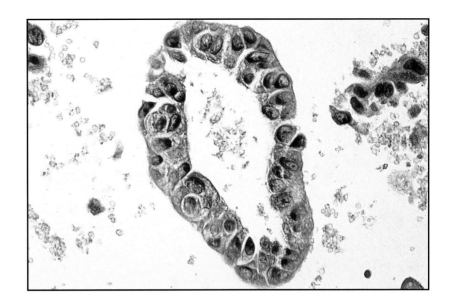

Image 14.17
Expression of progesterone receptor evidenced by nuclear staining in the same aspirate (Immunoperoxidase, 200X).

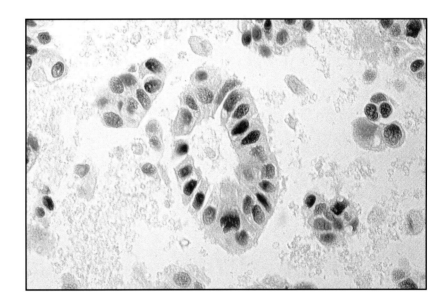

Image 14.18
Breast aspirate, direct smear: the expression of Ki-67 evidenced by nuclear staining indicates tumor proliferation (Immunoperoxidase, 200X).

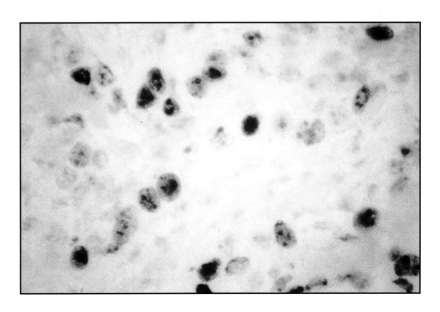

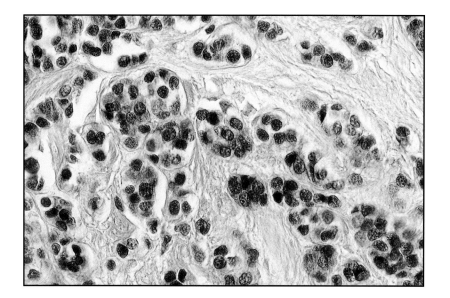

Image 14.19
Corresponding tissue section of the surgically excised lesion: Ki-67 expression similar to that in the fine needle aspirate (Immunoperoxidase, 200X).

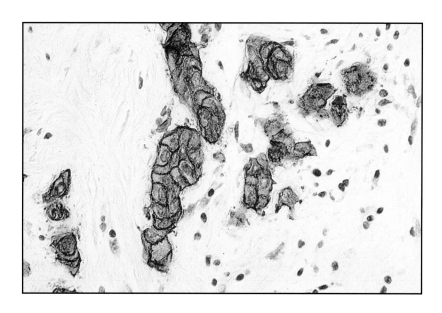

Image 14.20
Breast aspirate, cell block preparation: Expression of HER-2/*neu* oncogene evidenced by cell membrane staining in a patient with advanced breast cancer (Immunoperoxidase, 200X). Reproduced with permission from: Masood S: Prognostic factors in breast cancer: use of cytologic preparations. *Diagn Cytopathol* 13:388–395, 1995.

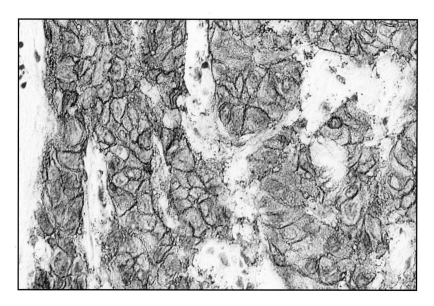

Image 14.21
Similar expression of HER-2/*neu* oncogene in the corresponding surgically excised lesion (Immunoperoxidase, 200X).

Image 14.22
Cell block preparation of a breast aspirate reveals clusters of neoplastic epithelial cells (H&E, 200X).

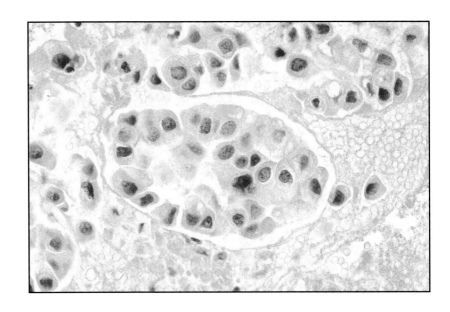

Image 14.23
Expression of p53 evidenced by nuclear staining in the same case (Immunoperoxidase, 200X).

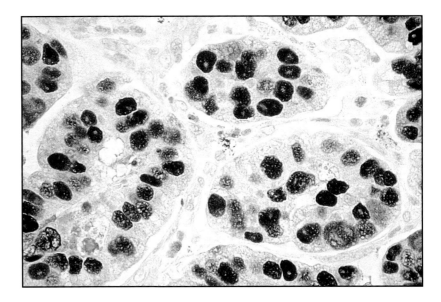

Image 14.24
Expression of nm23 in epithelial cells of normal breast (Immunoperoxidase, 200X). Reproduced with permission from: Barnes R, Masood S, Barker E, et al: Low nm23 protein expression in infiltrating ductal breast carcinomas correlates with reduced patient survival. *Am J Pathol* 139:245–250, 1991.

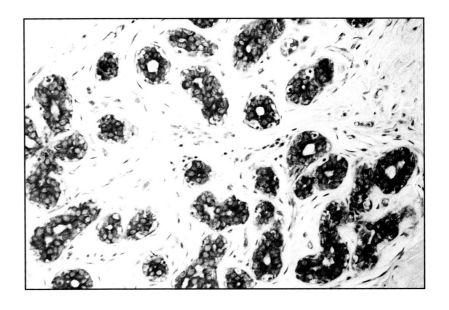

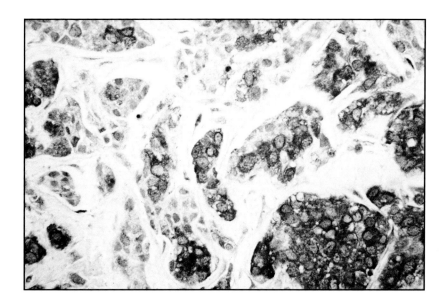

Image 14.25
Focal loss of nm23 in a patient with primary breast cancer (Immunoperoxidase, 400X). Reproduced with permission from: Barnes R, Masood S, Barker E, et al: Low nm23 protein expression in infiltrating ductal breast carcinomas correlates with reduced patient survival. *Am J Pathol* 139:245–250, 1991.

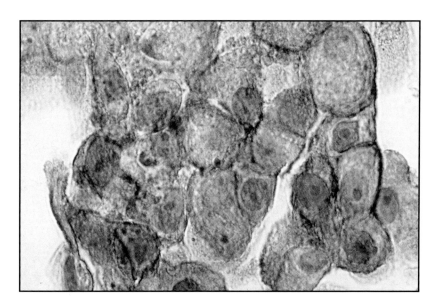

Image 14.26
Expression of epidermal growth factor receptor seen as membrane staining in tumor cells obtained from aspirate of a malignant breast lesion (Immunoperoxidase, 1000X). Reproduced with permission from: Masood S: Prognostic factors in breast cancer: use of cytologic preparations. *Diagn Cytopathol* 13:388–395, 1995.

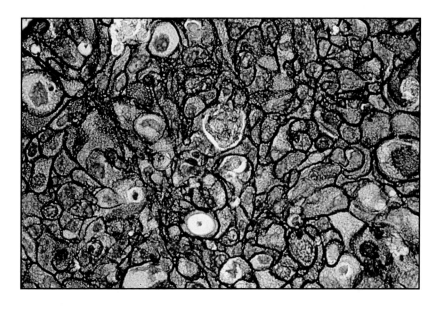

Image 14.27
Similar expression of epidermal growth factor receptor in the corresponding surigcal specimen (Immunoperoxidase, 1000X). Reproduced with permission from: Masood S: Prognostic factors in breast cancer: use of cytologic preparations. *Diagn Cytopathol* 13:388–395, 1995.

Image 14.28
Cathepsin D–positive tumor cells evidenced by cytoplasmic staining in a breast aspirate (Immunoperoxidase, 200X).

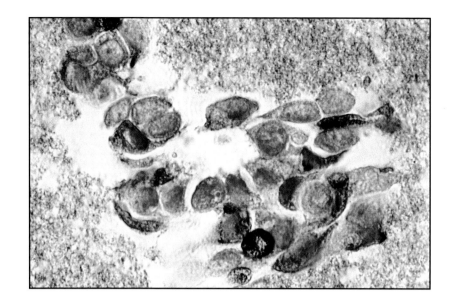

Image 14.29
Similar expression of cathepsin D in the corresponding surgically excised lesion (Immunoperoxidase, 400X). Reproduced with permission from: Masood S: Prediction of recurrence for advanced breast cancer. In: Bland K, ed. *Surgical Oncology Clinics of North America.* Philadelphia, Pa, WB Saunders Co, 1995, pp. 601–632.

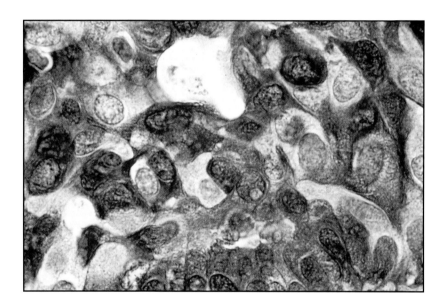

Image 14.30
Evidence of angiogenesis in a breast cancer. The presence of small vessels is highlighted by immunostaining for factor VIII (Immunoperoxidase, 200X). Reproduced with permission from: Masood S: Prognostic factors in breast cancer. *J Surg Pathol* 1:45–61, 1995.

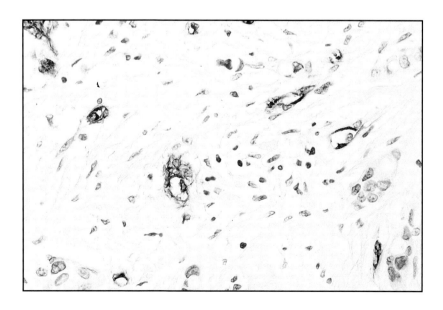

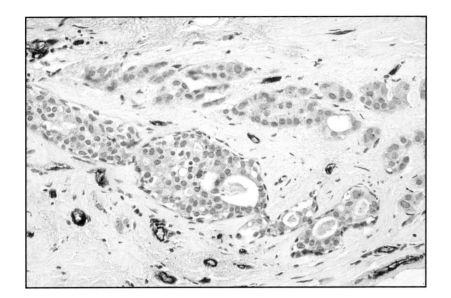

Image 14.31
Higher magnification of the same case reveals evidence of angiogenesis (Immunoperoxidase, 400X).

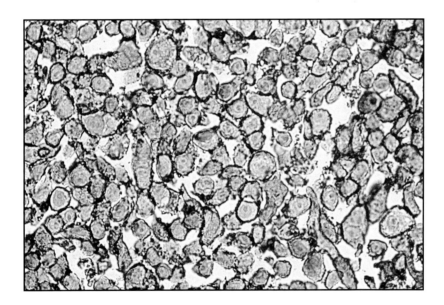

Image 14.32
Direct smear of a breast aspirate: membrane staining as expression of p-glycoprotein in tumor cells (Immunoperoxidase, 200X). Reproduced with permission from: Masood S: Prognostic factors in breast cancer: use of cytologic preparations. *Diagn Cytopathol* 13:388–395, 1995.

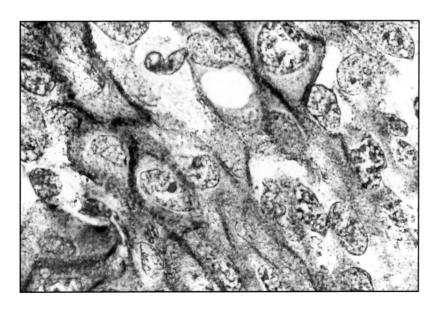

Image 14.33
Expression of multidrug gene resistance (p-glycoprotein) in surgically excised lesion from the same case (Immunoperoxidase, 1000X).

References

1. Early Breast Cancer Trialists' Collaborative Group: Effects of adjuvant tamoxifen and of cytotoxic therapy on mortality in early breast cancer: an overview of 61 randomized trials among 28,896 women. *N Engl J Med* 319:1681, 1988.

2. Bonadonna G, Valagussa P, Tancini G, et al: Current status of Milan adjuvant chemotherapy trials for node-positive and node-negative breast cancer. *Monogr Natl Cancer Inst* 1:45, 1986.

3. Fisher B, Costantino J, Redmond C, et al: A randomized clinical trials evaluating tamoxifen in the treatment of patients with node-negative breast cancer who have estrogen-receptor-positive tumors. *N Engl J Med* 320:479, 1989.

4. Fisher B, Redmond C, Dimitrov NY, et al: A randomized clinical trial evaluating sequential methotrexate and fluorouracil in the treatment of patients with node-negative breast cancer who have estrogen-receptor negative tumors. *N Engl J Med* 320:473, 1989.

5. Mansour FG, Gay R, Shatila AH, et al: Efficiency of adjuvant chemotherapy in high-risk node negative breast cancer. An intergroup study. *N Engl J Med* 320:485, 1989.

6. Bonadonna G: Karnofsky memorial lecture. Conceptual and practical advances in the management of breast cancer. *J Clin Oncol* 7:1380–1397, 1989.

7. Salmon SE: *Adjuvant Therapy of Cancer*, vol 6. Philadelphia, Pa, WB Saunders Co, 1990.

8. NIH Consensus Conference: Treatment of early stage breast cancer. *JAMA* 265:391–395, 1991.

9. Page DL: Prognosis and breast cancer. Recognition of lethal and favorable prognostic types. *Am J Surg Pathol* 15:334–349, 1991.

10. Wilson RE, Donegan WL, Mettlin C, et al: The 182nd National Survey of Carcinoma of the Breast in the United States by the American College of Surgeons. *Surg Gynecol Obstet* 159:309–318, 1984.

11. Fisher B, Slack N, Katrych D, et al: Ten year follow-up results of patients with carcinoma in the breast in a cooperative clinical trial evaluating surgical adjuvant chemotherapy. *Surg Gynecol Obstet* 140:528–534, 1975.

12. Atliyeh FF, Jensen M, Huvos AG, et al: Axillary micrometastases and macrometastases in carcinoma of the breast. *Surg Gynecol Obstet* 144:839–842, 1977.

13. Cutler SJ, Zipin C, Asire AJ: The prognostic significance of palpable lymph nodes in cancer of the breast. *Cancer* 23:243–250, 1969.

14. Bettelheim R, Price KN, Gelber RD, et al: International (Ludwig) Breast Cancer Study Group. Prognostic importance of occult axillary lymph node micrometastases from breast cancer. *Lancet* 335:1565–1568, 1990.

15. Neville AM, Price KN, Gleber RD, et al: Axillary node micrometastasis and breast cancer. *Lancet* 337:1110, 1991.

16. Trojani M, de Mascarel I, Bonichon F, et al: Micrometastasis to axillary lymph nodes from carcinoma of breast. Detection by immunohistochemistry and prognostic significance. *Br J Cancer* 55:303–306, 1987.

17. Wells CA, Herget A, Brochier J, et al: The immunocytochemical detection of axillary micrometastasis in breast cancer. *Br J Cancer* 50:193–197, 1984.

18. Kay S: Evaluation of Rotter's lymph nodes in radical mastectomy specimens as a guide to prognosis. *Cancer* 18:1441–1444, 1965.

19. Veronesi O, Cascinelli N, Bufalino R, et al: Risk of internal mammary lymph node metastasis and its relevance on prognosis of breast cancer patients. *Ann Surg* 198:681–684, 1983.

20. Urban JA, Marjani MA: Significance of internal mammary lymph node metastasis in breast cancer. *Am J Roentgenol* 111:130–136, 1971.

21. Fentiman IS, Lavelle MA, Caplan D, et al: The significance of supraclavicular fossa node recurrence after radical mastectomy. *Cancer* 57:908–910, 1986.

22. Papaionannou A, Urban JA, Scalene: Node biopsy in locally advanced primary breast cancer of questionable operability. *Cancer* 17:1006-1011, 1964.

23. Mambo NC, Gallager HS: Carcinoma of the breast. The prognostic significance of axillary disease. *Cancer* 39:2280-2285, 1977.

24. Donegan WL: Staging and primary treatment. In: Donegan WL, Spratt JS, eds. *Cancer of the Breast*. Philadelphia, Pa, WB Saunders Co, 1988, pp. 336–402.

25. Carter CL, Allen C, Henson DE: Relation of tumor size, lymph node status, and survival in 24,740 breast cancer cases. *Cancer* 63:181, 1989.

26. McGuire WL. Prognostic factors in primary breast cancer. *Cancer Surv* 5:527, 1986.

27. Fisher B, Slack NH, Brass IDJ, et al: Cancer of the breast: size of neoplasm and prognosis. *Cancer* 24:1071–1080, 1969.

28. Koscielny S, Tubiana M, Le MG, et al: Breast cancer: relationship between the size of the primary tumor and the probability of metastatic dissemination. *Br J Cancer* 49:709, 1984.

29. Rosen PP, Groshen S, Saigo PE, et al: A long term follow-up study of survival in stage I (T1N0M0) and stage II (T1N0M0) breast carcinoma. *J Clin Oncol* 7:355, 1989.

30. Rosen PP, Groshen S, Saigo PE, et al: Pathological prognostic factors in stage I (T1N0M0) and stage II (T1N0M0) breast carcinoma: a study of 644 patients with median follow-up of 18 years. *J Clin Oncol* 7:1239, 1989.

31. Bondeson L, Lindholm K: Aspiration cytology of tubular breast carcinoma. *Acta Cytol* 34:15–20, 1989.

32. Baker RR: Unusual lesions and their management. *Surg Clin North Am* 70:963–975, 1990.

33. Hunt CM, Ellis IO, Elston CW, et al: Cytological grading of breast carcinoma: a feasible proposition? *Cytopathology* 1:287–295, 1990.

34. Mouriguard J, Gozlan-Fior M, Villemain D, et al: Value of cytoprognostic classification in breast carcinomas. *J Clin Pathol* 39:489–496, 1986.

35. Schulte E, Wittekind C: The influence of the wet-fixed Papanicolaou and air-dried Giemsa techniques on nuclear parameters in breast cancer cytology: a cytomorphometric study. *Diagn Cytopathol* 3:256–261, 1987.

36. Sneige N: Nuclear grading in fine needle aspirates of the breast. In: Schmidt WA, ed. *Cytopathology Annual*. Baltimore, Md, Williams & Wilkins, 1992, pp. 161-171.

37. Ciatto S, Bonardi R, Herd-Smith A, et al: Prognostic value of breast cancer cytologic grading: a retrospective study of 213 cases. *Diagn Cytopathol* 9:160–163, 1993.

38. Dabbs DJ: Role of nuclear grading of breast carcinomas in fine needle aspiration specimens. *Acta Cytol* 37:361–366, 1993.

39. Mouriguard J, Pasquier D: Fine needle aspiration of breast carcinoma. A preliminary cytoprognostic study. *Acta Cytol* 24:153–159, 1980.

40. Dabbs DJ: Duct carcinoma of breast: nuclear grade as predictor of S-phase fraction. *Hum Pathol* 24:652–656, 1993.

41. Cajulis RS, Sneige N, El-Naggar A: Cytologic nuclear grading of fine needle aspirates of breast carcinomas: concordance with histopathologic and flow data. *Mod Pathol* 3:14, 1990. Abstract.

42. Masood S: Prognostic value of nuclear grading in breast cytology. *Mod Pathol* 8:21, 1994. Abstract.

43. Dabbs DJ, Silverman JF: Prognostic factors from the fine needle aspirate: breast carcinoma nuclear grade. *Diagn Cytopathol* 10:203–208, 1994.

44. Wallgren A, Zajicek J: The prognostic value of aspiration biopsy smear in mammary carcinoma. *Acta Cytol* 20:479–485, 1976.

45. Robinson JA, McKee G, Nichols A, et al: Prognostic value of cytological grading of fine needle aspirates from breast carcinomas. *Lancet* 343:947–949, 1994.

46. Howell LP, Gandour-Edwards R, O'Sullivan D: Application of the Scarff-Bloom-Richardson tumor grading system to fine needle aspirates of the breast. *Am J Clin Pathol* 101:262–265, 1994.

47. New NE, Howart AJ: Nuclear grading of breast carcinoma. *Acta Cytol* 38:969–970, 1994.

48. Howart AJ, Armstrong GR, Briggs WA, Nicholson CM, Stewart DJ: Fine needle aspiration of palpable breast lumps: a 1-year audit using the cytospin method. *Cytopathology* 3:17–22, 1992.

49. Elston CW, Ellis IO: Pathological prognostic factors in breast cancer: I. The value of histological grade in breast cancer: experience from a large study with long term followup. *Histopathology* 3:17–22, 1992.

50. Fisher ER, Redmond C, Fisher B: Histologic grading of breast cancer. *Pathol Annu* 15:239–251, 1980.

51. Harris J, Lippman M, Veronsi U, et al: Breast cancer. *N Engl J Med* 327:390–392, 1992.

52. Hortobagyi GN, Ames FC, Buzdar AW, et al: Management of stage II primary cancer with primary chemotherapy, surgery and radiation therapy. *Cancer* 62:2507–2516, 1988.

53. Beatson GT: On treatment of inoperable cases of carcinoma of the mamma. Suggestions for new method of treatment with illustrated cases. *Lancet* 2:104, 1896.

54. Huggins C, Hodges CV: Studies on prostatic cancer. The effect of castration of estrogen and androgen injection on serum phosphatase in metastatic carcinoma of the prostate. *Cancer Res* 1:293, 1941.

55. Huggins C, Bergenstal DM: Inhibition of human mammary and prostatic cancers by adrenalectomy. *Cancer Res* 12:134–141, 1952.

56. Luft R, Olivecrona H, Ikkos JD, et al: Hypophysectomy in management on metastatic carcinoma of breast. In: Currie A, ed. *Endocrine Aspects of Breast Cancer; Proceeding of Conference Held at University of Glasgow.* Edinburgh, Scotland, Churchill Livingstone, 1958, pp. 27–35.

57. Harris HS, Spratt JS: Bilateral adrenalectomy in metastatic mammary cancer: an analysis of sixty-four cases. *Cancer* 23:145–151, 1969.

58. Folca PJ, Glascock RD, Irving WT: Studies with tritium labelled hexestrol in advanced breast cancer. *Lancet* 2:796, 1961.

59. Toft D, Gorski J: A receptor molecule for estrogens: Isolation from the rat uterus and preliminary characterization. *Proc Natl Acad Sci U S A* 55:1574–1581, 1966.

60. Jensen EV: Pattern of hormone receptor interactions. In: Griffiths K, Pier-Repoint EG, eds. *Some Aspects of Aetiology and Biochemistry of Prostatic Cancer.* Cardiff, Wales, Alpha Omega Alpha, 1970, p. 151.

61. Mass H, Engle B, Hohmeister H, et al: Estrogen receptors in human breast cancer tissue. *Am J Obstet Gynecol* 113:337–382, 1972.

62. Engelsman E, Persijin JP, Korsten CB, et al: Oestrogen receptors in human breast cancer tissue and response to endocrine therapy. *Br Med J* 2:750–752, 1973.

63. Leung BS, Fletcher WS, Lindell TD, et al: Predictability of response to endocrine ablation in advanced breast carcinoma. *Arch Surg* 106:515–519, 1973.

64. Savlov ED, Wittliff WL, Hilf R, et al: Correlation between certain biochemical properties of breast cancer and response to therapy. Preliminary report. *Cancer* 33:303–339, 1974.

65. Harwitz KB, McGuire WL, Pearson OH, et al: Predicting a response to endocrine therapy in human breast cancer. A hypothesis. *Science* 189:726–727, 1975.

66. Clark GM, McGuire WL, Hubray CA, et al: Progesterone receptors as a prognostic factor in stage II breast cancer. *N Engl J Med* 309:1343–1347, 1983.

67. King WJ, Greene GC: Monoclonal antibodies localize estrogen receptor in the nuclei of target cells. *Nature* 307:747–754, 1984.

68. Press MJ, Greene GL: Localization of progesterone receptor with monoclonal antibodies to the human progestin receptor. *Endocrinology* 122:1165–1175, 1988.

69. Walter P, Green S, Greene G, et al: Cloning of the human estrogen receptor cDNA. *Proc Natl Acad Sci USA* 82:7889–7893, 1985.

70. Misrahi M, Atger M, d'Auriol L, et al: Complete amino acid sequence of the human progesterone receptor deduced from cloned cDNA. *Biochem Biophys Res Commun* 143:740–748, 1987.

71. Clark JH, Peck EJ, Scharader WT, et al: Estrogen and progesterone receptors: methods of characterization, quantification and purification methods. *Cancer Res* 12:367–417, 1976.

72. McGuire WL, Carbone PP, Wollmer EP, eds: *Estrogen Receptors in Human Breast Cancer.* New York, NY, Raven Press, 1975, pp. 1–8.

73. Greene GL, Jensen EV: Monoclonal antibodies as probes for estrogen receptor detection and characterization. *J Steroid Biochem* 16:353–359, 1982.

74. Lee SH: Cytochemical studies of estrogen receptor in human mammary cancer. *Am J Clin Pathol* 70:197–203, 1978.

75. Jacobs SR, Wolfson WL, Cheng L, et al: Cytochemical and competitive protein binding assays for estrogen receptor in breast disease. A comparative study of 62 cases. *Cancer* 51:1621–1624, 1983.

76. Lee SH: Validity of a histochemical estrogen receptor assay. *J Histochem Cytochem* 32:305–310, 1984.

77. Pertschuk LP, Tobin EH, Gaetjens E, et al: Histochemical assay of estrogen and progesterone receptors in breast cancer: Correlation with biochemical assays and patient response to endocrine therapies. *Cancer* 46:2896–2901, 1980.

78. Chen P, Mei Z, Yao X, et al: Selection of hormone responsive advanced breast cancer with a cytoplasmic estrogen receptor assay. *Cancer* 63:139-142, 1989.

79. Pertschuk LP, Eisenberg RN, Carter AC: Estrogen binding with FluoroCep estrogen. Correlation with biochemical assay, clinical endocrine response and disease-free interval. *Lab Invest* 56:59, 1987. Abstract.

80. McGuire WL, Horwitz KB, Pearson AH, et al: Current status of estrogen and progesterone receptors in breast cancer. *Cancer* 39:2936–2974, 1977.

81. Henson JC, Longeval E, Mattheiem WH, et al: Significance of quantitative assessment of estrogen receptors for endocrine therapy in advanced breast cancer. *Cancer* 39:1971–1977, 1977.

82. Lee SH: Coexistance of cytoplasmic and nuclear estrogen receptors. A histochemical study on human mammary cancer and rabbit uterus. *Cancer* 64:1461–1466, 1989.

83. Masood S: Use of monoclonal antibody for assessment of estrogen receptor content in fine needle aspiration biopsy specimen from patients with breast cancer. *Arch Pathol Lab Med* 11:26–30, 1989.

84. Masood S: Use of monoclonal antibody for assessment of estrogen and progesterone receptors in malignant effusions. *Diagn Cytopathol* 8:161–166, 1992.

85. Masood S: Estrogen and progesterone receptors in cytology. *Diagn Cytopathol* 8:475–491, 1992.

86. Masood S: Immunocytochemical localization of estrogen and progesterone receptors in imprint preparations of breast carcinomas. *Cancer* 70:2109–2114, 1992.

87. Masood S, Dee S, Goldstein JD: Immunocytochemical analysis of progesterone receptors in breast cancer. *Am J Clin Pathol* 96:59–63, 1991.

88. Masood S, Dee S, Hardy N, et al: Cytospin preparation for assessment of hormone receptors in fine needle aspiration. *J Histotechnol* 13:23–25, 1995.

89. Wilber DC, Willis J, Mooney RA, et al: Estrogen and progesterone detection in archival formalin-fixed, paraffin-embedded tissue from breast carcinoma: a comparison of immunocytochemistry with dextran coated charcoal assay. *Mod Pathol* 5:79–84, 1992.

90. Pertschuk LP, Kim DS, Nayer K, et al: Immunocytochemical estrogen and progesterone receptor assays in breast cancer with monoclonal antibodies. *Cancer* 66:1663–1670, 1990.

91. Elias JM, Cartun RA, England DM, et al: Interlaboratory comparison of estrogen receptor analysis in paraffin sections by a monoclonal antibody to estrophilin (H222). *J Histotechnol* 16:57, 1993.

92. Masood S: Standardization of immunobioassays as surrogate endpoints. *J Cell Biochem* 19(suppl):28–35, 1994.

93. Esteban JM, Battifora H, Warsi Z, et al: Quantitation of estrogen receptors on paraffin-embedded tumors by image analysis. *Modern Pathol* 4:53-57, 1991.

94. Esteban JM, Kandalaft PL, Mehta P, et al: Improvement on the quantitation of estrogen and progesterone receptors on paraffin-embedded tumors by image analysis. *Am J Clin Pathol* 99:32–38, 1993.

95. Masood S, Lu L, Rodenroth N: Potential value of estrogen receptor immunocytochemical assay in formalin fixed breast tumors. *Mod Pathol* 3:724–728, 1990.

96. Osborne CK, Yachmowitz MG, Knight WA, et al: The value of estrogen and progesterone receptors in the treatment of breast cancer. *Cancer* 46:2884, 1980.

97. Fisher ER, Osborne C, McGuire WL, et al: Correlation of primary breast cancer histopathology and estrogen receptor content. *Breast Cancer Res Treatt* 1:37, 1981.

98. Dressler LG, Seamer LC, Owens MA, et al: DNA flow cytometry and prognostic factors in 1331 frozen breast cancer specimens. *Cancer* 61:420, 1988.

99. Osborne C: Receptors. In: Harris JR, Hellman S, Henderson IC, et al, eds: *Breast Diseases*. Philadelphia, Pa, JB Lippincott Co, 1987, p. 210.

100. Fisher B, Redmond C, Fisher ER, et al: Relative worth of estrogen and progesterone receptor and pathologic characteristics of differentiation as indicators of prognosis in node-positive breast cancer patients: findings from National Surgical Adjuvant Breast and Bowel Project Protocol B-06. *J Clin Oncol* 6:1076, 1988.

101. McGuire WL, Clark GM: Prognostic factors for recurrence and survival in axillary node-negative breast cancer. *J Steroid Biochem* 34:145–148, 1989.

102. Clark GM, McGuire WL: Steroid receptors and other prognostic factors in primary breast cancer. *Semin Oncol* 15:20, 1988.

103. Leung BS, Fletcher WS, Lindell TD, et al: Predictability of response to endocrine ablation in advanced breast carcinoma. *Arch Surg* 106:515–519, 1973.

104. Allegra JC, Lippman ME, Thompson ME, et al: Estrogen receptor status is the most important prognostic variable in predicting response to endocrine therapy in metastatic breast cancer. *Cancer Res* 39:1973–1979, 1979.

105. Lippman ME, Allegra JC: Quantitative estrogen receptor analysis: the response to endocrine and cytotoxic chemotherapy in human breast cancer and the disease free interval. *Cancer* 46:2829–2834, 1980.

106. Bezwada WK, Esser J, Dansey R, et al: The value of estrogen and progesterone receptor determinations in advanced breast cancer. Estrogen receptor level but not progesterone receptor level correlates with response to tamoxifen. *Cancer* 68:867–872, 1991.

107. Tinnemans JGM, Beex VAM, Wobbes TH, et al: Steroid-hormone receptors in nonpalpable and more advanced stages of breast cancer. A contribution to the biology and natural history of carcinoma of the female breast. *Cancer* 66:1165–1167, 1990.

108. Seymour L, Bezwada R, Meyer K: Response to second line hormone treatment for advanced breast cancer. Predictive value of DNA ploidy determination. *Cancer* 65:2720–2724, 1990.

109. Nenci J: Receptor and centriole pathways of steroid action in normal and neoplastic cells. *Cancer Res* 38:4204–4207, 1978.

110. Waseda N, Kato Y, Imura M, et al: Effects of tamoxifen on estrogen and progesterone receptors in human breast cancer. *Cancer Res* 41:1984–1988, 1981.

111. Baak JPA: Mitosis counting in tumors. *Hum Pathol* 21:683–685, 1990.

112. Van Viest PJ, Baak JPA: The morphometric prognostic index is the strongest prognosticator in premenopausal lymph node negative and lymph node positive breast cancer patients. *Hum Pathol* 22:326–330, 1990.

113. Clayton F: Pathologic correlates of survival in 378 lymph node negative infiltrating ductal breast carcinomas. Mitotic count is the best single predictor. *Cancer* 68:1309–1317, 1991.

114. Meyer JS, Friedman E, McCrate M, et al: Predicition of early course of breast carcinoma by thymidine labelling. *Cancer* 51:1879–1886, 1983.

115. Tubiana M, Pejovic MN, Charaudra N, et al: The long term prognostic significance of the thymidine labeling index in breast cancer. *Int J Cancer* 33:441, 1984.

116. Meyer JS, McDivitt RW, Stone KR, et al: Practical breast carcinoma cell kinetics: Review and update. *Breast Cancer Res Treat* 4:79, 1984.

117. Kallioniemi OP, Blanco G, Alavaikko M, et al: Tumour DNA ploidy as an independent prognostic factor in breast cancer. *Br J Cancer* 56:637–642, 1987.

118. Kallioniemi OP, Blanco G, Alavaikko M, et al: Improving the prognostic value of DNA flow cytometry in breast cancer by combining DNA index and S-phase fraction. A proposed classification of DNA histograms in breast cancer. *Cancer* 62:2183–2190, 1988.

119. Clark GM, Dressler LG, Owens MA, et al: Prediction of relapse or survival in patients with node-negative breast cancer by DNA flow cytometry. *N Engl J Med* 320:627–633, 1989.

120. Lewis WE: Prognostic significance of flow cytometric DNA analysis in node-negative breast cancer patients. *Cancer* 65:2315–2320, 1990.

121. Keyhani-Rofagha S, O'Toole RV, Farrar WB, et al: Is DNA ploidy an independent prognostic indicator in infiltrative node-negative breast adenocarcinoma? *Cancer* 65:1577-1582, 1990.

122. Toikkanen S, Joensuu H, Klemi P: The prognostic significance of nuclear DNA in invasive breast cancer—a study with long-term follow-up. *Br J Cancer* 60:693–700, 1989.

123. Sigurdsson H, Baldetorp B, Borg A, et al: Indicators of prognosis in node-negative breast cancer. *N Engl J Med* 322:1045–1053, 1990.

124. Fisher B, Gunduz N, Costantino J, et al: DNA flow cytometric analysis of primary operable breast cancer. Relation of ploidy and S-phase fraction to outcome of patients in NSABP B-04. *Cancer* 68:1465–1475, 1991.

125. Johnson H Jr, Masood S, Belluco C, et al: Prognostic factors in node-negative breast cancer. *Arch Surg* 127:1386–1390, 1992.

126. Hedley DW, Clark GM, Cornelisse DJ, et al: Consensus review of the clinical utility of DNA cytometry in carcinoma of the breast. *Cytometry* 14:482–485, 1993.

127. Hedley DW, Rugg CA, Gelber RD: Association of DNA index and S-phase fraction with prognosis of node positive early breast cancer. *Cancer Res* 47:4729–4735, 1987.

128. Stal O, Wingren S, Carstensen J, et al: Prognostic value of DNA ploidy and S-phase fraction in relation to estrogen receptor content and clinicopathological variables in primary breast cancer. *Eur J Cancer Clin Oncol* 25:301–309, 1989.

129. Muss HB, Kute TE, Case LD, et al: The relation of flow cytometry to clinical and biologic characteristics in women with node negative primary breast cancer. *Cancer* 64:1894–1900, 1989.

130. Sigurdsson H, Baldetorp B, Borg A, et al: Flow cytometry in primary breast cancer: improving the prognostic value of the fraction of cells in the S-phase by optimal categorisation of cut-off levels. *Br J Cancer* 62:786–790, 1990.

131. O'Reilly SM, Camplejohn RS, Barnes DM, et al: DNA index, S-phase fraction, histological grade and prognosis in breast cancer. *Br J Cancer* 61:672–674, 1990.

132. Falleninis AG, Franzen SA, Auer GU: Predictive value of nuclear DNA content in breast cancer in relation to clinical and morphological factors. A retrospective study of 227 consecutive cases. *Cancer* 62:521-530, 1988.

133. Kute TE: Response to Beerman et al: Flow cytometric analysis of DNA stemline heterogeneity in primary and metastatic breast cancer. *Cytometry* 12:155–156, 1991.

134. Masters JRW, Camplejohn RS, Millis RR, et al: Histopathological grade, elastasis, DNA ploidy and the response to chemotherapy of breast cancer. *Br J Cancer* 55:455–457, 1987.

135. Remvikos Y, Beuzboc P, Zajdela A, et al: Correlation of pretreatment proliferative activity of breast cancer with the response to cytotoxic chemotherapy. *J Natl Cancer Inst* 81:1383, 1989.

136. Sulkes A, Livingston RB, Murphy WK: Tritiated thymidine labeling index and response in human breast cancer. *J Natl Cancer Inst* 62:513, 1979.

137. Baildam AD, Zaloudik J, Howell A, et al: DNA analysis of flow cytometry, response to endocrine treatment and prognosis in advanced carcinoma of the breast. *Br J Cancer* 55:553, 1987.

138. Seymour L, Bezwada WR, Meyer K: Tumor factors predicting for prognosis in metastatic breast cancer: the presence of p24 predicts for response to treatment and duration of survival. *Cancer* 66:2390–2394, 1990.

139. Hastschek T, Carstenson J, Fogorberg G, et al: Influence of S-phase fraction on metastatic pattern and post-recurrence survival in a randomized mammography screening trial. *Breast Cancer Res Treat* 14:321–327, 1989.

140. Paradiso A, Tommasi S, Mangia A, et al: 3H-Tdr-Li PgR status, ploidy and clinical outcome of ER and advanced breast cancer patients treated by hormonotherapy. *Proc Am Soc Clin Oncol* 9:48, 1990. Abstract.

141. Blanco G, Holli K, Heikkinen M, et al: Prognostic factors in recurrent breast cancer, female sex steroid receptors, ploidy and histological malignancy grading. *Br J Cancer* 62:142–146, 1990.

142. DeLena M, Romero N, Rabinovich M, et al: Metastatic pattern and DNA ploidy in Stage IV breast cancer at initial diagnosis relation to response and survival. *Am J Clin Oncol (CCT)* 16:245–249, 1993.

143. Hitchock A, Ellis IO, Robertson JF, et al: An observation of DNA ploidy, histological grade and immunoreactivity for tumor related antigen in primary and metastatic breast carcinoma. *J Pathol* 159:129–134, 1989.

144. Wintzer H-O, Sipfel I, Schulte-Monting J, et al: Ki-67 immunostaining in human breast tumors and its relationship to prognosis. *Cancer* 67:421–428, 1991.

145. Brown RW, Allred DC, Clark GM, et al: The prognostic significance of cell-cycle kinetics measured by Ki-67 immunohistochemistry in node-negative breast cancer. *Lab Invest* 64:10, 1991. Abstract.

146. Shahin AA, Ro J, Ro JY, et al: Ki-67 immunostaining in node-negative stage I/II breast carcinoma. Significant correlation with prognosis. *Cancer* 68:549–557, 1991.

147. Freeman JW, McGrath P, Bondada V, et al: Prognostic significance of proliferation associated nuclear antigen P120 in human breast carcinomas. *Cancer Res* 51:1973–1978, 1991.

148. Vielh P: *Guides to Clinical Aspiration Biopsy: Flow Cytometry.* New York, NY, Igaku-Shoin, 1991.

149. Masood S, Hart N: Use of fine needle aspiration biopsy specimens in DNA flow cytometry study. *Am J Clin Pathol* 92:535, 1989. Abstract.

150. Lopez F, Bello F, Lacombe F, et al: Modalities of synthesis of Ki-67 antigen during the stimulation of lymphocytes. *Cytometry* 10: 731–738, 1989.

151. Landberg G, Roos G: Flow cytometric analysis of proliferation associated nuclear antigen using washless staining of unfixed cells. *Cytometry* 13:230–240, 1992.

152. Rishi M, Schwarting R, Kovalich AJ, et al: Detection of growth fraction in tumors by Ki-67 monoclonal antibody in cytologic smears: a prospective study of 40 cases. *Diagn Cytopathol* 9:52–56, 1993.

153. Henry MJ, Stanley MW, Swenson B, et al: Cytologic assessment of tumor cell kinetics. Applications of monoclonal antibody Ki-67 to fine needle aspiration smears. *Diagn Cytopathol* 7:591–596, 1991.

154. Charpin C, Andrac L, Vacheret H, et al: Multiparametic evaluatoin (SAMBA) of growth factors (monoclonal Ki-67) in breast carcinoma tissue sections. *Cancer Res* 48:4368–4374, 1988.

155. Charpin C, Andrac L, Habib C, et al: Immunodetection in fine needle aspirates and multiparametric (SAMBA) image analysis. Receptors (monoclonal antiestrogen and antiprogesterone) and growth fraction (monoclonal Ki-67) evaluation in breast carcinomas. *Cancer* 63:863–872, 1989.

156. Masood S: Prognostic factors in breast cancer: use of cytologic preparations. *Diagn Cytopathol* 13:388–395, 1995.

157. Cline MJ, Battifora J, Yokota J: Proto-oncogene abnormalities in human breast cancer: correlations with anatomic features and clinical course of disease. *J Clin Oncol* 5:999–1000, 1987.

158. Slamon DJ, Clark GM, Wong SG, et al: Human breast cancer: correlation of relapse and survival with amplification of the HER-2/*neu* oncogene. *Science* 235:177–182, 1987.

159. Tandon AK, Clark GM, Chambness GC, et al: HER-2/*neu* oncogene protein and prognosis in breast cancer. *J Clin Oncol* 7: 1120–1128, 1989.

160. Paik S, Hazan R, Fisher ER, et al: Pathologic findings from the National Surgical Adjuvant Breast Project: prognostic significance of *erb*B-2 protein overexpression in primary breast cancer. *J Clin Oncol* 8:103–112, 1990.

161. Allred D, Clark GM, Tandon AK, et al: HER-2/*neu* in node negative breast cancer: prognostic significance of overexpression influenced by presence of in situ carcinoma. *J Clin Oncol* 10:599–605, 1992.

162. Masood S: HER-2/*neu* oncogene expression in atypical hyperplasia, carcinoma in situ and invasive breast cancer. *Mod Pathol* 4:12, 1991. Abstract.

163. Varley JM, Swallow JE, Brammar WJ, et al: Alterations to either C-*erb*B-2 (*neu*) on *c-myc* proto-oncogenes in breast carcinomas correlate with poor short-term prognosis. *Oncogene* 1:423–430, 1987.

164. Finlay CA, Hinds PW, Levine AJ: The p53 proto-oncogenes can act as a suppressor of transformation. *Cell* 57:1083–1093, 1989.

165. Bishop M: Molecular themes in oncogenes. *Cell* 64:235–248, 1991.

166. Osborne RJ, Merle GR, Mitsudemi T, et al: Mutations in p53 gene in primary human breast cancers. *Cancer Res* 51:6194–6198, 1991.

167. Thor AD, Moso III DH, Edgerton SM, et al: Accumulation of p53 tumor suppressor gene protein: an independent marker of prognosis in breast cancer. *J Natl Cancer Inst* 84:845–855, 1992.

168. Isola J, Wisakorpi T, Holli K, et al: Association of overexpression of tumor suppressor protein p53 with rapid cell proliferation and poor prognosis in node-negative breast cancer patients. *J Natl Cancer Inst* 84:1109–1114, 1992.

169. Thor AD, Moore DH, Edgerton SM, et al: Increased accumulation of the p53 suppressor gene product is an independent prognostic variable for breast cancer. *J Natl Cancer Inst* 84:845–855, 1992.

170. Allred DC, Clark GM, Brown RW, et al: Mutation of p53 is associated with increased proliferation and early recurrence in node-negative breast cancer. *Proceedings of the American Society of Clinical Oncology, 28th Annual Meeting.* 11:55, 1992.

171. Masood S, Barnes R, Villas B, et al: p53 oncosuppressor protein in carcinoma of the breast. *Mod Pathol* 6:80, 1991. Abstract.

172. Davidoff AM, Herndon JE, Glover NS, et al: Relation between p53 overexpression and established prognostic factors in breast cancer. *Surgery* 110:259–264, 1991.

173. Faille A, DeCremoux PD, Extra JM, et al: p53 mutations and overexpression in locally advanced breast cancer. *Br J Cancer* 69:1145–1150, 1994.

174. David AM, Kerns BJ, Iglehart D, et al: Maintenance of p53 alterations throughout breast cancer progression. *Cancer Res* 51:2605–2610, 1991.

175. Steeg PS, Bevilacqua G, Kopper L, et al: Evidence of a novel gene assocaited with low tumor metastatic potential. *J Natl Cancer Inst* 80:200–203, 1988.

176. Bevilacqua G, Sobel ME, Liotta LA, et al: Association with low nm23RNA levels in primary infiltrating ductal breast carcinomas with lymph node involvement and other histopathological indicators of high metastatic potential. *Cancer Res* 49:5185–5190, 1989.

177. Hennessey C, Henry JA, May FEB, et al: Expression of the anti-metastatic gene nm23 in human breast cancer: association with good prognosis. *J Natl Cancer Inst* 83:281–285, 1991.

178. Barnes R, Masood S, Barker E, et al: Low nm23 protein expression in infiltrating ductal breast carcinomas correlates with reduced patient survival. *Am J Pathol* 139:245–250, 1991.

179. Perez N, Pascual M, Marcias A, et al: Epidermal growth factor receptors in human breast cancer. *Breast Cancer Res Treat* 4:189–193, 1984.

180. Horne GM, Argus B, Wright C, et al: Relationship between oestrogen receptor, epidermal growth factor receptor, ERD5 and P24 oestrogen regulated protein in human breast cancer. *J Pathol* 155:143–150, 1988.

181. Sainsbury JR, Farnoon JR, Needham GK, et al: Epidermal growth factor receptor status as a predictor of early recurrence and death from breast cancer. *Lancet* 1:1398–1402, 1987.

182. Rochefort H, Augereau P, Capony F, et al: The 52K cathepsin-D of breast cancer. Structure, regulation, function and clinical value in breast cancer. *Cancer Treat Res* 40:207–222, 1988.

183. Thorpe SM, Rochefort H, Garcia M, et al: Association between high concentrations of Mr52,000 cathepsin D and poor prognosis in primary human breast cancer. *Cancer Res* 49:6008–6014, 1989.

184. Henry JA, McCarthy AL, Agnas B, et al: Prognostic significance of the estrogen-regulated protein, cathepsin-D in breast cancer. *Cancer* 65:525–527, 1990.

185. Spyratos F, Brouillet JP, Defrenne A, et al: Cathepsin D: an independent prognostic factor for metastases of breast cancer. *Lancet* 2:1115–1118, 1989.

186. Duffy MJ, Brouillet JP, Reilly D, et al: Cathepsin D concentration in breast cancer cytosols: correlation with biochemical, histological and clinical findings. *Clin Chem* 37:101–104, 1991.

187. Romain S, Muracciole X, Varette I, et al: Cathepsin D: an independent prognostic factor in cancer of the breast. *Bull Cancer* 77:439–447, 1990.

188. Namer M, Ramaioli A, Fontana X, et al: Prognostic value of total cathepsin D in breast tumors. *Breast Cancer Res Treat* 19:85–93, 1991.

189. Pujol P, Maudelonde T, Daures JP: A prospective study of the prognostic value of cathepsin D levels in breast cancer cytosols. *Cancer* 71:2006–2012, 1993.

190. Granata G, Coradini D, Cappelletti V, et al: Prognostic relevance of cathepsin D versus oestrogen receptors in node negative breast cancers [published erratum appears in *Eur J Cancer* 1992:28:246]. *Eur J Cancer* 27:970–972, 1991.

191. Domagala W, Striker G, Szadowska A, et al: Cathepsin D in invasive ductal NOS breast carcinoma as defined by immunohistochemistry: no correlation with survival at 5 years. *Am J Pathol* 141:1003–1012, 1992.

192. Cowan WK, Angus B, Henry J, et al: Immunohistochemical and other features of breast carcinomas presenting clinically compared with those detected by cancer screening. *Br J Cancer* 64:780–784, 1991.

193. Martin AW, Lear SC, Corrigna C: Immunohistochemical demonstration of cathepsin B and D in breast cancer and its relationship to prognosis. *Mod Pathol* 5:15, 1992. Abstract.

194. Kandalaft P, Chang K, Ahn C: Immunohistochemical analysis of cathepsin D in breast cancer: is it prognostically significant? *Mod Pathol* 5:14, 1992. Abstract.

195. Tetu B, Cote C, Brisson J: Cathepsin D in node-positive breast carcinoma: an immunohistochemical study of 400 cases. *Mod Pathol* 5:18, 1992. Abstract.

196. Sahin A, Sneige N, Ordonez N, et al: Immunohistochemical determination of cathepsin D in node negative breast carcinoma. *Mod Pathol* 5:17, 1992. Abstract.

197. Isola J, Weitz S, Visakorpi T, et al: Cathepsin D expression detected by immunohistochemistry has independent prognostic value in axillary node-negative breast cancer. *J Clin Oncol* 11:36–43, 1993.

198. Armas OA, Gerald WL, Lesser ML, et al: Immunohistochemical demonstration of cathepsin D in T2N0M0 breast carcinoma. *Am J Surg Pathol* 18:158–166, 1994.

199. Tandon AK, Clark GM, Chamness GC, et al: Cathepsin D and prognosis in breast cancer. *N Engl J Med* 32:297-302, 1990.

200. Coman DR, Scheldon WF: The significance of hyperemia around tumor implants. *Am J Pathol* 22:821–826, 1946.

201. Day ED: Vascular relationship of tumor and host. *Prog Exp Tumor Res* 4:57–97, 1964.

202. Folkman J: What is the evidence that tumors are angiogenesis-dependent? *J Natl Cancer Inst* 82:4–6, 1990.

203. Liotta LA, Kleinerman J, Saidel G: The significance of hematogenous tumor cell clumps in the metastatic processes. *Cancer Res* 36:889–894, 1976.

204. Weidner N, Semple JP, Welh WE, et al: Tumor angiogenesis and metastasis: correlation in invasive breast carcinoma. *N Engl J Med* 324:1–8, 1991.

205. Bosari S, Lee AKC, DeLellis RA, et al: Microvessel quantitation and prognosis in invasive breast carcinoma. *Hum Pathol* 23:755–761, 1992.

206. Horak E, Leek R, Klenk N, et al: Angiogenesis, assessed by platelet/endothelial cell adhesion molecule antibodies, as indicator of node metastasis and survival in breast cancer. *Lancet* 340: 1120–1124, 1992.

207. Weidner N, Folkman J, Pozza F, et al: Tumor angiogenesis: A new significant and independent prognostic indicator in early stage breast carcinoma. *J Natl Cancer Inst* 84:1875–1887, 1992.

208. Visscher DW, Smilanetz S, Drozdowicz S, et al: Prognostic significance of image morphometric microvessel enumeration in breast carcinoma. *Anal Quant Cytol Histol* 15:88–92, 1993.

209. Shurbaji MS, Pasternack GR, Kuhajda FP: Expression of hapto-globin-related protein in primary and metastatic breast cancer: a longitudinal study of 48 fatal tumors. *Am J Clin Pathol* 96:238–242, 1991.

210. Abbondanzo SL: Prognostic significance of immunocytochemically determined pS2 in axillary node-negative breast carcinoma. *Breast Cancer Res Treat* 16:182, 1990.

211. Schwartz LH, Koerneu FC, Edgerton SM, et al: pS2 expression and response to hormonal therapy in patients with advanced breast cancer. *Cancer Res* 51:624–628, 1991.

212. Gerlach JH, Kartner N, Bell DR, et al: Multidrug resistance. *Cancer Surv* 5:25–46, 1986.

213. Pastan I, Gottesman M: Multiple drug resistance in human cancer. *N Engl J Med* 316:1388–1393, 1987.

214. Kartner N, Riordan JR, Ling V: Cell surface p-glycoprotein associated with multidrug resistance in mammalian cell lines. *Science* 221:1285–1288, 1983.

215. Chen C-J, Chin JE, Veda K, et al: Internal duplication and homology with bacterial transplant proteins in the MDR 1 (p-glycoprotein) gene from multi-drug resistant human cells. *Cell* 47:381–389, 1987.

216. Dalton WS, Durie BGM, Alberts DS, et al: Characterization of a new drug resistant human myeloma cell line which expresses p-glycoprotein. *Cancer Res* 46:5125–5130, 1986.

217. Merkel DE, Fugua SAW, Tandon AK, et al: Electrophoretic analysis of 248 clinical breast cancer specimens for p-glycoprotein overexpression of gene amplification. *J Clin Oncol* 6:1129–1136, 1989.

218. Ro J, Sahin A, Ro JY, et al: Immunocytochemical analysis of p-glycoprotein expression correlated with chemotherapy resistance in locally advanced breast cancer. *Hum Pathol* 21:787–791, 1990.

219. Schneider J, Bak M, Efferth TH, et al: P-glycoprotein expression in treated and untreated human breast cancer. *Br J Cancer* 60:815–818, 1989.

220. Lonn V, Lonn S, Nylen V, et al: Appearance and detection of multiple copie of MDR1 gene in clinical samples of mammary carcinoma. *Int J Cancer* 51:602–682, 1992.

221. Gee JM, Robertson JF, Ellis IO, et al: Immunocytochemical localization of bcl-2 protein in human breast cancers and its relationship to a series of prognostic markers and response to endocrine therapy. *Int J Cancer* 59:619–628, 1994.

222. Hurlimann J, Larrinaga B, Vala DR: bcl-2 protein in invasive ductal breast carcinomas. *Virchows Arch* 426:163–168, 1995.

223. Johnston SR, MacLennan KA, Sacks NP, et al: Modulation of bcl-2 and Ki-67 expression in estrogen receptor positive human breast cancer by tamoxifen. *Eur J Cancer* 30:1663–1669, 1994.

224. Sierra A, Lloveras B, Castellsaque X, et al: bcl-2 expression is associated with lymph node metastasis in human ductal breast carcinoma. *Int J Cancer* 60:54–60, 1995.

225. Hellemans P, Van-Dam PA, Weyler J, et al: Prognostic value of bcl-2 expression in invasive breast cancer. *Br J Cancer* 72:354–360, 1995.

226. O'Reilly AM, Campeljohn RS, Barnes DM, et al: Node negative breast cancer: prognostic subgroups defined by tumor size and flow cytometry. *J Clin Oncol* 8:2040, 1990.

227. McGuire WL, Tandon AK, Allred DC, et al: How to use prognostic factors in axillary node negative breast cancer patients. *J Natl Cancer Inst* 82:1006, 1991

228. Masood S: Prognostic factors in breast cancer. *J Surg Pathol* 1:45–61, 1995.

229. Masood S: Prediction of recurrence for advanced breast cancer: traditional and contemporary pathologic and molecular markers. In: Bland K, ed. *The Surgical Oncology Clinics of North America.* Philadelphia, Pa, WB Saunders Co, 1995, pp. 601–633.

230. Masood S: Pathologists and breast cancer: a changing role. *Breast J* 1:1–2, 1995.

◙ Index

Page numbers in **boldface** indicate images, figures, and tables.

recurrence rate, 177
therapy, 177
Core needle biopsy
   disadvantages, 39–40
   fine needle aspiration biopsy differences, 3, 38–39
   long-throw needle, 39–40
   mammographic guidance, **39**
   tissue fragments, **40**
Cysts
   aspiration and mammogram, 78
   fluid
      blood in tumors, 77–78, **98–100**
      cellularity, 77
      cytomorphology, **96–98**
      indications for examination, 77–78
   medullary carcinoma, 78, **100–101**
   prevalence, 77

D

DCIS. *See* Ductal carcinoma in situ
Diff-Quik® stain, fine needle aspiration biopsy, 11, 13, **26**
DNA ploidy
   assessment, 382–383
   cell cycle, **383**
   histograms, 383, **384–385**
   prognostic significance, 174, **174**, 383–385, 393
Duct cell carcinoma. *See* Ductal carcinoma in situ; Infiltrating
      duct cell carcinoma
Ductal adenoma, diagnosis, 81
Ductal carcinoma in situ (DCIS). *See also* Comedocarcinoma;
      Noncomedocarcinoma
   cytomorphology, 176–178, **192–194**
   diagnostic accuracy, 173
   treatment, 179

E

Epidermal growth factor receptor, expression and prognostic
      value, 390, **406**
Epidermal inclusion cyst, cytomorphology, 54
Estrogen receptor
   activation, 377
   assays
      accuracy, 380–381
      dextran-coated charcoal assay, 378
      immunofluorescence assay, 378–379, **400**
      immunoperoxidase assay, 378–379, **380**, **400–403**
   endocrine ablation therapy indications, 376, 381–382
   gene, 377
   localization, 376–377, **377**
   prognostic significance, 380–382

F

Fat necrosis
   cytomorphology, 55–56, **71–74**
   differential diagnosis, **86**
Fibroadenoma. *See also* Juvenile fibroadenoma
   associated malignancies, 78–81
   cytologic atypia, 80, **105–109**
   cytomorphology, **43**, 80–81, **102–104**, 210, **239**
   differential diagnosis, 80–81, **109–110**, **111–113**, 149, 210,
      239
   fine needle aspiration biopsy, 78–79
   gross appearance, **79**
   immunostaining, 81, **110–111**
   lactational changes, 87–88
   prevalence, 78
   radiology, 78, **79**
Fibrocystic change
   breast cancer risk, 167
   cytomorphology, 167, **182**
Fibromatosis
   clinical presentation, 148
   cytomorphology, 148–149, **155–156**
   differential diagnosis, 148–149
   recurrence rate, 148
   tamoxifen therapy, 148
Fibrosis, fine needle aspiration biopsy, false–negative results, 32
Fine needle aspiration biopsy (FNAB)
   advantages, 4–5
   biopsy service
      establishment, 23–25
      justification, 24
      staff training, 23–24
   cart preparation, 22, **23**
   complications, 5
   core needle biopsy differences, 3, 38–39
   cost-effectiveness, 1, 4
   defined, 2–3
   diagnostic testing of cells
      accuracy, 29–30, **30**, 35
      aspirate, **6**
      techniques, 22
   grading system, 168, **168**, 171–173
   history, 1–2
   mammographic guidance, 15, **15–16**, 25, 35, **39**
   nonpalpable breast lesion
      false-negative results, 37–38
      false-positive results, 38
      management of patients, 41–42, **42**
      reporting of findings, 41–42
      sensitivity and specificity, 35–37, **35–37**
   palpable breast lesion
      false-negative results, 32

false-positive results, 32–33
  management of patients, 33, **34**, 35
  reporting of findings, 33
  technique, 11, **12**, 13
pathologist competence, 24, 30, 40–41
patient acceptance, 4
rapidity, 4
role in breast disease management, 29
smear preparation, 11, **13**, 31
specimen adequacy criteria, 31
stereotactic guidance
  instruments, 16–18, **17–19**, **38**
  limitations, 18
  sensitivity and specificity, 35–36
  techniques, 2, 18
stromal proliferation, 147
tumor sampling, **3**, 4–5
tumor spreading, 1, 5
ultrasound guidance
  accuracy, 35
  techniques, 19–20, **20–21**
FNAB. *See* Fine needle aspiration biopsy
Fungal infection, fine needle aspiration biopsy, 54–55

G

Granular cell tumor
  cytomorphology, 152, **159–160**
  gross description, 152
  ultrastructure, **153**
Granulocytic sarcoma
  cytomorphology, 318, **324–325**
  treatment, 318
Granulomatous mastitis
  cytomorphology, 53–55, **66–68**
  differential diagnosis, 53–55
  pathogens, 54–55, **69–70**
  sarcoidosis, 54, **68–69**
Gynecomastia, male
  cytomorphology, 360, **363–364**
  etiology, 359
  malignancy association, 360
  types, 359–360

H

Hemangiopericytoma
  cytomorphology, 297–298, **308–309**
  differential diagnosis, 309
Hepatocellular carcinoma, metastasis to breast. *See* Metastatic
  carcinoma

HER-2/*neu* oncogene
  expression and prognosis, 174–175, **175**, **188–189**, 387–388,
    393, **404**
  product, 387
Hodgkin's disease
  cytomorphology, 317–318, **323**
  types in breast, 317

I

ILC. *See* Infiltrating lobular carcinoma
Infiltrating duct cell carcinoma
  clinical presentation, 203
  cytomorphology, 204–205, **219–222**
  diagnostic accuracy, 204–205
  giant cells, 204
  histology, 203–204
  immunostaining, 204, **223–225**
  incidence, 203
  small cell variant, 204, **222–223**
Infiltrating lobular carcinoma (ILC)
  clinical presentation, 205
  cytomorphology, 205–207, **225–229**
  diagnostic accuracy, 206
  incidence, 205
  treatment, 206
Inflammatory carcinoma
  cytomorphology, 267, **279–280**
  incidence, 267
Intracystic carcinoma
  cytomorphology, 218–219, **250**
  gross features, **218**
  incidence, 217
  males, 360
  ultrasonography, 217, **217**

J

Juvenile carcinoma. *See* Secretory carcinoma
Juvenile fibroadenoma, cytomorphology, 79–80, **104–105**
Juvenile hypertrophy, cytomorphology, 147–148
Juvenile papillomatosis
  breast cancer risk, 84
  cytomorphology, 84–85, **118–119**
  differential diagnosis, 84

K

Ki-67, immunostaining and prognostic significance, 385–386,
  403–404

therapy decision process, 394–395, **394–395**
Proliferative breast disease with atypia
    chemoprevention of carcinoma, 180
    cytologic findings, **168**
    cytomorphology, 170, **185–188**
    differentiation from neoplasia
        diagnostic accuracy, 171–173
        DNA ploidy pattern, 174, **174**
        HER–2/*neu* oncogene expression, 174–175, **175,**
          188–189
        MAB B72.3 staining, 175–176, **189**
        muscle specific actin immunostaining, 176, **190–191**
        scoring system, 171–173
    fine needle aspiration, 168, **169**
    lesion heterogeneity, 173–174
Proliferative breast disease without atypia
    cytologic findings, **168**, 169
    cytomorphology, 169–170, 172, **184–185**
    fine needle aspiration, 168, **169**
Prostate carcinoma, metastasis to breast. *See* Metastatic carcinoma
pS2, prognostic value of expression, 391–392

R
Radial scar
    cytomorphology, 94–95, **136**, 208, **233–235**
    distinguishing from cancer, 94
    lesion association, 84–85
    tissue section, **135**
    tubular carcinoma similarity, 208
Radiation atypia
    cytomorphology, 89, **126–129**
    distinguishing from recurrent cancer, 89
    etiology, 88
    fine needle aspiration biopsy, 89–90
RDD. *See* Rosai-Dorfman disease
Renal carcinoma metastasis to breast. *See* Metastatic carcinoma
Rhabdomyosarcoma, cytomorphology, 299–300
Rosai-Dorfman disease (RDD), cytomorphology, 320

S
Sarcoidosis, cytomorphology, 54
Sarcoma, metastasis to breast. *See* Metastatic carcinoma
Secretory carcinoma
    cytomorphology, 269–270, **282–284**
    differential diagnosis, 269–270
    gross characteristics, 269
    histology, 269, **282**
    treatment, 269
Signet ring carcinoma
    cytomorphology, 213–214, **243–245**

differential diagnosis, 213
    incidence, 213
    prognosis, 211, 214
Silicone implant
    cytomorphology of silicone-induced changes, 91–92,
      131–133
    distinguishing from recurrent cancer, 91
Skin tumor, diagnosis, 361
Small cell carcinoma, metastasis to breast. *See* Metastatic carcinoma
Spindle cell lipoma
    clinical presentation, 153
    cytomorphology, 153–154
Squamous cell carcinoma
    cytomorphology, 263–264, **274–275**
    differential diagnosis, 264
    gross features, 263, **263**
    incidence, 263
    metastasis to breast. *See* Metastatic carcinoma
    prognosis, 263
Stereotactic guidance
    instruments, 16–18, **17–19, 38**
    limitations, 18
    sensitivity and specificity, 35–36
    techniques, 2, 18
Steroid receptor. *See also* Estrogen receptor; Progesterone
    receptor
    activation, 377
    assays
        accuracy, 380–381
        dextran-coated charcoal assay, 378
        immunofluorescence assay, 378–379, **400**
        immunoperoxidase assay, 378–379, **380, 400–403**
    endocrine ablation therapy indications, 376, 381–382
    prognostic significance, 380–382
Stromal sarcoma, cytomorphology, 299
Subareolar abscess
    cytomorphology, 53, **65**
    gross appearance, **54**
    pathogenesis, 52–53
Supernumerary breast lesion, cytomorphology, 361, **366**
Surgery-induced fibrosis, distinguishing from recurrent cancer,
    90
Suture granuloma
    cytomorphology, 90, **129–131**
    distinguishing from recurrent cancer, 90

T
Tamoxifen
    cost, 396
    side effects, 396